Working with Complexity in PTSD

This accessible, evidence-based book provides readers with a practical framework to understand, formulate, and treat PTSD using the cognitive model while creatively adapting for complexity.

Cognitive therapy for PTSD is a highly effective treatment, but aspects of clinical complexity can complicate treatment and limit its effectiveness. Trauma memories themselves can be complex, the associated meanings can resist change and people may struggle to engage with them without feeling overwhelmed. Problems that commonly arise alongside PTSD add to clinical complexity, such as comorbid psychological or physical disorders, social problems, and ongoing risks. Bringing together the science and art of therapy, this book demonstrates how to approach these issues by holding firm to the principles of CBT, whilst flexing and creatively adapting techniques for each unique circumstance. Rich case studies, top tips, and frequently asked questions are used throughout to demonstrate the approach.

Written by clinicians for clinicians, the book synthesizes the latest research into a practical treatment manual to help readers overcome obstacles in PTSD treatment and 'supercharge' their therapy skills.

Dr Hannah Murray is a Research Clinical Psychologist based at the Oxford Centre for Anxiety Disorders and Trauma, University of Oxford. She works clinically and in research to develop, test and disseminate treatments for Post-Traumatic Stress Disorder, particularly Cognitive Therapy for PTSD.

Dr Sharif El-Leithy is a Consultant Clinical Psychologist specialising in psychological reactions to life-threatening traumas. He has over 20 years of experience in using cognitive-behavioural therapy to treat PTSD arising from complex traumatic experiences, including victims of war, torture, and domestic and childhood abuse.

Working with Complexity in PTSD

A Cognitive Therapy Approach

Hannah Murray and Sharif El-Leithy

Routledge
Taylor & Francis Group
LONDON AND NEW YORK

Cover image: © Maryam Salehi

First published 2022
by Routledge
4 Park Square, Milton Park, Abingdon, Oxon OX14 4RN

and by Routledge
605 Third Avenue, New York, NY 10158

Routledge is an imprint of the Taylor & Francis Group, an informa business

British Library Cataloguing-in-Publication Data
A catalogue record for this book is available from the British Library

Library of Congress Cataloging-in-Publication Data
A catalog record has been requested for this book

ISBN: 9781032264424 (hbk)
ISBN: 9781032264080 (pbk)
ISBN: 9781003288329 (ebk)

DOI: 10.4324/9781003288329

Typeset in Joanna
by codeMantra

For Hannah's medical team, without whom this book would not have been written

Contents

Foreword

It is an honour to write this foreword, and to have had an early opportunity to read this book. As a clinician, researcher, and trainer in this field I have learned greatly from the questions I have been asked by supervisees, workshop participants, and most of all clients with PTSD with whom I have worked. These questions have typically revolved around issues of complexity of one sort or another. Both for myself and for others there is now a core text to which we can all turn to help address such questions.

The treatment that Hannah and Sharif describe is Cognitive Therapy for PTSD (CT-PTSD), originated by Anke Ehlers and David Clark, and developed further by them and others in their team since the late 1990s. There is excellent evidence for the effectiveness of this treatment both in randomised controlled trials and routine clinical practice, and it forms part of the many guidelines for the treatment of PTSD around the world. However, as clinicians, we are often working 'beyond the guidelines', with varying issues of complexity, some of which are not well covered by the existing evidence base. What to do in such situations? There are a number of risks we face. We risk simply throwing out the evidence base, claiming it doesn't apply for the people we work with. We risk pushing on in a rigid fashion, slavishly following a set recipe, in the face of no change or even deterioration. And we risk drifting away from the core principles underlying the model and treatment, into a conceptually incoherent eclecticism.

Hannah and Sharif guide us between these risks, providing example after example of 'flexibility within fidelity'. Many implicit myths about the use of CT-PTSD, in particular contexts, or with particular people, are gently but firmly busted throughout this text. They provide an extremely helpful framework for considering many types of complexity, and offer conceptual clarity to issues around the definition of complexity, which is not simply synonymous with 'Complex PTSD'. At heart remain the core maintaining processes of PTSD, the nature of the trauma memory, the meanings people have taken from their experiences, and the behaviours they use to cope. This provides the framework for many chapters that address 'memory complexity', 'cognitive complexity', and 'complexity in coping'. Further chapters address other contextual complexities inherent in this work. This framework will also help guide the gathering of further evidence in these areas.

Jo Nesbo, the Norwegian thriller writer, suggests that 'The art of dealing with ghosts is to dare to look at them long and hard until you know that is what they are. Ghosts. Lifeless, powerless ghosts.' This applies to the people with whom we work in facing their personal memories, but also applies to us as clinicians in recognising the ghosts of complexity, which, if we face, we can also tackle.

It has been my privilege to work with Hannah and Sharif in various capacities over time. They have many years of experience as practitioners, supervisors, and trainers of CT-PTSD. They have the crucial combination of clarity of thought allied to clinical skill that allows both a deeper understanding of the treatment of PTSD and most importantly its practical application. I have learned from them and you will too. I'm excited for you to be able to read this now, to come back to it as needed, and to use it as a catalyst for you and your client's clinical creativity aligned around the key principles of an effective treatment for PTSD. This is the book you know you always needed and here it is!

Dr Nick Grey,
Consultant Clinical Psychologist

Preface

From a treatment perspective, Post-Traumatic Stress Disorder (PTSD) is often associated with clinical complexity, such as comorbidity and lifelong or repeated traumas, which can present complications in delivering effective treatment. Yet, much of the treatment research and training literature is focused on treating PTSD following single-incident adult traumas, presenting without additional layers of problem complexity. In this book, we hope to do the opposite. We focus on the more complex problems you might encounter in treating PTSD, and address many of the common obstacles that can arise.

The approach we describe stems from Cognitive-Behavioural Therapy (CBT) and, specifically, Cognitive Therapy for PTSD (CT-PTSD; Ehlers & Clark, 2000). However, the issues we discuss are universal; where to start with someone who has multiple trauma memories or how to build trust with someone who has a history of interpersonal trauma, for example, are relevant whatever treatment model you are using. In the first chapter, we'll talk about why we think CT-PTSD is particularly suited to working with complexity, but we appreciate that other treatment models are also highly effective in working with PTSD.

CT-PTSD has an excellent evidence base for PTSD. One of its strengths is flexibility and, when we work with complexity, we often need to be creative and adaptable to overcome complications in treatment while remaining theoretically congruent. This balance of being tight to principles, but flexible to tactics and techniques (Whittington, & Grey, 2014) underlies our approach. For example, we may draw broadly on techniques developed in other treatment approaches, as well as on clinical experience and the thinking, writing, and teaching of other experienced PTSD practitioners we have learnt from over the years, but we should always be working within a formulation, and know which process we are targeting with each intervention. There are lots of examples of this 'flexibility within fidelity' approach throughout the book.

The book is written by clinicians, for clinicians. After the first chapter or two, we've tried not to get bogged down in too much theory or present lots of research data, because we want to focus on practical implementation. We've included the areas of complexity which arise most commonly in our clinical practice and which can create barriers to implementing evidence-based treatments. Throughout the book, you'll find case examples, transcripts, formulation diagrams, and examples of 'hot cognitions' which we hope will bring the treatment to life. These are all based on real cases, but have been modified to preserve anonymity. We've also included 'frequently asked questions', and 'top tips', based on the types of issues that commonly arise in supervision and training.

Acknowledgments

To our clients, who allow us into their lives with such courage and candour, we owe the biggest thanks for teaching us about everything we have written and so much more besides.

Also with enormous thanks and apologies to all our talented colleagues, supervisors, trainers, and researchers past and present whose ideas we have stolen and not credited. Special thanks to our trauma families at the Traumatic Stress Service in Tooting, London and the Oxford Centre for Anxiety Disorders and Trauma, University of Oxford.

We would like to thank individuals who took the time to advise us on early drafts of chapters in the book, particularly Amy Hardy, Kirsten Smith, Lucy Maddox, Rebecca Lockwood, Emma Černis, Emily Greenfield, Katherine Wakelin, Jo Billings, Adrian Whittington, Samia Ezzamel, Rowena Jopling, and Richard Stott.

Lastly, thanks to our supportive and patient partners and family for putting up with so much for so long, especially Glenn and Emelie, and to our companion beasts Frederica, Stacey, Phoebe, and Raffa.

PART ONE

Foundations

CHAPTER ONE
Understanding PTSD and complexity

Post-Traumatic Stress Disorder (PTSD) is a common and disabling condition that can arise after very threatening or catastrophic experiences. A substantial proportion of people who develop PTSD recover naturally but around a third are left with chronic, sometimes lifelong, psychological difficulties.

Many people with PTSD live outwardly normal, albeit restricted, lives. The avoidance, isolation, and detachment characteristic of the disorder means sufferers can be slow in seeking treatment and, when they do, the condition tends to be poorly recognised. Furthermore, PTSD is often intertwined with a wide range of adverse physical and social consequences, including higher rates of illness and premature death.

Over the last 20 years, research into the psychological impact of traumatic events has greatly furthered our understanding of PTSD (see Olff et al., 2019, for a review), and several highly effective treatments have been developed and disseminated globally. However, even with 'gold standard' evidence-based treatments, not everyone with PTSD recovers and a substantial proportion is left with residual symptoms. And, while textbooks that comprehensively review the 'state-of-the-art' in PTSD treatment are available (e.g. Friedman et al., 2021; Schnyder, & Cloitre, 2015), many questions remain about how best to implement treatments to maximise their effectiveness in 'real world' clinical settings (Bryant, 2019). In this chapter, we discuss the key principles that help us understand how PTSD is developed and maintained. We then consider the issue of complexity – what we mean by it and how we approach it clinically.

Principles and theories: A brief overview

Research into the key mechanisms involved in PTSD has coalesced around certain principles; these are important because they form the foundations of our treatment approaches.

PTSD IS A LEARNING EXPERIENCE

The symptoms people experience after trauma can be understood as the result of a highly aversive learning experience. Behavioural models of PTSD focus on both classical and operant conditioning processes (Mowrer, 1947, 1960). The intense fear experienced during trauma becomes associated with the memories of the event and with a range of previously neutral stimuli present at the time which, when encountered again, trigger the same emotional reaction. Avoiding memories and reminders prevents this conditioned reaction from being naturally extinguished (Keane et al., 1985). These models underpin exposure-based treatments which aim to reduce symptoms through habituation to fear-provoking reminders of the trauma.

Contemporary learning theories have built on classical and operant conditioning models to explain a broader range of emotional experiences after trauma, as well as the findings that

DOI: 10.4324/9781003288329-2

many people do not fully recover following exposure-based therapies (Arch, & Craske, 2009), or may appear to recover but experience a 'return of fear' later on (Craske, & Mystkowski, 2006). One possible explanation is that, during successful exposure, the original associations learned during traumatic conditioning are not erased or 'unlearned', but remain intact. Instead, new secondary inhibitory learning develops that the conditioned stimuli are 'safe' and no longer warn of a dangerous outcome. This new learning then competes with the old threat associations to extinguish the conditioned fear response. Hence, one potential reason for a failure to naturally recover after trauma, or to benefit from exposure therapy, could be deficits in inhibitory learning and inhibitory neural regulation during exposure. Michelle Craske and colleagues (2014) have developed these ideas into techniques that can enhance the inhibitory learning acquired during exposure therapies, for example, by testing out threatening predicted outcomes, varying the type and number of stimuli presented, and conducting exposure in multiple contexts (Craske et al., 2014).

Theories of learning also form part of cognitive models of PTSD. For example, Anke Ehlers and David Clark (2000) highlight the role of associative learning processes in explaining the persistence of PTSD symptoms. They suggest that intrusive memories in PTSD often relate to the moments immediately preceding, rather than during, the greatest threat because they act as learned 'warning signals' to impending danger. Trauma memories also become easily triggered because of strong perceptual priming. This is a form of implicit memory, whereby people develop a reduced perceptual threshold and heightened sensitivity for noticing stimuli in their environment that were present during the trauma.

PTSD IS A DISORDER OF MEMORY

Disrupted memories are a key feature of PTSD, and re-experiencing symptoms are so-called because they go beyond normal remembering. Instead, trauma memories are felt powerfully, with vivid sensory details, intense sensations, and an impression of 'nowness' unlike usual autobiographical memories. Alongside these vivid involuntary memories can be difficulties intentionally recalling aspects of the trauma, missing details, or a sense of blankness when reminded of it. Such symptoms indicate that a problem has occurred in how trauma memories are processed, encoded, stored, and/or retrieved.

Several theories have sought to explain PTSD through how trauma memories are processed. For Mardi Horowitz (1975), trauma memories remain in an active memory storage system as individuals attempt to integrate and store them alongside their existing knowledge and experiences. Persisting trauma-related intrusions then arise as the active memory system rehearses the traumatic content in failed efforts to complete this processing.

Peter Lang's (1977) concept of 'fear networks' in anxiety disorders was extended by Edna Foa and colleagues (1989) into their emotional processing theory of PTSD. This suggests that trauma memories are processed as networks of interconnecting nodes, representing perceptual and cognitive information about the event, alongside verbal, physiological, and behavioural responses. The network acts as a 'programme' for dealing with danger, so matching triggers activate the network, prompting escape or avoidance. In PTSD, the connections between nodes in the fear network are strong, over-inclusive, and have a low threshold for activation, meaning that the fear response is very easily triggered, leading to re-experiencing of the trauma memories, hyperarousal, and avoidance behaviour.

Chris Brewin and colleagues (Brewin et al., 1996, 2010) instead propose a dual memory processing system associated with different parts of the brain. Here, trauma memories are encoded into two types of representation. One type is a lower-level perceptual representation that includes sensory details and emotional states (S-reps, earlier called 'situationally accessible memories'). The other type is a higher-level contextual representation (C-reps, or 'verbally-accessible memories') that includes a conceptual description of the sensory memories alongside information about its context – in space, time, and in relation to the person's life.

In Brewin's model, PTSD re-experiencing symptoms arise from very strong S-reps, reflecting the intensity of the traumatic experience; from relatively weak C-reps (which may be completely missing for some parts of the memories) due to a breakdown in conceptual cognitive processing during trauma; and/or from loose associations between the two representations. In successful processing, strong and detailed C-reps are tightly bound to their matching sensory S-Reps, so are activated together, diminishing the vividness and nowness of the subjective memories. In treatment, we describe this as 'putting words to every detail of the trauma memories', but a strong C-rep does not necessarily have to be verbally encoded, as long as it structurally represents the S-rep well. Brewin (2006) also introduces the idea of 'retrieval competition'. He suggests that, in PTSD, S-reps are more easily triggered and accessed than C-reps, so win the retrieval competition when people are exposed to reminders of traumatic experiences. In terms of recovery from PTSD, this suggests that making C-reps more easily accessed than S-reps should mean they are preferentially retrieved.

We find that a useful way to illustrate Brewin's dual representation theory is through the metaphors of sound and music. Sound can be represented in both a raw 'sensory' form, the shape of a soundwave, and in a 'contextualised' conceptual form, the notes in a musical score. Trauma memories are intensely sensory and aversive, like being blasted with a very loud sound. Encoding this S-rep into a C-rep is like transcribing the soundwave into musical notes, with annotations to describe all the variations in pitch, tempo, and intensity. The content is the same but represented in a form that is easier for us to read, understand, and remember. In PTSD, some of this C-rep musical score is missing or does not 'line up' correctly with parts of the S-rep soundwave. Those parts are then easily triggered rather than inhibited, and remembering them is like 'hearing them again' rather than 'reading the musical score'.

Now imagine that the sound is not one instrument, but a piece of music being played by a whole orchestra. If every instrument is in tune and following the same score, the music sounds coherent. However, if there are gaps or some notes are incorrectly transcribed, or if whole lines of an instrument are missing, the music loses its coherence and sounds disjointed and jarring. Similarly, in PTSD, C-reps can be incomplete, missing important cognitive, emotional, physiological, proprioceptive, and/or sensory details. To be successfully processed, S-rep trauma memories therefore need to be fully represented across all these levels. They also need to be contextualised within time and space, like giving the musical score a title and date-stamp, and then fitted into the person's previous experiences and belief systems, like filing the sheet music alongside all the other musical scores in their library.

The nature of trauma memories is also an important part of Ehlers and Clark's (2000) cognitive model, which posits that cognitive processing at the time of the trauma is one of the factors that predict the development of PTSD by influencing the nature of trauma memories (and related appraisals – more on these later) via:

- Data-driven processing, i.e. perceptual rather than conceptual processing
- Lack of self-referent processing, i.e. difficulty in processing the experience within other autobiographical memories
- Dissociation (see also van der Kolk, & Fisler, 1995)
- Mental defeat, where people experience total loss of autonomy and a sense of 'giving up' during a trauma.

Beierl et al. (2020) found that all four of these processing deficits are linked with the 'disjointedness' of trauma memories, which itself strongly predicts PTSD symptoms.

PTSD IS DRIVEN BY EMOTIONALITY

At the core of the experience of PTSD is emotion – not just fear, but often shame, horror, anger, helplessness, hopelessness, guilt, sadness, and many others. These emotions can interact in complex ways, both peri- and post-traumatically, for example, feeling ashamed for feeling angry, or feeling fearful of feeling helpless again. People with PTSD also often experience emotional numbness and may fluctuate between strong feelings and blunted affect. This can be especially apparent for people who had early-life, multiple, or sustained traumatic experiences. Janina Fisher (1999) uses the metaphor of having an 'emotional thermostat' which usually prevents feelings from becoming too intense or 'hot' versus disconnected or 'cold'. For some trauma survivors, their thermostat no longer automatically regulates their emotional temperature, leading to extremes of heat and cold, so they need to learn how to 'manually' regulate their emotional thermostat.

Emotions are central to the maintenance of PTSD. Efforts to cope with, and escape, unpleasant emotions may be maladaptive because they inadvertently exacerbate or maintain PTSD symptoms, or are temporarily effective but lead to additional problems. Beliefs about emotions are also important, for example 'I must control this feeling or I will become overwhelmed', or 'showing my distress means I am weak'. Emotions are also clues to important meanings; when we 'follow the emotion' in treatment, it often leads us to the key problematic appraisals that underpin an individual's PTSD.

PTSD IS DRIVEN BY PERSONAL MEANINGS

Subjective appraisals of threat during trauma are as important to the development of PTSD as objective measures such as physical injury (Blanchard et al., 1995). After a trauma, people may develop a variety of negative, highly idiosyncratic explanations of the event, and their role in it, that portray the trauma as having global implications rather than it being a discrete and time-limited event (Ehlers, & Clark, 2000). We often refer to these appraisals as 'meanings', which may also incorporate an individual's pre-trauma beliefs. Meanings can focus externally, for example, that the world is dangerous or unpredictable; or internally, that the person was to blame, attracts disaster, or deserved to be victimised (Dunmore et al., 2001). Negative meanings associated with the persistence of PTSD also include catastrophic interpretations of emotional/physiological responses (e.g. 'I am weak for feeling terrified and wetting myself during the trauma'), traumatic stress symptoms ('these intrusive images mean that I'm losing my mind'), the consequences of the event ('I'll never get over this, my life is pointless now'), and of other people's reactions ('people think I'm pathetic for still being affected by it', 'no-one can, or wants to, understand').

Cognitive responses to trauma can be understood, fundamentally, as the individual's struggle to fit the traumatic experience into their world view. Jean Piaget (1970) first described the processes of assimilation, where new information is modified to fit with pre-existing schemas, and accommodation, where schemas themselves are altered in response to new information. Traumatic experiences can violently disrupt fundamental schemas regarding safety, trust, power, esteem, and intimacy (McCann, & Pearlman, 1990), and can lead to 'over-accommodation' where schema changes are extreme or over-generalised (Resick, & Schnicke, 1993), for example, 'nobody can be trusted'. Previous fundamental assumptions about the world as safe and benevolent and the self as worthy can be 'shattered' by the trauma (Janoff-Bulman, 1992). Conversely, previously held negative core schemas can be seemingly confirmed by the experience.

PTSD IS INADVERTENTLY MAINTAINED BY COPING EFFORTS

People with PTSD will understandably attempt to cope with their emotions and symptoms by deploying all their available resources based on what seems most natural, or what has worked for them in the past. And this will depend on their pre-existing coping repertoire, personal circumstances, and support networks. Some attempts to cope will be strategic, such as coping with feeling vulnerable by avoiding leaving the house, withdrawing from relationships, or taking excessive precautions to prevent danger (safety-seeking behaviours). Other coping may be habitual or automatic, such as emotional suppression, numbing, or dissociative detachment. Trying to understand and come to terms with a traumatic event can motivate rumination in a search for meaning, or brooding on injustice and what could have been done differently to prevent the trauma. Even strategies that don't appear overtly helpful, such as self-harm or risk-taking behaviours, can function as forms of emotional coping; a way of blocking or distracting from negative feelings.

Inadvertently, these coping strategies can prevent natural recovery after trauma and maintain PTSD. They may block the emotional processing needed to resolve the trauma memories and their meanings. They may restrict or distort new experiences that might otherwise help the person to access information that challenges their negative trauma-related beliefs. Some lead to additional problems and losses, by contributing to physical, social, and psychological comorbidities that often develop alongside PTSD. Examples include financial problems arising from being unable to work because of avoiding triggers, depression arising from social withdrawal and isolation, or health problems arising from alcohol misuse.

PSYCHOLOGICAL TREATMENTS

These principles have evolved into psychological treatments for PTSD, each with a differing emphasis. Learning theories have generated behavioural treatments for PTSD, which emphasise exposure to trauma-related stimuli. Prolonged exposure therapy (Foa et al., 2007; Foa, & Rothbaum, 1998), based on emotional processing theory, uses imaginal reliving of the trauma memories alongside in vivo exposure to reminders of the traumatic event, to reactivate the fear network and introduce new non-threatening information that is incompatible with the fearful associations. Cognitive processing therapy (Resick et al., 2016; Resick, & Schnicke, 1992) focuses on so-called 'stuck points', where negative cognitions about the trauma are identified and resolved and particular cognitive themes common in PTSD are addressed: trust, intimacy, power, safety, and esteem.

Our preferred approach is cognitive therapy for PTSD (CT-PTSD; Ehlers & Clark, 2000), which integrates all the principles discussed above, and which we explain in detail in Chapter 2. To explain why we prefer this approach, we need to first explain how we think about complexity in PTSD.

COMPLEXITY IN PTSD

WHAT DO WE MEAN BY COMPLEXITY?

Operationalising the concept of complexity in psychological disorders is tricky and some have argued that the term has been overused, becoming a proxy for a range of different clinical features such as severity, risk, and chronicity, for relapsing or 'resistant' treatment responses, and even applied by therapists post-hoc to explain away their treatment failures (Barton et al., 2017). In PTSD, there is also often a conflation of the concepts of complex trauma (often a short-hand for multiple, prolonged, and/or repeated traumatic events), a complex reaction (such as severe symptoms and multiple comorbidities), and a complex treatment (one with multiple components or which encounters obstacles).

Seeking a more precise clinical definition, Barton et al. (2017) suggest that complexity arises when a problem has 'multiple moving parts and sometimes behaves unpredictably'. Typically, these moving parts are the biological, psychological, and social factors that exist beyond the core problem of PTSD. We would extend this to include the multiple moving parts that can exist within an individual, in the interplay between their experiences, beliefs, symptoms, behaviours, and environment. It is these variations, and their interactions, which make clients with PTSD so diverse and fascinating to work with.

Barton et al.'s (2017) definition draws a useful distinction between complexity and its potential impact: complications in the delivery of treatment, or 'interactions of biological, psychological and social factors that create barriers to treatment, challenge therapeutic alliances and modify the usual maintenance of a disorder' (p. 2). Complexity does not necessarily lead to complications. We know, for example, that people often respond to treatment for PTSD even when they have significant comorbidity (Ehlers et al., 2013). And, indeed, therapy can be complicated for quite simple reasons that have nothing to do with clinical complexity, for example, being unable to afford travel to treatment sessions.

Whether 'complex PTSD', as originally proposed by Judith Herman (1992), constitutes a distinct diagnosis from PTSD has been subject to much debate. The most recent Diagnostic Statistical Manual (DSM-5; American Psychiatric Association, 2013) has not included the diagnosis but has broadened the criteria of PTSD to incorporate symptoms commonly associated with complex PTSD, such as reckless and self-destructive behaviour, persistent negative trauma-related beliefs and emotions, and a dissociative subtype characterised by marked depersonalisation and derealisation symptoms. In contrast, the latest International Classification of Diseases (ICD-11; World Health Organisation, 2018) now includes complex PTSD as a separate diagnosis, defined as the symptoms of PTSD (a narrower list compared to DSM-5) plus symptoms reflecting 'disturbances in self-organisation' in the form of dysregulated affect (both over- and under-activated), disturbances in relationships, and persistent negative self-concept.

In this book, we've tended not to refer to complex PTSD as we wanted to encompass a broader spectrum of complexity issues than just 'disturbances of self-organisation'. However, many of the clients we describe would likely meet ICD-11 criteria for complex PTSD. Our other reason for not focusing on complex PTSD is because, while it is a useful description of a clinical presentation, it doesn't tell us what may, or may not, make treatment complicated. In this book, we focus on the types of complexity associated with PTSD that commonly lead to complications in therapy delivery, with the aim of helping therapists understand those complexities better and adjust and refine their treatment to address them as needed.

As illustrated in Figure 1.1, we have structured the book to reflect the 'multiple moving parts' both within the individual and their system, with sections on complexity in:

- The memories, cognitions, and coping strategies that form part of PTSD
- The psychological, physical, social, and risk comorbidities that often surround PTSD
- The interplay with the therapeutic relationship and issues of diversity.

An additional, final chapter covers self-care for therapists.

TREATMENTS FOR COMPLEXITY IN PTSD

The lack, until recently, of a diagnostic definition of complex PTSD and the diversity of presentations that have been labelled 'complex', has hampered the development and testing of effective treatments. Indeed, people with the most complex presentations are often excluded from research trials, so it remains unclear whether current evidence-based treatments for PTSD are as effective for this group. Encouragingly, emerging research suggests that people with complex PTSD may benefit equally from existing evidence-based treatments (Hoeboer et al., 2021). Dissemination trials of trauma-focused treatments in routine clinical settings, including prolonged exposure (Foa et al., 2013), cognitive processing therapy (Chard et al., 2012), narrative exposure therapy (Gwozdziewycz, & Mehl-Madrona, 2013), and cognitive therapy

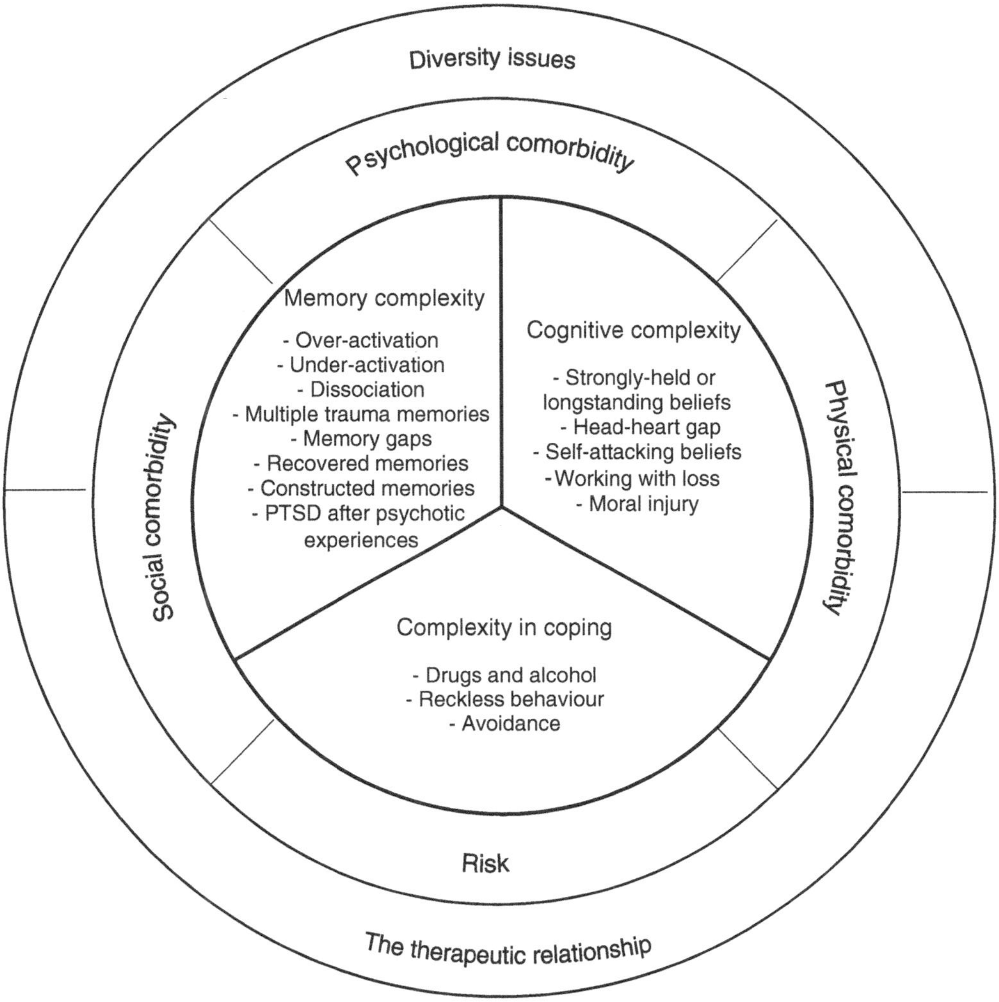

Figure 1.1 The multiple moving parts of complexity in PTSD

(Ehlers et al., 2013; Gillespie et al., 2002) have also demonstrated impressive effectiveness, including with people typically considered 'complex' such as those with significant comorbid difficulties or multiple and early life traumas.

Herman (1992) proposed a phase-based treatment approach for complex PTSD, comprising a distinct 'stabilisation' phase, before a trauma-processing phase, and a final phase of 'reintegration' with important areas of life such as relationships, socialising, and work. Despite high face validity, inclusion in expert consensus guidelines (McFetridge et al., 2017), and the development of effective treatment packages based on the phase-based model (Cloitre et al., 2002), there is limited evidence that phase-based approaches are superior to primarily trauma-processing interventions, with critics arguing that they are an unnecessary use of clinical time, neither improving outcomes nor reducing drop-out (de Jongh et al., 2016).

The reality of clinical practice may lie between these positions and recent guidelines no longer recommend a distinct stabilisation phase for all clients (International Society for Traumatic Stress Studies, 2019). Rather, they suggest that complexity is best approached with multi-component or modularised interventions, personalised to the needs of the client, that move beyond binary distinctions of phased versus non-phased treatments (Cloitre, 2021; Coventry et al., 2020). Our experience is that a distinct stabilisation phase is unnecessary for most clients, even those with complex presentations. However, where there is immediate risk, severe dissociation, interpersonal problems which are jeopardising the therapeutic relationship, or insufficient emotional regulation to tolerate work on the trauma memories, we implement stabilisation interventions before processing trauma memories, or 'as and when' needed during trauma processing. We also use additional modules as needed to address clients' specific goals or problems beyond core PTSD symptoms. We avoid 'one size fits all' stabilisation packages, because everyone has different needs, and we only do as much as needed to progress efficiently to trauma memory work. Nor do we generally depart from the CT-PTSD model, but use individualised CT-PTSD formulations to guide us in selecting from the many techniques available.

Why CT-PTSD works well with complexity

Given the other treatment approaches available, why have we chosen to focus on CT-PTSD? The NICE guidelines (National Institute for Health and Care Excellence, 2018), and indeed most other published guidelines (American Psychiatric Association, National Health and Medical Research Council, Institute of Medicine, International Society of Traumatic Stress Service; Forbes et al., 2010), recommend trauma-focused therapies for PTSD, specifically trauma-focused CBT and eye movement desensitisation and reprocessing (EMDR), rather than non-directive treatments such as counselling. But, within that range, there are still lots of different treatment models and many of them with a solid evidence base. Here are our top reasons for favouring CT-PTSD when we are working with complexity.

1. *The evidence base*

The evidence base for CT-PTSD is very strong, with randomised controlled trials (Ehlers et al., 2003, 2005, 2014), dissemination trials (Gillespie et al., 2002), and routine clinical practice audits (Ehlers et al., 2013) reporting very good effect sizes. The latter studies are important when we consider complexity, as the clients likely presented with many of the 'real world' features of complexity that we discuss in this book. In our clinic, we also routinely evaluate our treatments, which are based on CT-PTSD but include adaptations to meet the needs of our population, just like the approach we describe in this book, and we achieve comparable results. As we work in a specialist PTSD service, our clients usually present with psychological and physical comorbidities, as well as previous unsuccessful treatments in other services. The areas our clinic serves have high levels of social deprivation, so our clients generally present with social difficulties, exposure to multiple and sustained traumas, and ongoing threat. Many of our clients are refugees so treatment is often conducted through an interpreter.

2. *It's flexible*

CT-PTSD is a formulation-based rather than a protocolised treatment, which means that you don't have to follow all of the treatment elements in a specific order or deliver them in the same way for every client. Instead, you can respond to your client's needs and goals flexibly. Is your client using some risky behaviours? Start with the area of the formulation that addresses coping strategies. Are you stuck because your client feels too ashamed to talk about the trauma? Work on the cognitive appraisals associated with shame first. Working with someone whose main goal is to return to work, but gets too triggered by sitting in a shared office space? Use stimulus discrimination of the trigger first.

Flexibility is especially important when it comes to complexity issues, as it allows us to modify elements of the treatment and alter the order in which they are delivered to individualise the treatment. You can move between the areas of the model as needed, as long as you stick to your formulation and keep track of which process you are targeting with each intervention. This 'flexibility within fidelity' approach of sticking tightly to principles, while being adaptable and creative with techniques and tactics (Whittington, & Grey, 2014), is what we hope to demonstrate in this book.

3. *It's a parsimonious synthesis of other models*

There is a certain amount of overlap between the different models we've discussed in this chapter (see Schnyder et al., 2015 for a review). CT-PTSD provides an elegant synthesis of both the memory processing and social-cognitive models. Unlike treatment trials which have considered memory and cognitive work to be individual elements, or add-ons to existing treatment packages, in the CT-PTSD model they are interconnected. Memory work is used to access and activate appraisals, new meanings are integrated back into the trauma memories. As we will show you, CT-PTSD also has plenty of room to integrate novel techniques adapted from other approaches, where they fit with the principles of the CT-PTSD formulation, for example, using drawings, objects, and images instead of verbal narratives, to conceptually represent, process, and update key trauma memories, meanings, and emotions.

4. *It is a longitudinal, as well as maintenance, model*

The cognitive model includes the role of previous experiences and beliefs which, for many clients, is essential in understanding why a trauma has been processed in a way that has not led to natural recovery. Many people with PTSD have experienced earlier life traumas which may cause PTSD symptoms directly, or have been 'personality defining' through their impact on a person's core belief system. For example, someone who was neglected in childhood may not have particular memories that they re-experience from this time, but a strong sense of themselves as unworthy of love. This can leave a deep emotional scar which is re-opened by traumas in adulthood and compounds their impact. These prior beliefs are the lens through which the trauma is understood and guide how the person responds to their experiences. Using a treatment model that incorporates information about how a trauma has resonated with an individual in a particular way can be essential to working effectively with their trauma-related appraisals, particularly when they arise from multiple or sustained traumas, are longstanding, or difficult to change.

5. *It has experience and emotion at its centre*

The centre point of the cognitive model is the 'felt sense' experience of PTSD, including the strong and toxic emotions that trauma evokes. This is where we believe you should always start with clients – with the phenomenology of their emotional experience. From there, we can work outwards, through the processes which are leading to and maintaining the PTSD symptoms and the associated emotions.

Emotions are also often the guide to understanding someone's idiosyncratic appraisals. We sometimes find that the appraisals someone can access and verbalise do not match up with the feelings someone is experiencing. For example, if a client tells us that during their trauma they thought 'I am dying', but reports feeling guilty, we know we are missing something. There must be another appraisal or meaning attached, like 'I've let this happen, I'm not fighting back enough' or 'if I die, my children will be left alone', which leads to the emotion of guilt. It can be tricky for people to tell us all their appraisals because they may not have been experienced as clear thoughts during the trauma. This is partly why we use techniques to bring the trauma memories back to mind and then use the emotions as a guide through the layers of meaning.

It follows that CT-PTSD interventions are rooted in emotion. We need to access and evoke the trauma-related emotions through memory work, but also expose the client to different, corrective emotional experiences. This is why experiential techniques such as behavioural experiments, updating the memories while activated, and imagery rescripting are so useful.

6. *It is intrinsically validating and normalising*

Using a formulation-based approach means that, together with our clients, we are developing an understanding of where a problem has originated and what keeps it going. In doing this, we are showing that someone's experience is entirely understandable and makes sense. This is important because many people with PTSD have negative beliefs about having developed PTSD, such as that they are mentally weak, or that their mind or brain is permanently damaged. We use conversations about the nature of PTSD symptoms, their acquisition, and maintenance to show that the problem is caused by understandable processes rather than personal deficits. Creating order and bringing sense to a client's disparate experiences by sharing an individualised formulation is in itself an immensely therapeutic endeavour.

By explaining where an individual's PTSD comes from and what keeps it going, the CT-PTSD model also tells us how to treat it, by breaking the feedback loops that maintain it and prevent natural recovery. Every arrow in the model is a process, which means that making changes in one area will change the outcome in another. This provides structure to the treatment, helping make sense of every intervention and what it intends to target. It also provides the client with hope – if we understand what is happening to keep PTSD going, we have a chance to change it. Hope is important in PTSD treatment, as we ask clients to do things that are upsetting or that they prefer to avoid, like talking about their worst ever experience and accessing the difficult emotions it provokes.

7. *It is well-tolerated*

PTSD is a disorder that typically has high treatment drop-out rates (Imel et al., 2013), probably due to the challenges of working through painful material, the avoidance which is part of the disorder's diagnosis, and the challenging life circumstances that many clients face. CT-PTSD has shown far lower drop-out rates than other evidence-based treatments in its trials, and this has been replicated in routine clinical practice. There are probably various reasons for that, but we think that the flexibility in the approach is relevant. As there is not a specific protocol, therapists can tailor the treatment specifically to a client's goals, and adjust the delivery and timing of intervention strategies depending on individual need. Unlike prolonged exposure, work on the trauma memories is used to access problematic meanings, which are then immediately addressed through updating rather than requiring repeated re-exposures. Imaginal reliving therefore usually only takes place a few times, rather than every session. If clients find it challenging, it can also be adapted in a variety of ways while staying close to CT-PTSD principles. The emphasis on collaboration and flexibility hopefully helps clients to feel in control of the process. Taken together we think these features make the treatment less aversive, and so well-tolerated.

Recommended reading

Brewin, C. R., & Holmes, E. A. (2003). Psychological theories of posttraumatic stress disorder. *Clinical Psychology Review*, 23(3), 339–376.

Cloitre, M. (2021). Complex PTSD: Assessment and treatment. *European Journal of Psychotraumatology*, 12(sup1), 1866423.

Ehring, T., Kleim, B., & Ehlers, E. (2012). Cognition and emotion in posttraumatic stress disorder. In M. D. Robinson, E. Watkins, & E. Harmon-Jones (Eds.). *Handbook of cognition and emotion* (pp. 401–420). Guilford Press.

CHAPTER TWO
Cognitive Therapy for PTSD

Cian was assaulted on a night out with friends. He was having nightmares about the assault, ruminating angrily about his attackers, and feeling anxious in busy places. His therapist helped him to relive and update his memories of the trauma, and they used stimulus discrimination to address triggers to his memories, as well as behavioural experiments to address his beliefs about being assaulted again.

Ehlers and Clark's (2000) cognitive model of PTSD integrates many of the theories we discussed in the previous chapter into a single cognitive-behavioural formulation. It is distinctive both in its synthesis of theory and in several of its treatment techniques. The model provides a comprehensive but flexible framework for delivering an individualised cognitive-behavioural treatment.

In this chapter, we will summarise the model briefly, and the treatment which derives from it – cognitive therapy for PTSD (CT-PTSD). We recommend reading Ehlers and Clark's original (2000) paper describing the model, as it remains an excellent introduction. Do access further training if you are new to the approach, as this chapter is only a summary and refresher. The team who developed CT-PTSD have also made freely available some brilliant written and video training resources at www.oxcadatresources.com.

The cognitive model

Ehlers and Clark's (2000) model explains the core experience of PTSD as a sense of serious current threat that endures even though the trauma itself is in the past. They suggest that the sense of threat may be physical (e.g. feeling unsafe and in danger) or psychological (e.g. feeling a failure, defeated, or degraded). This sense of current threat is driven by three processes. Prior experiences, beliefs, and coping styles, alongside characteristics of the trauma itself, can influence all three processes.

The first process relates to excessively negative meanings that the person ascribes to the traumatic event or its consequences. For example, if they now perceive the world as unpredictable and other people as dangerous, or themselves as blameworthy or weak, this creates a persisting sense of threat.

The second concerns the nature of the trauma memories themselves. The model suggests that when the worst moments of the traumatic event are processed in a predominantly sensory or 'data-driven' way, their associated memories are poorly elaborated, disjointed, and lack context within the person's other autobiographical memories. As a result, when trauma memories are triggered, people struggle to access other information that could correct threatening impressions or negative beliefs they had at the time. In other words, the memories for these moments have not been 'updated' with what the individual knows now, such as that they survived, or that what

DOI: 10.4324/9781003288329-3

they believed during the worst moments may be inaccurate (e.g. the threatening and degrading words said to them by a perpetrator are not true). Powerful conditioning during the trauma, alongside a lack of contextualisation, also means the trauma memories and associated emotions become easily and unpredictably triggered by sensory cues which match those encountered at the time of the trauma. This adds to the sense of current threat.

Finally, cognitive and behavioural strategies intended to reduce the sense of threat inadvertently maintain the problem. These strategies can directly increase PTSD symptoms (e.g. memory suppression increases intrusions via the 'rebound effect') or the sense of threat itself (e.g. hypervigilance for danger increases feelings of being on edge). Avoidance and suppression of memories and reminders, safety-seeking behaviours, and rumination also prevent the person elaborating and contextualising their trauma memories, and disconfirming or reappraising negative trauma-related meanings.

The model is illustrated in Figure 2.1. This version is slightly adapted from the original model because we find that, with increasing complexity, there can be a great deal of relevant information in the top boxes of the model, so we have separated them to aid clarity. However, the original elements and their interactions remain the same. We have annotated it with some pointers about what goes in each box. The arrows are also labelled and explained underneath. We think the arrows are really important because they represent causal mechanisms, and therefore potential targets in treatment. It is the dynamic interaction between each element of the model which is key to understanding PTSD, i.e. the interacting functions and consequences of appraisals, coping strategies, and memory characteristics.

WHAT DO THE ARROWS MEAN?

A: Pre-trauma factors and experiences can affect how the traumatic event is cognitively processed, which will, in turn, affect both the nature of the trauma memory and trauma-related appraisals. For example, a survivor of childhood abuse may have learnt to cut off emotionally or dissociate in response to an inescapable situation. It follows that they will be prone to detach more readily when confronted with a later trauma and that the consequent low quality of cognitive processing during the trauma will contribute to a poorly elaborated memory, potentially with gaps. This may also lead to appraisals that the person's mind is failing them, or that something awful happened that they cannot recall. Prior beliefs are important in understanding how an event is appraised. Someone who has always seen themselves as able to manage any situation may have this belief shattered by a traumatic experience where they are completely out of control, leading to appraisals like 'I'm not the person I thought I was' or 'I can't control anything'. Conversely, someone who already had a very poor self-image may be more likely to perceive the trauma as further evidence that they are useless or worthless.

B: Event-specific factors can also affect cognitive processing and the nature of trauma memories and appraisals. For example, a traumatic event that is very sudden and unexpected, like being hit from behind in a traffic accident, will be very difficult to process, leading to trauma memories that are very sensory and lack context, as the person had no opportunity to make sense of the event as it happened. This kind of trauma may also lead to beliefs about unexpectedness and unpredictability, like 'something bad can happen at any time'. A trauma that is particularly prolonged and/or humiliating (such as torture) may lead to a sense of mental defeat, and an associated breakdown in conceptual processing as well as beliefs such as 'I gave up and let it happen' or 'I'm no longer human'.

C: The sequelae or consequences of a trauma also often affect appraisals. For example, significant life changes or losses such as permanent physical injury, death of a loved one, or forced migration may contribute to beliefs such as 'my life has been destroyed' or 'I am no longer the person I was'.

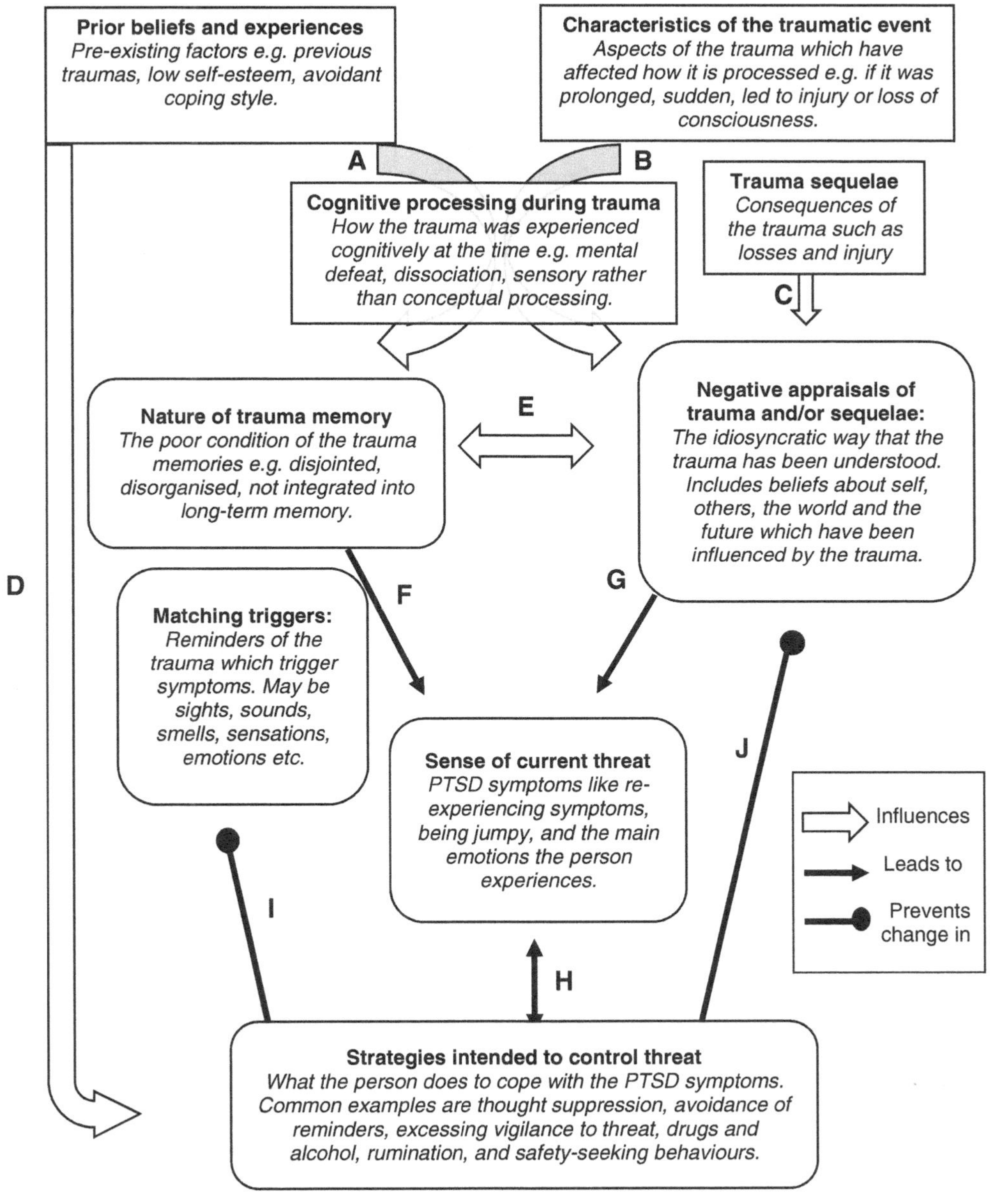

Figure 2.1 Adapted cognitive model of PTSD (reprinted from *Behaviour Research and Therapy, 38*(4), Ehlers, A. and Clark, D., A cognitive model of posttraumatic stress disorder, 319–145, (2000), with permission from Elsevier).

D: Previous coping styles are likely to influence how someone copes with PTSD. For example, a person who tends to deal with problems by ignoring them, self-medicating with drugs or alcohol, or dwelling on what they could have done differently may be more likely to cope in these ways following a traumatic event.

E: There is a reciprocal relationship between the nature of trauma memories and appraisals. The vivid, 'here and now' quality of trauma memories can lead people to conclude that the trauma is not in the past and they are still in danger, or that they have lost their mind. Appraisals can also affect how the trauma memories are recalled. For example, if a person has a strong belief that they are to blame for the trauma occurring, they are more likely to recall the moments in the trauma which support this appraisal and less likely to bring to mind those parts of the memories that do not.

F: Trauma memories that are poorly elaborated and not fully integrated into long-term memory are easily triggered, coming back in the form of intrusive, highly sensory recollections that feel as if they are happening in the 'here and now'. Triggers to re-experiencing symptoms often match an aspect of the trauma. These are sometimes obvious reminders, like returning to the place where the trauma happened or seeing someone who looks like the perpetrator, but triggers can be subtle, like a colour, smell, body sensation, or position that echoes a sensory detail present at the time of the trauma.

G: How the trauma has been appraised contributes to the sense of current threat and strong emotions which are central to the experience of PTSD. For example, if someone has appraised the world as more dangerous, themselves as less capable, and/or other people as less trustworthy following a traumatic event, they will continue to feel under threat. Internal threats also arise from appraisals about the effects of the trauma, e.g. 'I'm damaged goods', 'I have lost my mind', or 'I'll never get over this'. Specific appraisals are often highly idiosyncratic and key to understanding why PTSD persists for a given person.

H: Coping strategies are the client's understandable responses to the symptoms of PTSD. The arrow back up represents the direct effects that some of those coping strategies can have on PTSD symptoms. For example, trying to suppress intrusive memories often leads to a rebound effect, where they intrude even more. Excessive vigilance to threat can make an individual feel more on edge and under threat, by drawing their attention to ambiguous signs of danger.

I: Coping strategies can contribute to the maintenance of PTSD via two other processes. Firstly, avoidance of thinking and talking about trauma memories (using distraction, suppression, drugs or alcohol, avoidance of triggers, etc.) means that they remain disjointed and unintegrated into autobiographical memory systems. Avoiding the memories means that details are not filled in, they are not updated with new information, or linked to memories of other experiences that would help contextualise them.

J: The other maintenance cycle is via trauma appraisals. Some coping strategies prevent appraisals from being tested and updated. For example, if a person feeling under threat avoids going to busy places or uses safety-seeking behaviours such as avoiding eye contact with strangers, they never find out whether these precautions have actually kept them safe or whether they would have been safe anyway. Withdrawing to avoid triggers feeds the belief that life is permanently ruined. Isolating from others prevents people testing out their beliefs about others' judgements of them. Rumination is often an attempt to make sense of what has happened but instead tends to consolidate negative appraisals rather than challenge them. Self-attack can follow on from responsibility appraisals, e.g. 'it was my fault' or 'I deserved this to happen' and, while intended to improve future performance or make amends, instead strengthens those beliefs. Worry may similarly function to plan for future threats, but instead strengthens beliefs about danger and the need to take precautions.

Cognitive therapy for PTSD

The model forms the basis of CT-PTSD and leads to three main aims in treatment:

- To modify the threatening appraisals (personal meanings) of the trauma and its consequences

- To reduce re-experiencing by elaborating and contextualising the trauma memories, and by discriminating triggers
- To reduce the cognitive and behavioural coping strategies that maintain the sense of current threat, prevent memory elaboration or meaning reappraisal.

BASIC PRINCIPLES

CT-PTSD has as its foundation the important principles of CBT, including being formulation-derived, collaborative, structured, and based on empirical evidence (see Westbrook, 2014, for a reminder). Like other CBT models, it uses guided discovery to identify and address idiosyncratic appraisals. The therapist takes a position of curiosity rather than attempting to change the client's mind about their beliefs. Together, they examine the beliefs and the evidence supporting them, before considering potential alternative perspectives.

CORE TECHNIQUES

Collaborative case conceptualisation

The early sessions of CT-PTSD include gathering information, providing some psychoeducation, and creating a formulation to explain the key cycles maintaining the person's PTSD. This is usually summarised as a few key points by the end of session one.

Reclaiming or rebuilding your life

In the first session, the therapist asks about areas of life that the client has disengaged from since the trauma. It is common for people to withdraw from activities and relationships that used to give their life meaning and pleasure, which contributes to beliefs that their life has permanently changed for the worse.

'Reclaiming your life' involves a gradual reintroduction of these activities and continues throughout treatment, with the therapist encouraging the client and helping them to overcome barriers to returning to previously valued activities. Where the client is unable to re-engage with previous activities, for example, due to a change in circumstances such as moving country, because of a permanent physical injury, or where they have no healthy 'baseline' because of a lifetime of trauma, the focus may be on 'claiming' what they never had and/or 'rebuilding' a life that they want.

Imaginal reliving/narrative writing

Imaginal reliving involves accessing trauma memories in imagination. Usually, the client is asked to close their eyes and speak in the first person, present tense to aid emotional engagement with the memories and to reduce distractions. The client is asked to describe the traumatic event in detail, including their perceptions, thoughts, feelings, and bodily sensations.

An alternative to imaginal reliving is to create a written narrative of the trauma. This is preferable for some clients, especially where they are prone to dissociation, if the trauma was very protracted, or the memories are very disorganised. There is no evidence to suggest that imaginal reliving is more effective than narrative writing or vice versa, so the techniques can be used interchangeably or in combination. The written narrative is usually prepared with the therapist, with a similar level and range of detail as reliving.

FAQ: How many times should I do imaginal reliving?

The goal of reliving in CT-PTSD is to create a more complete version of the trauma memories and reduce disjointedness, to aid their integration into autobiographical memory, and to identify hotspots and their key personal meanings. This might be achieved in the first reliving session, or it might take a couple of attempts. On average, imaginal reliving of the whole of one traumatic event usually takes place only 2–3 times in CT-PTSD.

Some clients experience an immediate positive effect on their symptoms after reliving, probably because they spontaneously update the problematic appraisals by fully accessing the trauma memories. Traumas where the main emotion was fear or horror often update quickly and one or two reliving sessions may lead to big changes. When the peritraumatic emotions are more complex, like guilt, shame, anger, humiliation and so on, it is best to move on to addressing the hotspots immediately, as the related appraisals will be less likely to update spontaneously so will need cognitive restructuring. Imaginal reliving can be used again to update the hotspots once new appraisals have been accessed.

Following reliving or writing out the trauma memories, the client is asked to identify the moments which are associated with the highest levels of distress, known as 'hotspots'. These usually have important personal meanings attached to them and are therefore a focus for further work.

FAQ: How do I tell what are hotspots?

After a reliving or narrative writing session, we ask clients which moments in the trauma memories felt most distressing, vivid, or like they were happening 'right now'. It helps to do this as soon as possible after going through the trauma memories, while the experience is still fresh. The therapist can also sometimes spot hotspots during reliving, for example, when the client seems most emotional or distant, where they physically flush or shake, or moments the client seems to skim past or avoid mentioning. Another way to identify likely hotspots is by finding out which parts of the trauma are most frequently re-experienced in intrusions, flashbacks, and nightmares, as this will reflect the trauma memories which are particularly poorly processed and most easily triggered.

Updating trauma memories

Once the hotspots have been identified, the therapist and client explore the emotions and meanings attached to those moments and begin to identify new information which might 'update' problematic meanings. In some cases, these updates are easily identified and can be added into the trauma memories immediately. Others will need further exploration using guided discovery. Adding additional details to the updates, and introducing ways of making them feel meaningful, can help the updates to 'stick' when they are then introduced back into the trauma memories.

Once meaningful updates have been generated, they are integrated back into the trauma memories. This can be done during imaginal reliving by pausing and holding the memory at the point at which the hotspot is activated while bringing in the new updating information. If a written narrative has been created, the updates can be written into the account at the appropriate point in a different colour. Imagery can also be used to enhance updates. For example, people might be asked to bring to mind an image of their wounds healing to update a hotspot where they believed they had been permanently disfigured.

Cassie thought she was going to die during a traumatic birth. Cassie's therapist asked what would have been the worst thing about that and Cassie said, 'that I'd never get to meet my daughter'. As well as reliving and updating the hotspot where she believed she would die with the new information 'I survived', Cassie was encouraged to add further details to address this additional layer of meaning. Cassie said 'I know now that I see my daughter every day. I took her to pre-school this morning and she was really excited because it started snowing'. Cassie's therapist encouraged her to hold the hotspot in mind, then look at a photo of her daughter playing happily in the snow to reinforce this new meaning.

Some hotspots may take more work to find meaningful updates and a range of cognitive restructuring techniques can be used as required. For example, if someone has a strong belief that the trauma was their fault, some time may be needed to examine the evidence for this belief using techniques such as surveys and responsibility pie charts. If someone believed during the trauma that they were worthless, and this feels like a confirmation of a belief they have long held about themselves, it may require several sessions to explore a meaningful alternative, using techniques like positive data logs, behavioural experiments, and a historical review of evidence.

FAQ: What is the difference between imaginal reliving and imagery rescripting?

Imaginal reliving involves revisiting trauma memories in imagination and putting words to the moment-by-moment details of the event. Imagery rescripting often starts the same way, but the memories are rapidly altered, moving away from what occurred in reality towards imagining the events unfolding or ending differently. Usually, the new version is imagined in a way that feels better, for example, 'rewriting' the memories by bringing a friend in to help, so the person feels less powerless or alone than they did at the time. Imagery rescripting has been used as a stand-alone treatment for PTSD (Arntz, 2012), but in CT-PTSD we generally use it as an adjunct to imaginal reliving to help 'super-charge' new meanings or updates. So, from a CT-PTSD perspective, imagery rescripting is a version of memory updating, for example, to bring in the information that, although they were alone then, they are not alone now.

We use imagery rescripting a lot, as we find it a very effective and creative way of helping clients update complex, rigid, and multi-layered meanings, and gain control over otherwise overwhelming imagery and memories. Imagery rescripting can activate thoughts, feelings, and sensations all at once, so it helps in bridging the 'head–heart gap' (Chapter 14). There are endless variations on how to use imagery rescripting, some of which are described in this book, such as bringing in the adult self (page 85, 162, 224), conversations with the deceased (page 171-2), consulting a moral authority (page 184-5), afterlife imagery (page 119), and strength and mastery imagery (page 82, 152).

Cognitive work

As well as developing updating information to address peri-traumatic appraisals, cognitive restructuring techniques are also used with trauma-related beliefs which have developed since the trauma (or which pre-date it and appear confirmed) and which lead to negative emotions such as guilt, shame, anger, or an over-generalised sense of danger. As before, a wide range of cognitive techniques can be employed, usually focused on guided discovery and behavioural experiments. These are described in more detail in Chapter 12.

Stimulus discrimination

Stimulus discrimination or 'then versus now' is a technique to address triggers to intrusive memories. It is based on the idea that triggers match trauma memories in some way, for example, the colour red may trigger memories of blood, the smell of smoke may trigger memories of fire. However, many other details of the triggering situation will be different, details which highlight the person is safe and the memory is in the past, and stimulus discrimination involves drawing attention to these differences.

The therapist first helps the client identify triggers to intrusive memories. Some triggers will be obvious, but others may be more subtle. It can feel as if intrusive symptoms like flashbacks come out of the blue, but there is usually a trigger that can be identified with some detective work. Keeping an intrusions diary can be very helpful for this. For each trigger, the client and therapist list the matching features, as well as the differences between the triggering situation and the trauma.

> Gilberto was in a road traffic accident where his car was struck by a speeding driver in a blue car. Intrusions to the memories were triggered when he saw blue cars on the road. His therapist asked for a recent example of this trigger and together they listed the similarities and differences.

Once the differences have been discussed, the next step is to deliberately encounter the triggers and practise noticing all the differences. This can be done in the therapy session, either using electronic resources like pictures, videos, or sound files, or by going 'out and about' to locate the trigger in vivo. With the example above, Gilberto and his therapist first practised the technique by looking at photos of blue cars online, and then went to a busy road nearby to practise with actual cars. Gilberto also practised using the technique between sessions when he was driving. The more familiar the technique becomes, the easier it will be to implement when triggers are unexpectedly encountered.

Reduce/replace unhelpful coping strategies

The strategies that the client uses to cope with the sense of current threat associated with PTSD are identified and, where they appear to maintain the problem, clients are encouraged to drop or replace them. Guided discovery is used, including reviewing the costs and benefits of different strategies, followed by behavioural experiments to test the effects of dropping coping strategies. There is lots more on this topic in Part 4.

Site visits

Towards the end of treatment, the therapist and client return to the scene of the trauma. The therapist encourages the client to notice all the differences between the site as it was at the time of the trauma ('then') and how it is in the present day ('now'). Sometimes obvious changes have happened at the site and there will be other differences, such as the time of day, date, presence of the therapist, weather, and so on, which can be highlighted. Seeing the difference between the trauma site in the present day compared to at the time of the trauma helps make the memories feel more like they are in the past (Murray et al., 2016).

The therapist and client can also reconstruct the trauma while at the site by walking through what happened. This can lead to further information being revealed which may fill gaps in memories or aid in understanding the experience, which sometimes addresses misappraisals.

Table 2.1 Gilberto's stimulus discrimination table

THEN – car accident	Same or different?	NOW – seeing a blue car
Blue car	✓	Blue car
Model of car - Audi	✗	Model of car – Toyota
Rainy, cold day	✗	Weather is sunny
October 2015	✗	June 2020
Driving on the M25	✗	Driving south on M40
Alone in the car	✗	Wife next to me
Other driver was speeding	✗	Other driver not speeding
Dangerous situation	✗	No danger
Wearing jeans and jumper	✗	Wearing shorts and t-shirt

Hazel hit and killed a pedestrian while driving at 30 mph, and always blamed herself for reacting too slowly. At the site, she and her therapist worked out where her car had been when the pedestrian had stepped into the road and then looked up her stopping distance online on the Highway Code website. They concluded the stopping distance made it impossible to avoid the crash, even if she had braked immediately.

Specific behavioural experiments can be planned before the site visit; others emerge during it. It can be useful to speak to relevant people while at the site, which may require advance arrangement. For example, during site visits to hospitals or maternity units, it can be helpful to speak to staff who were present and can provide some more information about what happened.

Where it is not possible to return to the scene of the trauma for safety reasons or because it is impractical, a virtual site visit using tools like Google Street View or Google Earth can achieve many of the same aims as an in vivo site visit. For a therapist's guide to conducting site visits, read Murray et al. (2015).

Notes from the therapy room: Cian

Cian developed PTSD after being assaulted on a night out with friends. A group of men confronted Cian's friend at the bar, claiming he had pushed in, and Cian stepped in to defuse the argument. He was punched by one of the men and then kicked by others as he lay on the floor. He briefly lost consciousness and came around when the bouncers dragged him outside. No one was prosecuted for the assault.

Cian came to treatment after encouragement from his parents and girlfriend. He was having nightmares about being attacked, and flashbacks often triggered in busy places and by sudden movements near his face. He ruminated about the assault and felt angry that the perpetrators had 'got away with it'. He had stopped going out with his friends as he felt uncomfortable and jumpy in crowded places. He was irritable and rowing with his girlfriend. His formulation is in Figure 2.2.

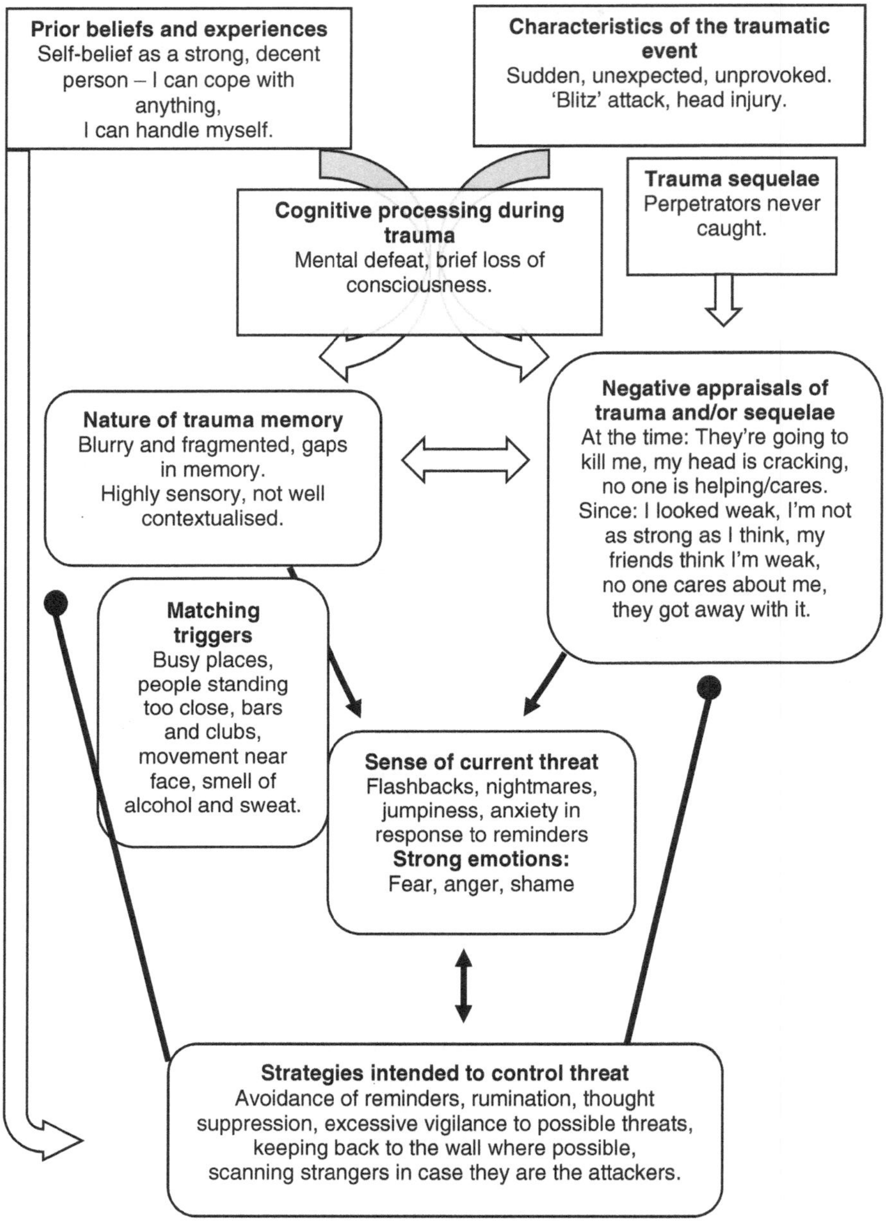

Figure 2.2 Cian's formulation

In the first session, Cian and his therapist discussed his problems and developed a preliminary formulation and treatment rationale. They also agreed treatment goals and began discussing 'reclaiming your life' activities. Cian used to like going to the gym and socialising with his friends but now felt anxious in busy places. They set some initial, manageable tasks towards reclaiming these activities including starting to exercise at home, taking a short walk every day, and messaging some friends.

Cian described the assault briefly in the first session and, in the second session, the trauma memories were elaborated further through imaginal reliving. Two hotspots were identified: the moment he glimpsed a fist coming towards his face and could do nothing to stop it and a moment of hopelessness and humiliation as he was kicked on the floor. For homework, Cian agreed to write a narrative of the trauma. A further hotspot emerged from when Cian was waiting in hospital later that night. He remembered feeling lonely and upset that there was no one there to comfort him.

Cian and his therapist discussed the emotions experienced in his hotspots and what had gone through his head at the time. They began to identify some updating information. Some updates were easy to establish, for example, that he was not seriously hurt, although he believed he would be at the time. Further information was revealed from working through the trauma story. For example, Cian remembered that he had told his friends not to come with him to the hospital and his girlfriend had met him there within an hour, which made him feel less angry and lonely.

Other updates required some cognitive restructuring. For example, Cian believed that his friends now saw him as weak and had avoided them since the assault, so had not had the opportunity to learn if this was true. With the encouragement of his therapist, Cian invited some of his friends over to his flat and they talked about the night of the assault. His friends expressed anger at the attackers and gave no indication that they thought Cian should have responded differently, or that they now saw him as weak. Cian's friends were pleased to see him and invited him to come round the following weekend to one of their houses. This helped further with Cian's belief that people didn't care about him. These updates were then added into the trauma story during reliving, and written into Cian's written account. A summary of Cian's hotspots and updates is in Table 2.2.

By the midpoint of treatment, Cian's symptoms had significantly reduced. Following a progress review with his therapist, goals for the second half of treatment were agreed. Cian continued to feel anxious in crowded places and wanted to start going out again at night. He was also still feeling angry about his attackers not being punished. Cian and his therapist planned a series of behavioural experiments to test his beliefs that he would be attacked again if he were in a busy place and didn't take measures to protect himself. They also reviewed the 'then versus now' technique and practised in session by bringing things close to his face to reduce this trigger.

Cian and his therapist also talked through the pros and cons of ruminating about his attackers. Cian concluded that dwelling was making him feel bad, was affecting his relationship with his girlfriend, and wasn't punishing his attackers in any way. He also believed in karma and realised that his attackers would probably be punished in some way for their bad actions, even if he wasn't there to see it. He resolved to stop dwelling on them and put his attention into his future.

Table 2.2 Cian's hotspots and updates

Hotspot	Main emotions	Main appraisals	Updates
Being punched in the face	Shock Fear	This is going to hurt	It did hurt, but there was no permanent damage. My face is fine now.
Being kicked on the floor	Humiliation Hopelessness	I'm getting beaten up and I should be fighting back. Everyone will think I am weak.	I was outnumbered and there was nothing I could do. I'm not weak, and my mates don't think that.
Waiting alone in A&E	Lonely Angry	No one cares enough to come with me	I told my mates not to come – they would've if I'd asked. Dani arrived after an hour.

As he was beginning to feel more comfortable out and about, Cian continued reclaiming his life by returning to the gym, initially during quiet times of day, and later during busy periods. He arranged to meet friends at a local pub and practised using the 'then versus now' technique if he felt uncomfortable. Gradually his confidence returned. Before finishing treatment, Cian prepared a therapy blueprint with the help of his therapist, which summarised his learning during treatment and planned for his continued progress as well as how to handle any setbacks.

Recommended reading

Ehlers, A., & Clark, D. M. (2000). A cognitive model of posttraumatic stress disorder. *Behaviour Research and Therapy*, 38(4), 319–345.

Grey, N. (2007). Post-traumatic stress disorder: Treatment. In S. Lindsay & G. Powell (Eds.). *The handbook of clinical adult psychology* (pp. 185–205). Routledge.

CHAPTER THREE

Assessment and formulation

Fatimah was experiencing recurrent headaches after being mugged at knifepoint in her local area. She was frightened of leaving the house and reported strong beliefs that her neighbourhood was dangerous. As well as assessing Fatimah for PTSD, her therapist gathered further information about Fatimah's headaches using diaries to establish any triggers and reviewed objective data about the safety of Fatimah's local area to understand whether she was at risk.

How we approach an assessment and what we cover depends partly on the goals of the assessment and the context in which we are working. For example, in a research setting, we often pay close attention to measuring symptoms, as the assessment may represent our baseline data point. In a medico-legal context, we may be instructed as an expert witness and asked to assess issues of causality, prognosis, and reliability. In this chapter, we'll focus mainly on assessments in clinical settings, where our usual aim is to establish the following:

- Our client's presenting problems and needs
- The presence of psychological disorders and comorbidities
- The suitability of psychological therapy and/or a particular clinical pathway
- Information to guide an individualised formulation and treatment plan
- Laying the groundwork for therapy.

Depending on the goals of our assessment, we use a variety of tools including clinical interviews, structured assessment tools, self-report measures, symptom diaries, and observation. This is the case whether assessments are straightforward or more complex but, as we'll discuss in this chapter, complex assessments may involve some additional methods to enable more detailed analysis and tracking of symptoms.

Making the assessment comfortable and useful for the client

Whatever the context of our assessment, our first priority is to ensure our clients feel comfortable and are treated with dignity, humanity, and respect. Although it is familiar to us, the process of a psychological assessment might be new to our clients, added to which they are facing the prospect of talking to a stranger about the most awful experiences of their life – no wonder many people feel anxious! Some of our clients have been controlled, deceived, exploited, and abused by others, so trusting us and forming an interpersonal connection immediately might be hard. From the outset, we do our best to build a working alliance that will lay the foundation for therapy (see also Chapter 24). Here are some areas to consider:

- *Physical safety*: Some aspects of the physical environment can be triggering for clients, such as small rooms, closed doors and windows for someone who has been imprisoned, or being

DOI: 10.4324/9781003288329-4

seated with their back to a door or window for someone who has been assaulted. Ask if there are any ways you can make the environment more comfortable and be prepared to rearrange the room or use another one. Where you can, try to limit extraneous noise such as banging doors.

- *Introductions and explanations*: Welcome the client, acknowledge their achievement in coming, introduce yourself, and ask how they wish to be addressed. Be as clear as possible about your role, the purpose of the assessment, confidentiality, and its limits. Remember that it is hard for clients to take in lots of information when they are anxious, so be prepared to go slow and repeat things if needed.
- *Demonstrate your compassion*: Use verbal and non-verbal behaviour to express empathy and compassion when your client is talking. Of course, we do this for all clients, but those with PTSD may be particularly sensitive to signals of threat, rejection, or judgement, so we need to demonstrate unconditional positive regard even more clearly.
- *Validate and normalise*: Wherever possible, summarise using your client's own words to show you are listening. Make comments which validate both their distress and difficult experiences. We often start sentences with 'given what you've experienced, it's no wonder that you've been …' to show that we view their reactions or behaviours as understandable. During the assessment we usually provide some information about PTSD and its prevalence, to normalise our client's symptoms as a common reaction to awful events.
- *Cultural considerations*: As we discuss in Chapter 25, understandings of psychological problems, the role of the psychologist, and expressions of distress will differ across cultures. We also need to consider how we use language, including using interpreters and translated measures as needed, to enable effective communication in an assessment.

FAQ: What do I do if my client brings another person to the assessment?

Ideally, we meet with a client alone for their assessment (and treatment). There are various reasons for this. Clients might feel the need to protect the other person and censor what they say or defer to the other person when we really want their perspective. There is also the (rare) possibility that the other person is abusive or coercive, and has insisted on being present to monitor what the client says.

However, our first goal at the assessment is to make our client feel comfortable so we invite others in if the client so wishes. If possible, we then ask to have part of the assessment session (or a second session) alone with the client. There are also benefits to including partners, friends, and family members as they often provide a useful perspective on a client's difficulties and may be an important source of support during treatment. If the client agrees, we invite them to join the feedback session, when we discuss a formulation and treatment plan.

What to cover in a clinical assessment

Detailed accounts of conducting clinical assessments are available elsewhere, but here is a quick recap of what to cover:

- Current life circumstances (e.g. work/studies, living situation, relationship status)
- The client's main problems, and their history (when they started, how they have progressed, what triggered them)

- The impact of problems on important areas of functioning (relationships, work etc.)
- Developmental and personal history of important life events including traumatic events
- A brief account of the main traumatic events and how they relate to their PTSD symptoms
- Risk (to self, to others, and from others)
- Drugs, alcohol, medication
- Physical health problems
- Treatment history and treatment goals.

One goal of clinical assessment is often to ascertain whether the treatment offered in a particular setting is suitable for the client's needs. This will vary depending on the setting, for example, the professional composition of the team and whether shorter- or longer-term interventions are offered. Measures to assess suitability of short-term CBT are available (e.g. the 'Readiness for Therapy Questionnaire'; Ghomi et al., 2020). However, to our knowledge, there are no published measures that specifically predict outcomes of PTSD treatment. When making treatment decisions, we therefore also consider the severity of known moderators of treatment outcome (Novakova, 2019) to guide treatment pathway decisions; for example, the amount of perseveration or detachment during the assessment, historical difficulties with engagement, and overall symptom burden (full list available on request). The presence of these features doesn't preclude treatment but can indicate potential treatment complications, many of which are the subject of this book.

FAQ: How much should I ask about the trauma at assessment?

Many clients come to the assessment expecting to talk about their traumas and will be willing to give a brief account of what happened. Others are, understandably, initially reluctant to discuss them, but may be willing to once in treatment.

Although referrals normally include some information about people's trauma history, we think it is important to ask about traumatic experiences as part of a PTSD assessment, both to confirm that they meet criterion A and to relate them to the content of any re-experiencing and avoidance symptoms. Asking about traumas also helps us determine the suitability and tolerability of a trauma-focused treatment approach, and can provide information relevant to the formulation. Lastly, it allows us to check for experiences the client may not have mentioned because they feel too ashamed, were not explicitly asked, or do not consider them traumatic. A trauma exposure questionnaire, such as the Life Events Checklist for DSM-5 (LEC-5; Weathers et al., 2013a) provides a quick way to check for the full range of traumatic events, and a gentle opening to asking for more details.

We do not insist on obtaining a full account of the index (worst) traumas at assessment, so we don't ask lots of follow-up questions, or delve into cognitive themes. We usually say: 'we don't need to talk in detail about your traumatic experiences at this stage, but would it be okay to ask you very briefly what happened? Only tell me as much as you are comfortable.' In most cases, this elicits sufficient information, while supporting the client to retain full control over their disclosures. If a client starts to give a detailed account and becomes upset or dissociated, we gently stop them, telling them we will return to the story later in treatment. We always praise our client's courage for talking about their traumas, validate their experiences, and their distress.

Measures of PTSD

There are various measures of PTSD available and here we've highlighted a few that we use most often. The website for the US Department of Veterans Affairs (https//:www.va.gov) is a good source of assessment tools and information. PTSD measures form part of a clinical assessment but are not sufficient in themselves to develop a treatment plan.

SELF-REPORT SYMPTOM QUESTIONNAIRES

We most commonly use the PTSD Checklist for DSM-5 (PCL-5; Weathers et al., 2013b), a 20-item measure that aligns with the DSM-5 PTSD criteria and is freely available. This should be used together with the LEC-5, which assesses for criterion A events. For ICD-11, a self-report questionnaire has been developed and is available in 27 languages: the International Trauma Questionnaire (Cloitre et al., 2018), used together with the International Trauma Exposure Measure (Hyland et al., 2020).

CLINICIAN-ADMINISTERED INTERVIEWS

Clinician-administered semi-structured interviews, which check the client's symptoms against the diagnostic criteria for PTSD, are considered the best way of establishing a PTSD diagnosis. The most commonly used are: the Structured Clinical Interview for DSM-5, Clinician Version (SCID-5-CV; First et al., 2016) and the Clinician-Administered PTSD Scale for DSM-5 (CAPS-5; Weathers et al., 2013c). These both diagnose PTSD according to DSM-5 criteria, including the dissociative subtype. The corresponding clinical interview for ICD-11, the International Trauma Interview, is currently in development (ITI; Cloitre, 2020).

COMPLEX PTSD ASSESSMENT TOOLS

Complex PTSD (as defined in ICD-11) can be assessed using the ITQ and ITI. Alternatively, a complex PTSD item set from ICD-11 can be added to the CAPS-5 to allow both sets of diagnostic criteria to be assessed concurrently (Lechner-Meichsner, & Steil, 2021).

FAQ: How do I tell what is an intrusion and what is rumination?

It can be tricky to tell intrusions from rumination. If your client says, 'I think about it all the time', they could mean either. To complicate matters further, intrusions can trigger rumination and vice versa, and it is very common for someone to experience both. A good place to start is to explain the difference between intrusions and rumination to your client. Intrusions are re-experiencing symptoms, they have a sense of 'nowness' (this might include the re-experiencing of strong trauma-related emotions without a clear memory attached, so-called 'affect without recollection'), whereas rumination involves thinking 'in circles' about the trauma, and doesn't have the same 'here and now' quality. We also ask our clients 'what were you doing when it started?'. Intrusions usually appear suddenly, triggered by a trauma reminder. Rumination is a more effortful thinking process, often involving the client trying to work out some aspect of the trauma, or fixating on an aspect of it that bothers them.

COGNITIVE ASSESSMENT

If the assessment immediately precedes treatment, one of our goals is to gather information relevant to the formulation, so we want to find out about the following:

- Current coping strategies (responses to intrusions and strong emotions, avoidance, other ways of feeling safe or managing symptoms)
- Content of intrusions (what is re-experienced in nightmares and flashbacks), which is often the starting point for identifying the main memory hotspots
- Cognitive themes, both those associated with hotspots (e.g. 'I thought he was going to kill me'), and those which have developed since (e.g. 'I'm losing my mind')
- Relevant previous experiences, and pre-trauma beliefs and coping styles
- Triggers (reminders that bring back memories or strong feelings).

Questionnaires can be used to investigate these areas, provide information for your formulation, and track progress during treatment. We find them particularly useful when a client is struggling to identify their thoughts, behaviours, or coping strategies, as they list common examples which we can then explore further. The following are available for free on the OxCADAT resources website:

- Post-Traumatic Cognitions Inventory (Foa et al., 1999)
- Trauma Memories Questionnaire (Ehlers et al., 2005)
- Response to Intrusions Questionnaire (Clohessy, & Ehlers, 1999)
- Safety Behaviours Questionnaire (unpublished).

ASSESSING COMPLEXITY

Assessment for complexity follows the same principles and structure as we have discussed so far. We also hold in mind the model on page 9 as a reminder of the areas we may want to investigate.

Multiple traumas

Multiple trauma histories can raise certain issues at assessment, not least how to make sense of their cumulative effects. For example, people may have experienced many traumas, but only have PTSD symptoms related to one or two of them, or may report delayed-onset re-experiencing symptoms of an earlier trauma which only started after a later trauma or event. Often memories of multiple traumas become blurred and entangled with one memory triggering another, nightmares may combine elements or themes from different traumas, and triggers can relate to multiple events.

In the assessment, we document the trauma history, drawing on questionnaires such as the LEC-5, and then try to identify which of the traumas relate to the client's PTSD symptoms (or vice versa). Clinical assessment tools like the CAPS-5 and self-report measures like the PCL-5 ask the respondent to anchor their symptoms to one trauma at a time, usually the identified index or worst event. However, in practice, it can be challenging for clients to identify the 'worst' trauma or which symptoms relate to which traumas, so sometimes it helps to complete separate measures for each trauma or type of traumas (sometimes referred to as a trauma cluster). Re-experiencing symptoms are usually easiest to relate to particular memories, because the content of intrusions, flashbacks, and nightmares should reflect specific parts of the events, and triggers should match sensory features present at the time. Avoidance and vigilance for trauma reminders should be similarly related to triggers but can become highly generalised over time.

Symptoms such as negative changes to cognitions and emotions, and chronic hyperarousal symptoms may be harder to link to a particular trauma, so it is useful to map their onset to relate them temporally to specific traumas. Bear in mind, however, that some symptoms have a delayed onset, sometimes triggered by further trauma, or other life events. Creating a timeline and keeping an intrusions diary can help match symptoms to particular traumas (Chapter 7).

Sonja developed PTSD after an abusive relationship. She had been married to her husband for 12 years and he had physically, emotionally, and sexually abused her on multiple occasions. At assessment, Sonja's therapist asked her which of these incidents caused Sonja the most distress and which she regularly re-experienced in the form of intrusive memories and nightmares. Sonja identified three particular 'worst' events. They also mapped the development of Sonja's other symptoms, including a heightened startle response and her negative self-beliefs. Sonja reported that she had always had low self-esteem, but this gradually worsened after her husband began making demeaning comments early in her marriage. Her startle response began after the first time Sonja was physically assaulted but got much worse after she escaped the relationship and feared he would find her.

Psychological comorbidity

Most people with PTSD will have symptoms of other psychological disorders, and many will also have physical health problems and social difficulties. It can be helpful to map these out to develop a full picture of the client's problems, as well as to establish whether any comorbidities may present complications to treatment (these issues are covered in more depth in Part 5).

At initial assessment, screening tools such as the QuickSCID-5 (First, & Williams, 2021) or the Brief Symptom Inventory (Derogatis, 1993) can be used to identify potential psychological comorbidities, followed by more detailed assessment, such as with the relevant SCID-5-CV module. Where extensive, fluctuating, or unusual symptoms are reported, comprehensive multidimensional assessment tools help screen for a broad range of psychological disorders and important clinical features, for example, the Personality Assessment Inventory (Morey, 2003).

Where a client's symptoms meet criteria for more than one disorder, we need to consider the severity and impact of the different problems and how they interact, to develop a treatment plan. As described in Part 5, sequential, concurrent, or integrated treatment plans may be required to address different issues, either within a single treatment setting or in collaboration with other professionals and teams.

Ginny was raped by a man who broke into her house. After the attack, Ginny developed PTSD symptoms including nightmares and hypervigilance. She also experienced some psychotic symptoms, including hearing the voice of her attacker saying that he was watching her, and believing that she was being followed and monitored. She sometimes self-harmed in response to the voices. The psychotic symptoms appeared secondary to PTSD, but were highly distressing to Ginny and were triggering risky behaviour, so Ginny's mental health team suggested a trial of an antipsychotic medication before beginning treatment for PTSD. In early sessions, they also discussed how to manage and more safely respond to the voices. As Ginny's PTSD symptoms improved during treatment, the voices also subsided and Ginny gradually reduced the medication with careful monitoring from her team.

Additional associated symptoms

Some people with PTSD develop post-traumatic reactions which go beyond those described by the PTSD diagnosis, such as somatic symptoms, chronic pain, seizures or muscle weakness, eating or sleeping disorders, and compulsive behaviours. These symptoms can have other causes, so if the onset coincides with the development of PTSD, and other explanations are not apparent, they require careful assessment.

We take a collaborative approach to understanding such symptoms with our clients, using techniques such as chain analysis (a version of functional analysis; Rizvi, & Ritschel, 2014) to look at the sequence of events (including situations, thoughts, and emotions) leading up to a symptom or behaviour, vulnerability factors, and any consequences. We review recent examples as part of the assessment and also ask the client to keep a diary of the symptom and its triggers (Chapter 21).

A normalising explanation for why unusual symptoms arise after trauma is often a helpful part of the assessment. In some cases, it is unclear whether the symptoms are indeed trauma-related, or the client may be unconvinced by the hypothesised link. We may then present PTSD treatment as an experiment: if the additional symptoms resolve alongside the PTSD symptoms, we can conclude that they were probably related. If PTSD is successfully treated, and the other symptoms remain, then further exploration and an alternative treatment plan may be considered, having ruled out PTSD as the cause.

Interpersonal problems

Difficulties in forming and sustaining relationships can have an impact on the development of a therapeutic alliance. The process of assessment provides an opportunity to establish whether a collaborative therapy will be possible and to lay the groundwork for a therapeutic relationship. Problems with trust, hostility, perceived judgement, and avoidance of difficult feelings are all common, and can 'play out' in the assessment. The therapist can take this opportunity to non-confrontationally identify and 'go public' with their observation of these issues, discuss their origins and impact, both on the client's life and prior treatment experiences, then negotiate how they can be managed in therapy and whether they should form a treatment target.

Social problems

In Chapter 22, we'll describe how to work with clients who have significant social problems in addition to their PTSD, such as issues with housing, money, employment, or legal cases. When identified at assessment, a decision is made collaboratively about whether treatment for psychological problems is currently possible, or whether it should be deferred until after the client has received the necessary support for their social problems.

To assess this, we consider the level of the client's preoccupation with, and the impact of, their social problems. It can be useful to demonstrate this visually, for example, by drawing a pie chart to illustrate the client's current problems (including PTSD), with an appropriately sized 'slice of the pie' allocated to each problem. This helps to determine whether PTSD is currently their main problem. The assessment process itself is also a useful measure of preoccupation and interference from non-PTSD problems, for example, whether our client can maintain a focus on discussing PTSD rather than other issues during the assessment sessions and whether they attend regularly and complete homework tasks (such as keeping a symptom diary between sessions). We also need to consider the imminence of any major life events, such as upcoming court cases, housing evictions, or deportation, to plan how and when we can find a 'window' of stability to deliver treatment.

Risk

As discussed in Chapter 23, PTSD is often associated with risks of various kinds, which require careful assessment. Some clients present with self-harm and suicidal ideation, some pose a risk to others because of difficulties with controlling anger or a preoccupation with revenge, some are at risk from others, such as living nearby or being stalked by someone who has abused them. Occasionally, a client discloses a crime that has not previously been reported and, if the perpetrator potentially presents a continued risk to others, we need to consider safeguarding procedures.

Risk assessment and management is a standard part of clinical practice, so we won't repeat the basics here, except to note some additional considerations associated with PTSD. Firstly, for some clients (although not all), accessing the trauma memories in treatment temporarily increases their PTSD symptoms and, consequently, some risks. However, persisting PTSD symptoms also increase risks in the longer term, so often we are balancing short-term risks against potential benefits of treatment. Chapter 23 covers how to decide whether and how risks can be best managed during PTSD treatment.

A second consideration is that clients with PTSD tend to have a heightened perception of threat, so they may feel they are at risk when they are not. Others *are* objectively at risk, for example, they are being threatened by someone who has previously assaulted them, or have a job that puts them in dangerous situations. At assessment, we try to get an accurate estimate of risk by collecting objective data about the nature of the risk and make safety plans as appropriate.

> Bradley was assaulted by a man who lived in his local area. The police had been involved but the charges were dropped. Bradley avoided leaving his flat as he feared the man or his friends may attack him again. He was, therefore, reluctant to travel for weekly treatment sessions.
>
> To gather data about the risks to Bradley, his therapist asked about recent incidents when he had seen the man who assaulted him, including when and where he had seen him, and what had happened. Since the assault a year ago, Bradley had seen his attacker on three occasions, always on the local high street. Each time, Bradley had turned and walked away, and his attacker had not followed. There had been no other contact from the man or his friends online, by phone, or in person, and no threats had been made.
>
> Reviewing this information, they concluded there was a relatively low risk of the man assaulting Bradley again if he encountered him in public. They agreed a safety plan for how to cope if Bradley saw the man in a public place (walk away) and what to do if the man approached or threatened him (move to a busy area and call the police).

Pre-trauma mental health

Many people with PTSD have psychological problems which pre-date the trauma and may have worsened since. At assessment, we check whether PTSD is the main problem or whether other issues should take priority. If PTSD is the client's preferred focus, we let them know that pre-existing problems may persist even if PTSD is effectively treated. A further assessment and treatment plan can be considered following PTSD treatment.

Additional measures

It can be helpful to use additional questionnaires to learn more about, and track through treatment, symptoms which aren't covered by the standard PTSD measures. There are many available, but we've chosen some here which are readily available, well-validated, and clinically descriptive:

- Dissociation: The Dissociative Experiences Measure, Oxford (DEMO; Černis et al., 2018) or Trait State Dissociation Questionnaire (TSDQ; adapted from Murray et al., 2002, available at oxcadatresources.com)
- Grief: The International Prolonged Grief Disorder Scale (IPGDS; Killikelly et al., 2020)
- Moral injury: Moral Injury Outcome Scale (MIOS; Yeterian et al., 2019)
- Mental contamination: Posttraumatic Experience of Mental Contamination Scale (Brake et al., 2019)
- Recklessness: Posttrauma Risky Behaviours Questionnaire (Contractor et al., 2020).

Treatment planning and formulation

Typically towards the end of the assessment, we feed back our opinions on diagnosis, offer a provisional formulation, and agree a treatment plan. Here are some areas to include:

- *Agreeing a focus*: We review the client's goals and agree the aims for treatment, discussing what is achievable in the proposed course of treatment. If we decide not to offer trauma-focused therapy, we discuss alternative treatment plans.
- *Psychoeducation*: We typically offer some basic information about PTSD, including a psychoeducational leaflet which the client can share with others if they choose. Depending on the nature of their presenting problems, we may give more detailed information, for example, to normalise troubling symptoms or explain the common effects of certain types of trauma.
- *Drawing out a basic formulation*: This is idiosyncratic to the client but may be a simple 'vicious circle' diagram of how PTSD symptoms maintain each other or how different aspects of the client's symptoms interrelate. We do not generally share a full formulation based on the Ehlers and Clark (2000) model, as this can be overwhelming at an early stage, but we do draw out key maintenance cycles from it, for example, how avoidance prevents memory processing.
- *Getting feedback*: We ask for the client's feedback on the assessment process, how we have worked together, and what has been discussed. We leave enough time for any questions and provide the opportunity to contact us if they have further questions.

Notes from the therapy room: Fatimah

Fatimah was referred for psychological therapy by the neurology department of her local hospital, where she had been assessed for recurrent severe headaches. The neurology team could find no physical cause for her headaches, but had identified symptoms of depression and anxiety, and concluded that they were likely to be stress-related.

Fatimah attended the assessment with her daughter, who joined the assessment at Fatimah's request. Her therapist made introductions, explained the purpose of the assessment, and asked if there was anything that would make the assessment easier for Fatimah. Although English was not Fatimah's first language, she had previously said she did not require an interpreter, so the therapist encouraged her to ask for clarification if there was anything she didn't understand.

Fatimah said that her main problems were headaches and a fear of going out alone. She reported that she lived in a 'dangerous area' and that she had been mugged at knifepoint near her flat. She was now very wary of young men and did not leave the house unless accompanied by a family member. Her daughter remarked that Fatimah's anxiety had started after the mugging and, before this, she had been confident to travel in the local area alone. Fatimah also confirmed that the headaches had started after she was mugged.

Fatimah described some of her personal history. She had grown up in Eritrea, moving to the UK in the 1980s shortly after her marriage. She had four children, three of whom still lived at home. Fatimah had experienced several traumatic events during the war in Eritrea, including seeing dead bodies, deaths of family members, and being forced to flee her home village which came under aerial attack. However, Fatimah did not report PTSD symptoms relating to any of these incidents.

Fatimah was assessed for PTSD in respect to the mugging. She hadn't been seriously harmed but had believed her life was in danger. She reported nightmares of being chased by men in hoods and intrusive memories of seeing the knife. She avoided going out alone and tried hard not to think about the incident. There had been a significant change in her beliefs about her safety both in and out of the house, so she now felt frightened most of the time. Fatimah also reported hyperarousal symptoms such as jumpiness, hypervigilance, difficulty sleeping, poor concentration, and irritability, all of which had started after she was mugged. Fatimah also reported significant symptoms of depression which had started at the same time as her PTSD symptoms.

Fatimah reported no risks to herself or others, but she did feel very much at risk in her neighbourhood and had repeatedly asked the council to move her. Her therapist tried to gather some objective data on the risks in her neighbourhood. There had been some problems with antisocial behaviour locally, including drug-dealing and excessive noise. Fatimah knew of another woman who had been mugged at the local bus stop. However, in the 30 years that Fatimah and her family had lived in the area, Fatimah had only been affected by crime on one occasion, and her husband and children reported that they felt safe on the estate. Thus, there seemed little objective data that Fatimah was currently at serious risk, but rather her PTSD symptoms seemed to drive her sense of threats in her neighbourhood.

They gathered more details on Fatimah's headaches by asking her to keep a diary of her headaches and subjective stress levels, to test the hypothesis that the two were related. At the following session, Fatimah had partly filled in the diary and reported that she had three headaches but couldn't be sure if they were linked to stress, as she was stressed all the time. They used the chain analysis technique to look at a recent headache. Fatimah reported possible triggers including sleeping badly, her daughter's baby crying, and reading an article about knife crime, all of which had made her feel more stressed a short while before the headache started. They agreed that stress seemed one possible cause of the headaches.

Fatimah's therapist gave her some information about PTSD and shared a provisional formulation in bullet points. They also drew up a couple of maintenance cycles to demonstrate some of the points. A full formulation is shown in Figure 3.1.

- Fatimah's experience of being mugged had made her feel less safe in her local area. It might be that her earlier experiences of war and needing to flee Eritrea had left her vulnerable to beliefs about unsafety. She had believed herself to be safe in the UK, but these beliefs had been shattered by her recent experience.
- The local area had some problems but hadn't become objectively less safe since the mugging, although it felt that way to Fatimah, probably because the memories of the mugging weren't properly stored, so felt very current and kept coming back in intrusions and nightmares, making her feel unsafe. Trying to avoid thinking and talking about it meant the memories stayed stuck.

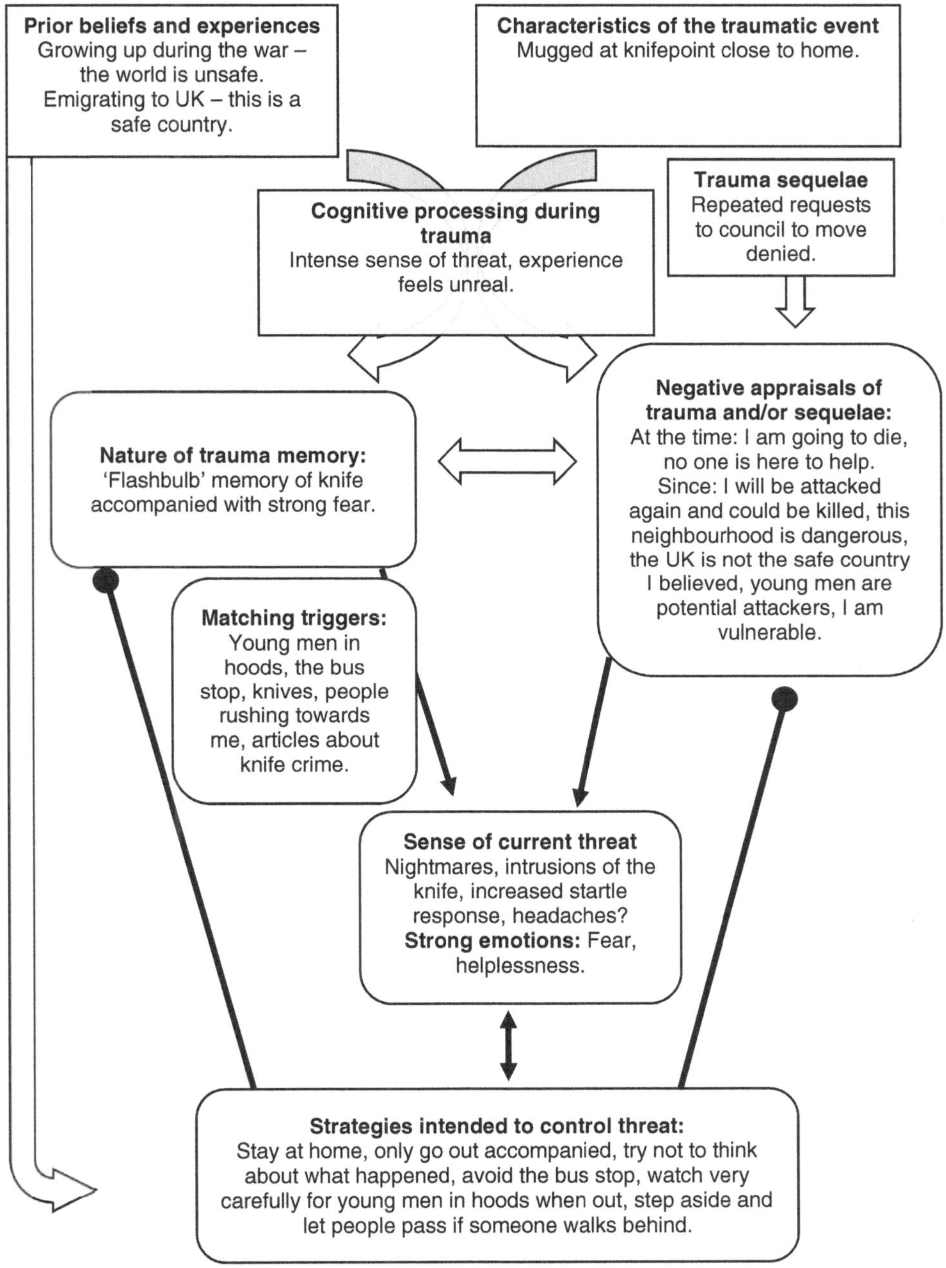

Figure 3.1 Fatimah's formulation

- Her beliefs about safety were being maintained by avoiding going out alone, as she never got the chance to find out whether something bad would happen again.
- Fatimah's headaches might be linked to stress and her PTSD symptoms. Treatment would be an opportunity to find out if they got any better when Fatimah was feeling less stressed and anxious.

They discussed a possible treatment plan. Fatimah was willing to try trauma-focused treatment to address her goals of having fewer headaches, feeling less anxious when going out, and sleeping better. Fatimah's final goal was to move out of her flat, and her therapist agreed to write a letter to the housing department on Fatimah's behalf. Fatimah felt she would be able to focus on treatment in the interim and the evidence from the assessment suggested she was able to form a working alliance, maintain a trauma focus, and work within the structure of therapy.

Recommended reading

Doyle, A. M., & Thornton, S. (2002). Psychological assessment of sexual assault. In P. Petrak & B. Hedge (Eds.). *The trauma of sexual assault: Treatment, prevention, and practice* (pp. 99–134). Routledge.

Grey, N. (2007). Post-traumatic stress disorder: Investigation. In S. Lindsay & G. Powell (Eds.). *The handbook of clinical adult psychology* (pp. 164–184). Routledge.

PART TWO

Complexity in memory work

CHAPTER FOUR

Over-activation of trauma memories

Carla developed PTSD following an assault. In therapy, she would become highly distressed and have a panic attack when she talked about the trauma, before asking to stop the session. Her therapist worried she would drop out of therapy, as she had done previously. The challenge in treatment was to understand what was driving the over-activation of the trauma memories and help her stay within the therapeutic window.

THE THERAPEUTIC WINDOW

To identify and change strong beliefs and emotions in therapy, we often need our clients to access them by bringing their trauma memories into mind. This is because some feelings and appraisals are context-dependent; they are embedded with the trauma memories and so activated in particular situations where the memories are triggered. It follows that making changes to thoughts and feelings occurs most easily when those memories are activated. However, if trauma memories are activated too strongly, they can overwhelm our clients' ability to think clearly, verbalise, and update their thoughts and feelings. This is the concept of the therapeutic window; it is the optimal level of emotional arousal in which to 'process the memory' – that is, convert the sensory details into verbal and conceptual representations, and restructure related meanings and feelings. Goldilocks had a similar idea when tasting porridge: not too hot, not too cold – just right!

When we work with trauma memories, we want our clients to re-experience the emotions that they felt at the time, but not feel overwhelmed by them or lose track of the fact that they are in a safe environment. We tell our clients to keep 'one foot in the present, one foot in the past' but, for some people, this is easier said than done. Lots of factors affect an individual's ability to stay in the therapeutic window, and it is these issues that we will discuss in this chapter.

Figure 4.1 shows how a good reliving session might look in terms of the therapeutic window. As the memories are activated, some distress and arousal arise, but remain within the therapeutic window and decrease by the end of the session.

Another way of thinking about the therapeutic window is by using the music metaphor we introduced in Chapter 1. If trauma memories are over-activated in a session, they become like an overwhelming noise. If a noise is too loud, we can't make sense of it or think straight. Imagine trying to sit an exam while music blares out loudly. You would want to turn the noise off or escape from it in some way. If your client is overwhelmed by trauma memories, they will try to do the same.

On the other hand, if the memories haven't been sufficiently activated, it's like the music is too quiet to hear all of the details. If we don't properly access trauma memories in a session, our client won't be able to recall and verbalise all the important somatic, sensory, and emotional details to make that elaborated, contextualised version which will then hopefully get stored alongside the sensory version in autobiographical memory.

DOI: 10.4324/9781003288329-6

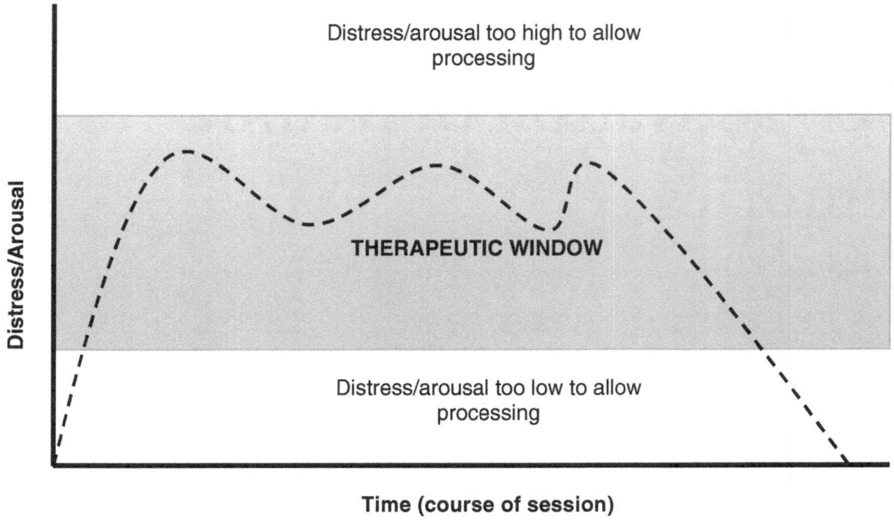

Figure 4.1 The therapeutic window

So, we want our Goldilocks level – just right. This means that, as therapists, we need to be alert throughout reliving (and other parts of the session too) to the volume of trauma memories and keep our client in the therapeutic window. This is important for several reasons. Firstly, it is the most effective level for changes to occur. Secondly, we are helping the client to gain control over their memories by teaching them how to adjust the intensity. Finally, it means the distressing memory work will be tolerable for our client.

FAQ: Should I take SUDs ratings during memory work in CT-PTSD?

In CT-PTSD, we don't usually take SUDs (subjective units of distress) ratings during imaginal reliving or other forms of memory work. Taking SUDs ratings pulls the client's attention away from the memories, which isn't usually helpful. Instead, ratings are taken afterwards, usually of distress, vividness, and 'nowness'. Classically, in therapies based on exposure therapy, the aim is to habituate to the anxiety that trauma memories cause, so exposure continues until SUDs ratings drop to a certain level. However, in CT-PTSD, our main interest is the meanings associated with the memories and we work on the hotspots associated with the highest distress. 'Nowness' gives a useful indication of whether memories feel more in the past, so helps us check on how well the memories are being processed.

There are, however, times when SUDs ratings are useful. If someone is experiencing over-activation or dissociation, taking SUDs ratings can help you track where they are in the therapeutic window and when to apply 'volume down' techniques. Taking a rating also brings attention into the here and now, and distracts briefly from the memories, which itself helps turn the volume down. Lastly, asking for ratings helps give the client greater control over the process.

Here, we draw a thermometer on the whiteboard, labelled 0–100 degrees, and take regular 'temperature checks'. If the temperature goes over an agreed limit, we pause the narrative and try to 'cool it down'. This turns monitoring into a shared responsibility which requires the client to view their emotions objectively, helping distance them slightly and see emotional arousal as a process they can control.

What is over-activation of trauma memories?

When trauma memories are over-activated, they become very vivid and intrusive and people feel overwhelmed with emotions and sensations. Usually, it will be apparent in the therapy room when this happens, as clients become extremely upset, agitated, or annoyed, may show physiological signs like shaking or vomiting, and may want to discontinue memory work or the session. On our graph of the therapeutic window, over-activation looks like Figure 4.2.

Over-activation of trauma memories is undesirable for various reasons. Firstly, it is aversive for our clients, as they will feel highly distressed and potentially more symptomatic for some time afterwards. This can damage their faith in therapy being helpful and may lead to disengagement and drop-out. Secondly, it is unhelpful for trauma memories to be over-activated as it inhibits useful processing. The client will struggle to develop or access any updating information or to stay with the memories long enough to become aware of extra details that might elaborate them.

Why does over-activation happen?

Understanding the reasons for over-activation can help focus your intervention. Here are some common underlying processes.

NATURALLY HIGH IMAGERY CAPABILITY

Various factors affect someone's ability to form mental images (James et al., 2016). Some people struggle to bring images to mind, while others find images form readily. For people with naturally high imagery capability, memories we access during treatment may be more intense and vivid, leading to higher distress. You can spot people with super-charged imagery capability as they will tell you they have 'photographic' memories, are artistic, or have a good 'eye for detail'. Asking them to do a neutral imagery task, such as imagining walking to the shops, will produce highly detailed and multi-sensory descriptions and they will report feeling 'really in it'.

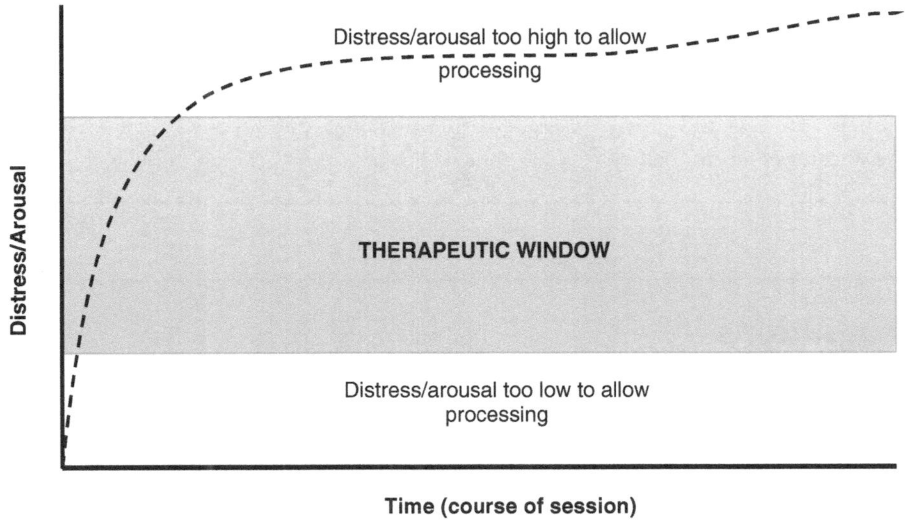

Figure 4.2 Over-activation of trauma memories

THE MEANING OF THE TRAUMA IS TOO PAINFUL

Distress may arise when the meaning of the trauma is extremely negative and strongly held, so accessing the memories generates painful emotions.

Bahram had been a member of the Iranian Police. During his career, he was aware of the police tactics becoming increasingly extreme, with severe punishments being inflicted on people who committed minor crimes which contradicted religious doctrine.

One day, Bahram and his colleagues were sent to arrest a group of women who reportedly opposed the government. They were ordered to take the women to some woods and execute them. Bahram was horrified, but he didn't know what to do. If he protested, he believed he would also be executed. Instead, he ran away and left the country soon after with his family. Recalling the memories of arresting the women was highly distressing for Bahram, as his appraisal was 'I left them to die; I'm as good as a murderer'. Bahram had joined the police because he wanted to do good, so this belief was incredibly painful to him. As soon as he recalled the memories, he felt an overwhelming flood of shame and anger which he found intolerable and he would discontinue the memory work.

THE MEANING OF HAVING THE MEMORIES IS TOO PAINFUL

Sometimes the most painful meanings lie not in the appraisals of the trauma itself, but its consequences, like the person's interpretation of having PTSD symptoms. If the meaning of the memories experienced is too painful, it will trigger toxic emotions, and prevent useful processing of the trauma memories.

Patience was trafficked to the UK as a teenager and forced into prostitution. To keep her from running away, her traffickers carried out juju rituals ('black magic') which placed a curse on her if she tried to escape. Patience had grown up in rural Cameroon and her community believed strongly in juju. When Patience was rescued from her traffickers, she refused to talk about what had happened to her, for fear that the juju would kill her. The intrusive memories were intensely distressing, as Patience interpreted them as a sign that the curse had been activated, that anyone she told would also be cursed, and that she would never escape her captors.

Hot cognitions

- The trauma shows I am a terrible person
- Re-experiencing the memories means something awful is happening/going to happen
- I couldn't breathe/nearly died at the time – the same thing could happen again when I remember it
- My feelings are uncontrollable
- My feelings won't be taken seriously unless I express them strongly

COMORBID PANIC DISORDER

Some people with PTSD also have panic disorder, or experience panic attacks in response to trauma reminders (Chapter 20). Distress and physiological arousal in response to reminders are common PTSD symptoms and people may feel panicky. However, a panic attack also involves a catastrophic misinterpretation of panic symptoms. For example, someone sees a person who looks like their ex-partner who assaulted them and physiological arousal is triggered. They feel hot and sweaty, and their heart rate increases. So far, this is typical of PTSD. However, if they then think 'there must be something wrong with my heart, I'm going to have a heart attack and die', triggering the panic cycle (Clark, 1986), the anxiety caused by the trigger spirals into a panic attack, fuelled by the catastrophic misinterpretation.

Sometimes panic symptoms, and coping behaviours, are also reminders of aspects of the trauma, perhaps because the person was also feeling or coping in that way during the trauma. For example, a very common physiological reaction to torture is hyperventilation. When a client then activates the trauma memories, and they get panic symptoms and feel breathless, they may start breathing very fast and hard, which then both worsens the sensation of chest tightness and also retriggers the memories of hyperventilating. In this way, the panic symptoms and trauma memories 'fold over' each other in a rapidly spiralling feedback loop (Otto, & Hinton, 2006).

Panic attacks that only occur in response to trauma triggers don't meet criteria for panic disorder (according to DSM-5). However, if someone is also having panic attacks out of the blue or triggered by experiences unrelated to the trauma, this might constitute an additional diagnosis of panic disorder (assuming the other criteria are also met). This distinction is important because it will help you decide whether to just help the person with the trauma triggers using stimulus discrimination, or whether you will also need to draw on panic disorder treatments.

UNDERSTANDING EMOTION

A low ability to understand and describe emotions, or alexithymia, has been associated with PTSD (Frewen et al., 2008). In CBT, we often ask clients to name and rate their emotions and there is some evidence that simply helping people put words to emotions (affect labelling) enhances treatments for anxiety (Kircanski et al., 2012). However, this is difficult for some of our clients.

Alexithymia can lead to problems with the therapeutic window. When it is difficult to understand your emotions, triggering trauma memories will give a strong sense of distress, which is hard to put into words. When we ask some of our clients how they are feeling, they tell us 'bad' and rate their distress as 100/100. It can be difficult to differentiate between emotions and to notice the gradations in levels of affect. Some people struggle to create detailed representations of their thoughts and feelings during their trauma, which makes updating them more difficult. Others have a limited vocabulary for emotion, for example, if they grew up in an environment where emotions weren't talked about.

For all these clients, finding a language and a scale for quantifying emotion can be invaluable. As well as helping communication throughout therapy, it will help emotions to feel less overwhelming and keep people in the therapeutic window. Furthermore, having alexithymia, or just having trouble talking about feelings, tends to impact other areas of peoples' lives, like their relationships, so learning some skills in this area helps outside the therapy room too.

EMOTIONAL DYSREGULATION

For some people, modulating emotion is a huge challenge and they find themselves frequently hurled between extreme emotions. This is common for people who had early life trauma, especially those who grew up in environments where emotional states were not recognised or responded to appropriately, or even punished as unacceptable. Emotions may be felt powerfully, easily triggered, and slow to subside. Some of these patterns are 'hard-wired' from early life and can present problems for working on trauma memories, as there is a high chance of someone being pushed above the therapeutic window, perhaps also triggering extreme or risky coping behaviours.

Managing over-activation of memories

Over-activation of trauma memories is upsetting and unpleasant for our clients, so we want to maximise their control, and appraisals of control, over their feelings. There are various ways to do this, depending on your assessment of what is causing the over-activation. If, during the first attempt at memory work, your client became intensely distressed and you needed to stop the session, help them develop some tools to manage their activation before you have another go. It isn't a good idea to give memory work as homework at this stage, as you won't be there to help them manage their distress, so give them skills practice homework instead (see 'top tips' for examples). Wherever possible, set skill development up as a behavioural experiment by asking your client to predict and then test how helpful the skills will be. Potentially this gives them data to update negative beliefs about emotions, such as how uncontrollable they are, which may be contributing to the over-activation.

Note, however, that a significant degree of distress is normal. Someone who is tearful, flushed and restless, but can stay with trauma memories with encouragement and get to the end of the reliving session, doesn't need extra intervention. Optimal memory activation is usually only one or two steps below unbearable. These techniques are for people who can't stay in the therapeutic window at all and are so intensely distressed that they can't tolerate working on trauma memories or react in unsafe ways.

MEASURE AND RECOGNISE EMOTIONS

First, offer your client a way of measuring and recognising their emotions. Help your client learn to rate their emotions by asking for SUDs ratings at different points in a therapy session. Agreeing an acceptable maximum SUDs rating before you implement a 'volume down' tactic will also hopefully empower your client to feel safer in approaching the memories.

If someone has a very limited vocabulary for emotion, practise naming emotions outside the trauma memories. Together, write a list of many different emotions. When someone tells you they are feeling 'bad', help them be more specific by choosing words from the list that match their feelings. Another good exercise (which we heard in a workshop by Martina Mueller) is to ask your client to watch a TV programme (soap operas work well) and try to name which emotion each character is feeling in each scene. They can do this together with a family member, friend, or partner to start with if they prefer. Talking about emotions can start the process of making them more understandable and easier to handle.

ADDRESS PANIC ATTACKS

Where memory work triggers panic attacks, you need to address these as no processing will happen if someone is in the midst of a panic attack and it may prompt them to disengage from therapy. If the panic attacks are triggered only by trauma reminders or are part of the trauma memories, practise stimulus discrimination with your client, and get them well-rehearsed at discriminating 'then versus now'. Approach memories gradually, for example, by first writing down a few keywords about what happened, and then gradually building up a narrative, switching to using 'then versus now' whenever your client needs to lower the volume. For most people, this is sufficient to get them through PTSD treatment and, if the panic attacks are secondary to PTSD, they should resolve by themselves. Where some of the panic symptoms and coping behaviours are also embedded within the trauma memories (e.g. they hyperventilated at the time), focus on these specifically in stimulus discrimination.

However, if someone has panic disorder, driven by catastrophic appraisals of their arousal symptoms, then further work may be required, drawing on techniques from cognitive therapy for panic disorder (Clark, 1986). These include developing a shared formulation for what is maintaining panic attacks, cognitive work on the threatening interpretations of symptoms, and behavioural experiments in interoceptive exposure tasks and with dropping safety-seeking behaviours. Where panic disorder developed after the trauma, we recommend only doing as much work on the panic attacks as is needed for you to work on the trauma memories as, once PTSD is successfully treated, the panic disorder may well resolve without needing further intervention. Of course, if it doesn't, that can be a further target for treatment.

AID EMOTION REGULATION

For people who have considerable emotion dysregulation difficulties, some stabilisation work may be required before addressing the trauma memories. Again, we would recommend doing just enough to make the memory work tolerable, as successful treatment of PTSD should have a positive knock-on effect on emotion dysregulation problems. Where possible, do this in parallel with the memory work. Learning emotion regulation skills shouldn't imply that expression of emotion is unwanted, but some tools can help with managing difficult and overwhelming feelings, and make treatment more tolerable and safer if the client uses risky coping strategies.

Top tips: Aiding emotion regulation

Often, the work done in early sessions of PTSD treatment in normalisation and formulation helps to provide a non-threatening understanding of the difficult feelings that arise after trauma. Here are some other techniques to try:

- *Teach stimulus discrimination early*: Getting a clearer idea of triggers, and learning a strategy to deal with them, helps to gain a sense of control over intrusions.
- *Monitor emotions and coping strategies*: Emotion diaries can be used to monitor emotions, learn triggers, and identify which coping strategies are most effective.
- *List helpful and unhelpful strategies*: Most people are aware of which strategies help with difficult feelings, and which do not, so ask clients to list them, practise the helpful ones in session, and in response to mildly challenging events.
- *Develop additional strategies*: For people who struggle to find helpful strategies, use some session time to practise new ones, such as safe place imagery, grounding techniques, breathing, and relaxation exercises. We also encourage prioritisation of good self-care, such as eating, sleeping, and exercising.
- *Coping with extremes of emotion*: Developing a (written) plan to cope with extremes of emotion is helpful, especially in the context of risky behaviour (Chapter 18). Strategies such as distraction and 'time outs' can be useful.
- *Formulating emotional responses*: Using basic CBT formulations, such as the 'five areas' model (Greenberger, & Padesky, 1995), can help to increase understanding of emotional responses and lead to activities such as thought challenging to address triggering thoughts.
- *Borrow from DBT*: Originally developed for borderline personality disorder, dialectical behaviour therapy (DBT; Linehan, 1987) includes a skills training component for regulating emotion, which has application to many disorders where emotion dysregulation is a feature. To read more, try Linehan et al. (2007).

WORK ON THE APPRAISALS

If the cause of over-activation seems to be beliefs related to either the meaning of the trauma or the meaning of having intrusive memories, these appraisals should be identified and addressed before revisiting the trauma memories.

Painful appraisals about the trauma or the experience of PTSD, such as beliefs about memories or emotions, will also form a central part of the client's formulation, as they are likely to be driving a lot of distress and sense of current threat. Once the worst meanings have been identified, the therapist can decide which cognitive restructuring techniques to use.

> James believed that his experiences of being groomed and sexually abused as a teenager meant that he was 'damaged' and that future partners would reject him. His therapist explored these beliefs using guided discovery techniques such as reviewing evidence and discussing what James would say to other people about the same beliefs. They developed a survey to test his beliefs about how others viewed people who had been sexually abused.

PRE-EXISTING BELIEFS

Pre-existing beliefs about emotions can underlie a pattern of memory over-activation. For example, someone may have previous experiences where becoming emotional felt overwhelming, or they were criticised or punished for showing distress. These earlier memories and the thought of them happening again adds further 'petrol to the fire' of their emotions during memory work. Others have had childhood experiences where their needs were not fully met, so fear that you will only take their distress seriously if they express it very strongly. Discussing these types of experiences and beliefs and normalising them often goes a long way to helping people feel more in control of their emotions, as they can label the process being triggered. Other times, the underlying beliefs and their associated memories may require some additional work.

TURN DOWN THE VOLUME

Whatever the cause of over-activation, you can use strategies during memory work to keep your client within the therapeutic window. We call these 'volume down' techniques because the aim is to reduce the intensity of the memories. If you are using the temperature metaphor with your client, call them 'cool down' techniques.

Volume down reliving

The typical instructions for imaginal reliving include shutting your eyes, speaking in the first person, present tense, and including as much detail as possible. This aims to help people connect with every detail of the trauma memories and minimises distractions. For people who tend to get overwhelmed by memories, we want to decrease the intensity, so we give different instructions. We conduct imaginal reliving with the eyes open, in a brightly lit room, and speaking in the past tense. If necessary, the first few attempts can include only brief details. We pause frequently to take 'temperature' ratings and to give encouragement. We speak more often and ask clarifying questions that bring our client's attention back into the room. We limit long silences and instead break the narrative up by summarising and checking our understanding. In this way, we can also track their activation level.

Depending on how memory work is going, we can increase the intensity again later on but, for early reliving sessions, we aim to get through an account of the trauma without our client having to stop. Getting to the end, which means reaching a point in the narrative where the client was in a position of (relative) safety, is a powerful demonstration that trauma memories are tolerable.

Focus on higher-order processes

Distress often occurs when the client is overwhelmed by sensory, physiological, and emotional elements of trauma memories. Imagine the orchestra where some of the instruments are playing too loudly, drowning out the others. If we try to bring attention to the other elements of the memories, it can help balance the recollection and reduce its intensity. Instead of asking lots of questions about internal details such as emotions, sensations, smells, or tastes, try asking more about external sensory elements in the memories, such as what they can see around them. We also focus on higher-order cognitive processes as prompts, e.g. 'what was going through your mind at that moment?', 'what did that tell you about what was going on?' (these questions are in the past tense, as we are using 'volume down' reliving). These engage the parts of the brain associated with more complex conceptual processing, rather than focusing on processing sensations. We sometimes refer to this as directing the 'flashlight' of our client's attention 'up' their nervous system, away from the gut and into the head.

Narrative writing rather than imaginal reliving

Writing an account of the trauma is generally less immersive than imaginal reliving. It slows things down, plus the additional cognitive and physical task of writing helps keep attention in the here and now. It is also easier to gradually build up the trauma account. You can start with just a few bullet points and, as your client gets better at monitoring and managing their arousal, gradually add further detail until the narrative is complete. If your client speaks a different language to you or cannot read, you can use pictures to create a narrative or ask them to write it in their language, with an interpreter helping to translate it for you. It is possible to move on to imaginal reliving after narrative writing if it becomes helpful to 'turn the volume up' on the memories.

Another alternative is to create a timeline of the memories (Chapter 7). This is created together with the therapist and maps the temporal order of events.

Different perspective reliving

Another alternative is to relive the memories from different perspectives. Usually, reliving takes place from the 'field perspective', i.e. through the client's eyes as they experienced it at the time. However, taking an 'observer perspective' such as reliving the event as a bystander or from a bird's eye view, often helps to distance people slightly from memories, which can be helpful to keep them within the therapeutic window.

We particularly like what we call 'board game reliving'. We put a whiteboard or a sheet of flipchart paper on the floor and, together with our client, draw a rough map of the trauma site as if we are looking down on it from above. We then use handy items (e.g. bits of stationery, or bottles of essential oils) to represent key people and objects and use them to re-enact the trauma as if we are observing it from above, while also re-telling the narrative. Moving around and using an observer perspective are useful ways of distancing slightly. For some clients, like ex-service personnel, it may also helpfully match a technique they are familiar with, like using a map to plan for a surveillance operation. We also stick Post-It notes, with key thoughts, feelings, and updates written on them, onto the trauma map so these can be incorporated into the narrative. As with other adaptations to reliving, we can build up to more immersive reliving if needed, and as the client becomes more able to tolerate the trauma memories and the emotions they provoke.

Imagery exercises for distancing

Another way of creating distance from the memories is via imagery manipulation exercises. These can be particularly helpful for people with higher imagery abilities. Practise first with a neutral image, so your client gets used to controlling images. Ask your client to imagine being in a large room with a television in the corner which is playing a film. They can manipulate the film in various ways in imagination, such as using a remote control to pause, rewind, or turn it off, muting the volume, and then gradually increasing it, changing the picture from colour to black and white and back again, shrinking it to a dot, and replacing it or putting another picture alongside it. Once your client has got used to the technique of manipulating the image, change the 'film' to the trauma memories. The client can manipulate it as before by pausing, rewinding, fast-forwarding to the end, changing the colour, volume etc. As they feel able, they can then imagine moving gradually closer to the screen until they are watching it closely in its entirety.

This exercise can help in various ways. It places control over the intensity of the trauma memories into your client's hands; they can mute or pause when it feels overwhelming, or move closer or further away depending on how they feel. It adds an extra cognitive task to the reliving, which reduces immersion in the memories. It also helps convey the message that trauma memories can be controlled.

Notes from the therapy room: Carla

Carla developed PTSD after being assaulted by her sister. Carla's sister had problems with drug addiction and asked Carla for money. When Carla refused, she began screaming at her, slapping, and choking her. They were in a shopping centre at the time and Carla saw people watching but not intervening. She also ran into a shop for help and was ignored. She believed at the time that no one cared enough to help. Carla began to experience PTSD symptoms soon after, including intrusive memories and flashbacks of the assault and panic attacks when she encountered reminders. She became highly avoidant, barely leaving the house for fear of encountering trauma triggers.

When Carla started PTSD treatment, she attempted to tell the story of the assault, but became highly distressed and had a panic attack. She had dropped out of a previous attempt at therapy as she felt unable to talk about the assault and believed it made her symptoms worse. Her therapist was wary of this happening again, so spent several sessions trying to unravel Carla's formulation (Figure 4.3).

Carla's history was particularly important in understanding her presentation. As a child, Carla had been looked after by her aunt after her mother died. Carla's aunt had other children and Carla felt that she was an unwanted inconvenience. When she was upset about something, she tended to push the feelings away rather than seek help for them, as she didn't believe others would care for her. In this way, she never learned how to effectively self-soothe. Now, faced with difficult emotions as an adult, Carla felt out of control and unable to cope. This amplified her emotionality when confronted with the memories. The felt-sense of being uncared for, and unworthy of care, was re-triggered during the trauma when others failed to help Carla.

The nature of the trauma was also relevant, particularly as Carla had been choked. Reminders made her feel as if she couldn't breathe, which quickly spiralled into a panic attack.

Carla's PTSD was maintained by avoidance. She tried not to think about the assault, for fear of having a panic attack, and pushed away her feelings as she struggled to know what to do with them. This meant that the trauma memories remained in an unprocessed, highly sensory, and

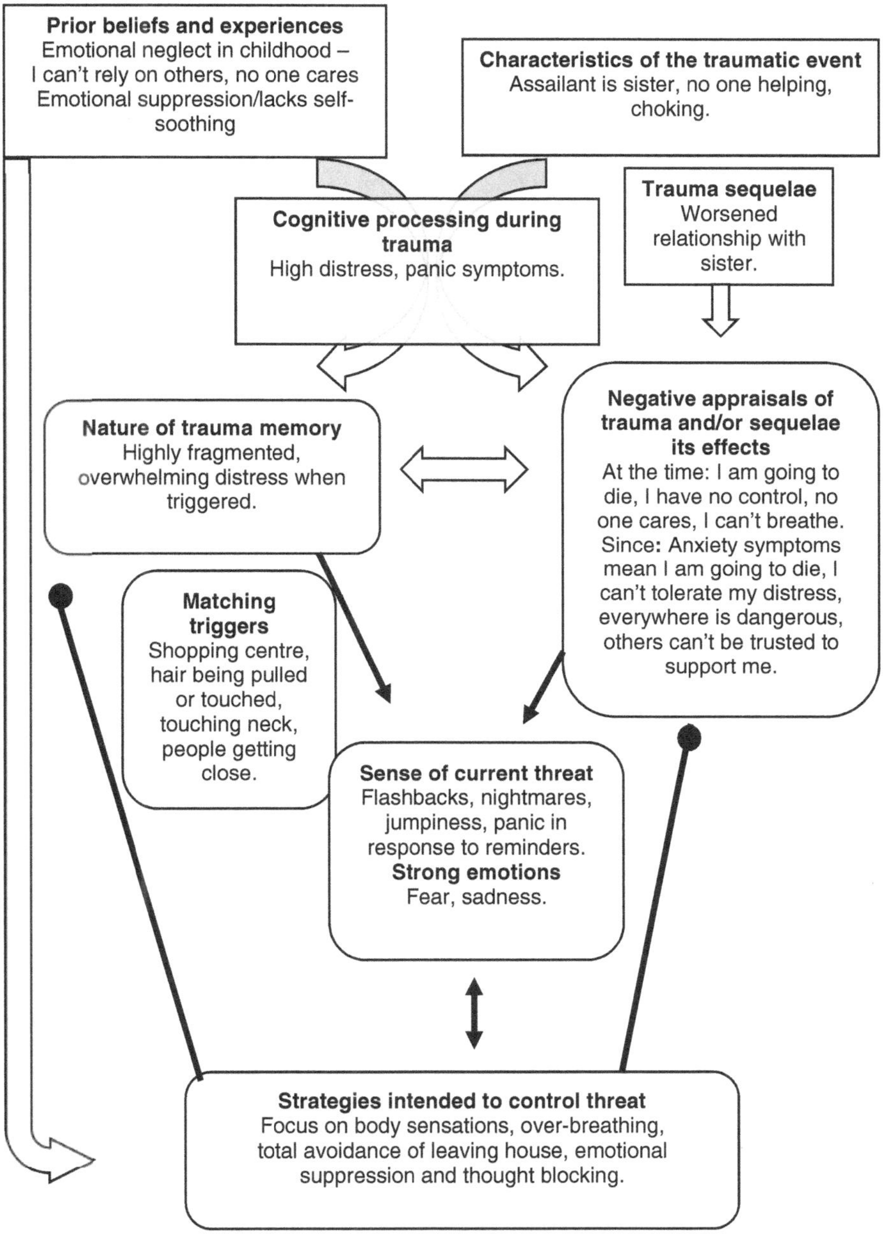

Figure 4.3 Carla's formulation

easily triggered form. She also avoided triggers to her memories, which resulted in her becoming very withdrawn, and inhibited any opportunities to find out that her worst fears would not come true.

A simplified version of this formulation was discussed with Carla. This helped to normalise her symptoms and provided an alternative explanation to what was going on during a panic attack.

At the time, it felt to Carla as if she couldn't breathe and was suffocating, but she accepted the possibility that she was re-experiencing what had happened during the trauma.

Carla and her therapist worked on stimulus discrimination to differentiate the trauma memories of being choked from the experience of having a panic attack. They practised ways to make this discrimination clearer, such as touching her neck to show there was nothing there. They also discriminated other reminders of the trauma, including people standing nearby. Carla began to feel less anxious in public places and was having fewer panic attacks.

Carla and her therapist also discussed different ways to help Carla calm down if she was feeling upset. She identified several, such as stroking her dog, playing games on her phone, and smelling an essential oil. For homework, Carla practised rating her emotions several times a day. If her distress increased over 60, she used one of her calming techniques to bring the emotion down. These were discussed as behavioural experiments, to test whether her feelings were controllable.

After six sessions, Carla felt able to think about the trauma. She agreed to start creating a timeline of what happened, initially with minimal detail. Carla's therapist asked for regular SUDs ratings, and they paused and used a coping strategy if her ratings went over 80/100. This also helped to test Carla's beliefs about whether her therapist could be trusted to support her.

Over the next few sessions, Carla and her therapist added further detail to the timeline, as well as updating information, e.g. that she did not die. They also worked on an update for the belief that people did not step in because they did not care, by imagining the scene from the perspective of a bystander. Carla realised that people would have been shocked and surprised and might not have known how to help. She also recalled that a security guard from a shop had approached her shortly after the assault to check if she was alright.

Developing a detailed account of the trauma memories led to a marked improvement in Carla's re-experiencing symptoms. The nightmares and flashbacks stopped. Carla still felt anxious in public places but was no longer having panic attacks. In the later stages of treatment, she and her therapist revisited the shopping centre where the assault happened. Carla experienced some panic symptoms but was able to remind herself that she was experiencing anxiety triggered by the trauma memories and was not in any physical danger.

Carla's sister was serving a prison sentence for burglary at the time of Carla's treatment, and Carla did not feel ready to visit her. She decided to write her a letter to express some of her feelings about the assault and wait a little while before deciding whether or not to send it. She knew that her sister loved her, but that the addiction made her behave in a hurtful way. She wished her sister the best in the substance abuse programme that she was undertaking in prison. Carla also wrote about their childhood. She had realised that they had both felt unwanted and unloved and that it was hard to shake off those feelings, even as adults. Writing the letter made Carla realise that there were people in her life who loved her, including her husband and her other siblings. In her therapy blueprint, Carla identified that an ongoing task after therapy would be noticing and recording evidence that people did care about her using a positive data log. She also reflected on what the process of learning to trust her therapist taught her about herself, others, and the future.

Recommended reading

Briere, J. N., & Scott, C. (2014). *Principles of trauma therapy: A guide to symptoms, evaluation, and treatment (DSM-5 update)*. Sage.

Liness, S. (2009). Cognitive therapy for post-traumatic stress disorder and panic attacks. In N. Grey. (Ed.). *A casebook of cognitive therapy for traumatic stress reactions*, (pp. 147–163). Routledge.

CHAPTER FIVE

Under-activation of trauma memories

Nelson had been working as a prison officer for ten years when he was taken hostage during a riot. In therapy, he would cover his face with his hands and hold back from remembering the trauma. He was ashamed of his reactions at the time of the trauma and didn't want to look weak in front of his therapist. Therapy focused on understanding and addressing his beliefs about emotions to stop him from holding back from the trauma memories.

Some clients struggle to activate trauma memories or connect with the associated thoughts and feelings. On a graph, a therapy session with under-activated trauma memories would look like Figure 5.1. Not reaching the therapeutic window in these sessions makes it very difficult to access or change the meanings embedded within the trauma memories. Our clients might be able to logically understand an update, for example, that a trauma wasn't their fault, but cannot link it with the memories themselves, meaning that this new information isn't accessible when they have re-experiencing symptoms, and leaving them feeling guilty and ashamed when they are reminded of the trauma.

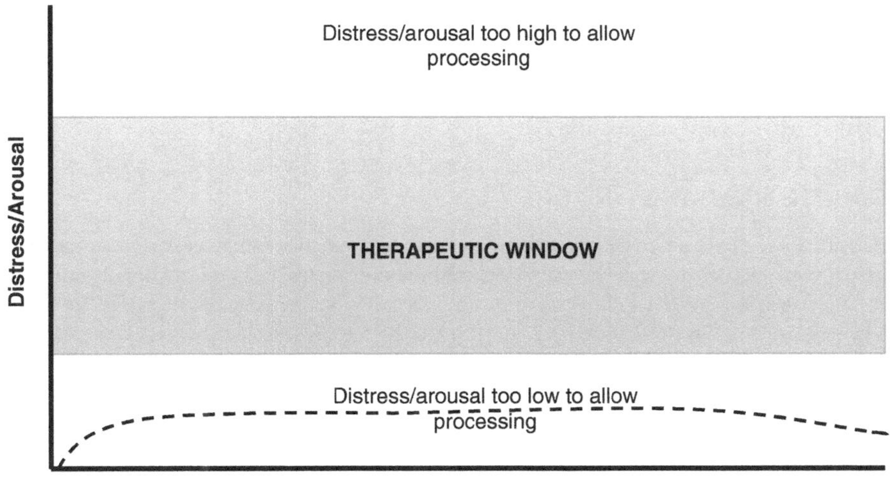

Figure 5.1 Under-activation of trauma memories

DOI: 10.4324/9781003288329-7

Why does under-activation happen?

There are a few reasons why it might be hard to activate the trauma memories, and understanding why will help guide your intervention.

IT ISN'T ACTUALLY PTSD

If someone experiences very little distress or arousal when they relive the trauma memories, it is worth checking that they have re-experiencing symptoms of PTSD (vivid intrusive and unwanted memories, flashbacks, nightmares and/or emotional and physiological arousal when confronted with reminders). If someone is having terrifying nightmares about the trauma but doesn't experience distress when they talk about the trauma, then it is very likely a case of under-activation. However, if they aren't having re-experiencing symptoms, it may be that they ruminate about the trauma or their feelings, but PTSD is not the most fitting understanding of their problem (see page 28 for the difference between rumination and intrusions).

Of course, they may be struggling with another type of problem, because traumatic events can trigger, and worsen, many other disorders (like depression, psychosis, eating disorders, personality disorders, and so on). Your client may still benefit from treatment, and knowing their trauma history will be important in formulating their problems. However, treatment should be based on the best available option for their primary presenting problem. Some CT-PTSD techniques can be interwoven with treatment of other disorders where relevant, such as imagery rescripting to target trauma memories in social anxiety disorder (Wild, & Clark, 2011) and depression (Wheatley et al., 2007).

LOW IMAGERY ABILITY

Just as some people have unusually high imagery ability, around 10% of the population struggle to generate mental images (Faw, 2009). This makes treatment techniques that rely on imagination, including reliving, very difficult, frustrating, and unlikely to be helpful. You can check imagery ability by asking your client to generate a neutral image (e.g. a sunrise), relive a recent memory like their journey to therapy that day, or by using a measure of imagery ability (Pearson et al., 2013). If they struggle to bring visual images to mind or to relive memories with sensory details, they may have low imagery ability. In this eventuality, you may need to use forms of memory work that rely less on imagination.

PERI-TRAUMATIC NUMBING

If someone felt numb at the time of the trauma, they may feel numb when accessing the trauma memories. The problem here is not that they can't activate the memories, but that the peri-traumatic numbness is being re-experienced. Clients can sometimes recall whether they felt numb at the time of the trauma or not. Another way of checking is to monitor the feelings attached to re-experiencing symptoms. If, when a client has flashbacks or nightmares, they re-experience a sense of numbness, this is probably how the memories were stored (and how they felt peri-traumatically). If they feel emotions when having re-experiencing symptoms that they cannot retrieve during imaginal reliving, the numbing is more likely post-traumatic rather than peri-traumatic.

BELIEFS ABOUT EMOTIONS

A common reason for under-activation is avoidance of the trauma memories due to beliefs about the emotions associated with it, for example fearing being overwhelmed by unbearable feelings. For some people, this avoidance is conscious and deliberate, but often it happens automatically. We all have emotional schemas – belief structures that we hold about our emotions, typically linked to our upbringing and cultural influences (Leahy, 2002, 2007). If we grew up in a family where emotions were never expressed, or we were taught that emotionality was dangerous in some way, our automatic reaction to strong negative emotions will often be to suppress or avoid them in some way.

A good place to start is some guided discovery about your client's views on emotions. You can ask them what they think will happen emotionally if they let themselves remember the trauma and how long they think they will feel that way (Leahy, 2007). This will help identify any catastrophic fears about becoming emotional. Sometimes, you will need to ask 'downward arrow' questions, such as 'what would be the worst thing about that?' and 'where would that lead?' to get to the worst meanings. You may also want to ask about past experiences, for example, 'how did your family express feelings?' and 'have there been times in the past when your feelings were out of control?'.

Connor grew up in a military family, was in the cadets at school, and joined the army aged 17. His father had been strict and had taught Connor not to complain if he was upset about something as a child. Connor's mother had suffered a severe depressive episode when Connor was in his teens and spent time in a psychiatric facility.

When Connor developed PTSD after a series of traumatic experiences in the army, he began to feel like his emotions had gone 'haywire'. He coped by avoiding and burying his feelings. He had learnt in the army to focus his mind on blankness when he had endured physical pain on marches and he used this tactic now when he felt negative emotions. In therapy, he presented as very calm and controlled, but he was also reporting terrifying nightmares and occasional multi-sensory flashbacks.

Connor's therapist gently explored his beliefs about emotions. Connor viewed them as dangerous and expressed the view that his mother had become unwell because she had lost control of her emotions and allowed them to overwhelm her. He was afraid the same thing would happen to him, that he would end up sectioned and 'rocking in the corner'.

BELIEFS ABOUT THE THERAPIST'S REACTION

Sometimes the beliefs that emerge through discussions about the emotional impact of memory work relate to the therapist. Some of our clients believe that we will judge them negatively if they tell us about the trauma or if they become emotional in sessions. Others feel protective towards us and don't want us to hear something unpleasant in case it causes us harm.

Again, the best place to start is by exploring these beliefs. You could say 'some of our clients worry about what we might think when they are talking about the trauma memories. Is that something which is on your mind at all?' or 'do you worry about how other people might be affected if you tell them your story in all its details?'. If, during reliving or another form of memory work, your client skims over a difficult part of the memories or seems to be suppressing their feelings, you can ask them 'what was holding you back just then?' or 'what might happen if we talked about that part in more detail?'.

Hot cognitions

- It is unsafe for me to get upset
- I am not an emotional person
- I can't bear to think about the trauma
- My therapist will think I am crazy/weak if I get emotional

BELIEFS ABOUT THE MEANING OF THE TRAUMA

The final type of beliefs that can contribute to under-activation is those related to the meaning of the trauma. For some people, the trauma has such a painful personal meaning that their only means of coping is to numb themselves or find another way of suppressing the memories. Again, this can be a very deliberate process, can be more like a habit, or feel entirely automatic and outside their control.

> Aliki was abducted by her ex-boyfriend and tied up in the boot of his car. She had terrifying nightmares about the incident but, when she talked about it, she experienced almost no emotions. At one point, her therapist realised that Aliki always talked about the event as if she was giving a statement and used the same 'stock' phrases each time. Aliki had made a statement to the police and had developed a 'safe' version of events which she recounted if needed. She was able to talk in this way without experiencing much emotion. When her therapist asked about this, Aliki realised that she often thought about the incident as if it happened to someone else or as if she had seen it in a movie. This was a way of protecting herself from accepting how much danger she had been in. When her therapist asked Aliki what it would mean to her if she did accept the trauma had happened to her, Aliki became tearful and responded that it would mean that someone she had loved and trusted actually hated her enough to want her dead, and that others could therefore behave in the same way. This meaning had been too painful for Aliki to accept, so she had found a way to retell the events without them being about her. She realised that she had done this so many times that she now did it without thinking.

MANAGING UNDER-ACTIVATION OF TRAUMA MEMORIES

It helps to be transparent and collaborative about the therapeutic window. Some of the techniques to 'turn up the volume' on the trauma memories amount to deliberately trying to increase the emotions your client feels, so having a good understanding of the rationale is more likely to promote engagement. Psychoeducation about the therapeutic window (e.g. using the music metaphor) and explaining the importance of fully accessing the trauma memories and their related meanings and emotions is therefore important, as it means working within the therapeutic window becomes a shared task. It will also reassure our clients that we do not want to over-activate the trauma memories so that the experience becomes overwhelming.

WORK WITH THE BELIEFS

Where beliefs about emotions, the therapist's reactions, or the meaning of the trauma are part of the reason for under-activation, these can be identified and addressed. The primary technique is guided discovery, to learn about an individual's beliefs and to identify and test potential alternatives. Psychoeducation is also helpful, for our clients to understand that their feelings, and other symptoms, are a normal and understandable part of PTSD.

Where the beliefs concern emotions, the therapist can help the client to understand that we all think about our emotions differently, probably as a result of previous experiences. It is understandable and normal to have developed ways to protect ourselves from difficult feelings. The beliefs can then be examined. For example, reviewing evidence for and against a belief such as 'if I become upset, I will lose all self-control, become hysterical and not be able to calm down'. Does the client have experiences of this happening to them or someone else? Has this happened when they experience intrusive trauma memories (which are likely to be more intense than accessing the memories deliberately using imaginal reliving)? What are the advantages and disadvantages of having emotions? What helpful functions might they have in certain situations? Behavioural experiments can be conducted to test out specific beliefs. For example, to test the effects of not suppressing emotion, we could allow emotions to increase to a certain level (e.g. a SUDs rating of 30/100) by deliberately thinking of something upsetting, and then monitoring what happens if the emotion is not suppressed.

Trudie believed that having emotions was dangerous because she was severely punished as a child for crying. Her therapist encouraged Trudie to consider alternative theories, including that they could sometimes be acceptable and beneficial and that negative emotions, although unpleasant to experience, usually passed in time and did not always lead to negative outcomes. With prompting, Trudie was able to identify times when she had experienced emotions, both positive and negative, without dire consequences. They also considered alternative explanations for why she was punished as a child, including that it reflected parenting beliefs that Trudie did not hold. She agreed to try some behavioural experiments in reducing her emotional control and review the consequences. She watched a sad movie with her partner, went to a comedy show with a friend, and attended her nephew's birthday party. On each occasion, Trudie tried to reduce the control she normally exerted over her emotions and found that she did feel more, but there were no serious negative consequences.

Where beliefs concern the therapist's reactions, it can help to provide some information about the therapist's context and training; for example, that therapists have regular supervision that addresses technical aspects of their work and also provides them with emotional support. Clients may be reassured to hear that their therapist has worked with many other people who have experienced traumatic events and has heard about a wide range of experiences, including very disturbing material. We sometimes use the metaphor of therapy as a 'laboratory', with 'psychological protective equipment' and systems in place designed to make the work safe for both of us, just as if we were handling toxic substances. It can also help to remind clients about confidentiality, and that upsetting details they choose to tell us will not be repeated elsewhere. Be aware that clients who are embarrassed or ashamed may be closely monitoring us for signs of distaste, judgement, and distress. We need to clearly signal unconditional positive regard for our clients, both verbally and in our manner, to model that we are not shocked by, or critical of, what they tell us. This doesn't mean that we need to keep a poker face and not respond with our normal emotional reactions, just be aware that our clients might be sensitive to signs of perceived negative judgement. It can be helpful to model this, validating a disturbing detail by saying 'what an awful experience' or 'that sounds really distressing' while remaining composed and keeping the structure of the session.

FAQ: Is it okay for me to show emotion in a therapy session?

Therapists aren't robots, and it is easier for our clients to connect with us when we show that we are humans, with our own experiences and emotions. Of course, the focus of therapy should be the client, not the therapist, so we draw boundaries around how much we disclose, and try to avoid our clients feeling responsible or protective over us.

If you hear something upsetting in a session, it is fine to show that it has affected you. We were told once 'it's fine to cry with your client, but make sure you start after they do, and finish before them'. In other words, we can show emotions, but we still need to contain our client's distress and demonstrate that we are capable of hearing, and helping with, whatever our clients have experienced.

Lastly, where beliefs relate to the meaning of the trauma, working on these meanings before revisiting memory work can be beneficial.

Aliki, who found it difficult to accept the painful meanings associated with her trauma, benefitted from identifying and discussing her belief that someone she had loved was capable of hurting her and therefore others could do the same. This was addressed initially through some Socratic dialogue, including asking Aliki to consider what she would say to a friend who had experienced the same trauma. A historical review of evidence was also used, considering all the other people Aliki had trusted, and how many of them had hurt her. Other than one friend who had spread nasty rumours about Aliki, she was able to conclude that most people she had been close to had been trustworthy. Exploring the belief in this way led to a decrease in Aliki's belief ratings, and she felt more able to connect with the emotions of fear and betrayal that she had been avoiding.

TURN UP THE VOLUME

Once the shared goal of activating the memories within the therapeutic window has been established and any blocking beliefs have been addressed, the therapist and client can jointly experiment with 'turning up the volume' on the memories to access the full details and the associated emotions.

Increase the intensity of reliving

For people who are easily distracted, struggle with imagery, or have difficulty connecting emotionally with the trauma memories, it can help to increase the intensity of imaginal reliving by asking the client to speak in the first person, present tense, closing their eyes, dimming the lights in the therapy room, and reducing any distractions, like closing the window blinds and turning off the screen of a computer. The therapist should intervene minimally, to avoid distracting the client from the memories, and only take ratings after reliving. Some of our clients feel self-conscious and prefer the therapist to turn away or close their own eyes during reliving.

Focus on emotions and sensations

Through questions that direct their attention, encourage your client to focus on the emotions and physical sensations they experienced at the time of the trauma. Be vigilant to the client avoiding difficult moments, slipping into the past tense, or giving a very rehearsed or matter-of-fact account of the trauma that minimises the emotionality. Gently prompting them to describe their feelings and physical sensations (e.g. what they feel in their gut at those worst moments, plus tastes, smells, and touch) should increase the intensity of the experience.

Introduce triggers

Especially for our clients who struggle with generating images, it is possible to activate the trauma memories by introducing triggers in the session. Combinations of triggers can be used for a stronger response (and has also been found to prevent relapse when used as part of exposure therapy; Craske et al., 2014).

Jasmine developed PTSD after a pedestrian bridge she was crossing collapsed. She experienced strong emotions when she saw similar bridges or walked on unstable surfaces. However, she struggled with imagery, and could not connect with the emotions that she felt at the time of the trauma through imaginal reliving.

With her therapist, Jasmine found pictures of the bridge online and used these to access some of her peri-traumatic emotions. They also re-enacted parts of the trauma in the therapy room, with Jasmine demonstrating her body position after she fell. The most effective intervention was finding a similar pedestrian bridge at a train station near the treatment centre and practising walking over it. This allowed Jasmine to access how she had felt at the time of the trauma. With encouragement from her therapist, they talked through the trauma while standing on the bridge and included updates to the trauma narrative.

Site visits

An even more powerful way of introducing triggers is to revisit the trauma site. Although usually undertaken towards the end of therapy, under-activated trauma memories are a good example of when to use a site visit earlier in treatment. This can be done virtually if necessary, but an in vivo site visit is usually more effective if possible, as there will be many triggers to the trauma memories.

Notes from the therapy room: Nelson

Nelson was a prison officer who was held hostage in a cell by a prisoner during a riot. The prisoner held a blade to Nelson's throat and threatened to kill him. Nelson was terrified and begged the prisoner for his life. Afterwards, Nelson described feeling ashamed that he had been so scared and felt humiliated in front of the prisoners and his colleagues. He believed he had 'lost face' at work, and wanted to leave the job. When he started therapy, Nelson struggled with imaginal reliving, saying that he was 'just talking' about what happened, rather than reliving it.

Nelson's therapist was concerned that he was holding back from fully accessing the memories and initiated a conversation about emotions. She also noticed that Nelson would cover his face and turn away while talking about the trauma. Nelson described himself as an unemotional person who liked to keep himself to himself. Various factors in his background seemed relevant. Nelson was originally from Jamaica and explained that in Jamaica 'men are men', meaning that they do not get upset or show weakness. This belief had been maintained within his family, with his father instructing Nelson and his brother to 'be strong' and not to cry or complain as children. The family moved to the UK when Nelson was ten, and he was bullied at school. Nelson said that he learnt 'to handle himself', standing up to the bullies and not letting them see he was upset. Overall, Nelson's childhood experiences had left him with beliefs that emotions were unacceptable for a man to feel or express, and that other people would view him as weak and take advantage of him if he did so. This was maintained through his work in the prison, as there was a culture amongst the guards of not showing vulnerability in front of the prisoners and, amongst prisoners, of relentlessly teasing guards they perceived as 'soft'.

Nelson and his therapist added this information to his formulation (Figure 5.2). His therapist validated that it was not surprising that Nelson found it difficult to relive the painful emotions from the trauma, given that he had been taught that it was 'unmanly' to be distressed. It also made sense of why the trauma was so difficult for Nelson to think about as, to him, begging for his life meant that he was 'soft' and weak. She normalised that anyone who felt this might then feel ashamed to disclose it. This helped Nelson acknowledge that he felt embarrassed in front of his therapist, believing she would judge him negatively for how he behaved during the trauma and if he became emotional in the session.

Nelson's therapist explained the idea of the therapeutic window and the importance of accessing the memories in a way that felt safe. She also explained that, as a trauma therapist, she had heard about similar traumatic experiences before and was there to support Nelson, not judge him. They discussed the differences between their work environments – in prison, expressing emotion was seen as a weakness but, in therapy, it was seen as important progress. Here is an extract from their session:

THERAPIST: How did you find talking about what happened just now?

NELSON: It's just not me, you know, all the emotional stuff.

T: Yes, I can see that. Does it make you feel uncomfortable?

N: Oh yes, I am a fish out of water!

T: What would it mean to you if you did get emotional?

N: I wouldn't like it.

T: Would it say something about you as a person?

N: It's just not me. I know people say different but, to me, it isn't something for men to do.

T: Getting emotional isn't something men do?

N: Some do maybe, but not men like me, like working men, strong men.

T: Okay, so some men do get emotional, but not working men or strong men. Can you give me an example of a strong man?

N: Soldiers, policemen. You know – people whose job it is to be strong.

T: Let me check I am understanding. So men who have certain jobs, who need to be strong in their jobs, never get emotional? Do they ever cry?

N: No! No way.

T: Okay, I wonder if we can do a little experiment. If I search in Google Images here for a picture of a soldier crying, what am I going to find?

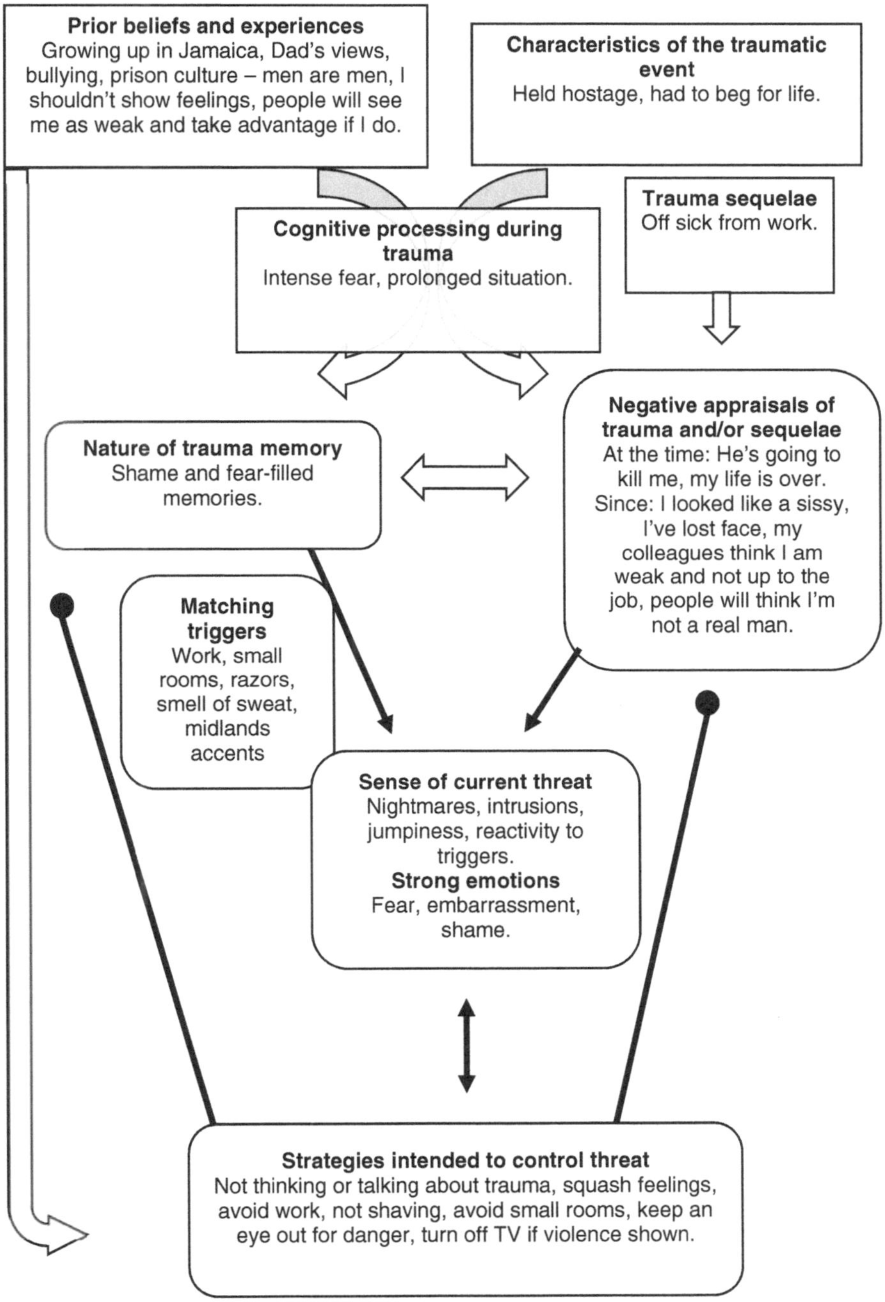

Figure 5.2 Nelson's formulation

N: No real soldiers. Actors in a film maybe.

T: Let's try it [types 'soldier crying' into Google Images and scrolls down the page]. What do you think of this?

N: There's a lot, I'm surprised.

T: There are lots, aren't there? What do you notice?

N: Lots of different people – men, women, different armies, black, white.

T: What does this mean in terms of your belief about strong men crying?

N: Soldiers cry, I guess sometimes they cry. But I don't think they would cry in a battlefield.

T: When do you think they might cry?

N: Some of these pictures look like funerals, so maybe their friend died. Some of them are crying when they see their families, maybe they've been away a long time. Some of them look like they are in pain, maybe something bad has happened.

T: So is it okay for strong men to cry sometimes? Like if something bad has happened?

N: Ha, I see what you are saying! That, if a soldier can cry, it is okay for me to cry.

T: Yes, well that is something I think. I've worked with lots of men – policemen, soldiers, really strong men, who've had a bad experience. Sometimes they cry and I don't think that means they aren't strong.

N: Everyone feels pain sometimes.

T: Yes, exactly. We are all human, so we have pain sometimes. You're doing really well talking about all this. How do you feel?

N: Okay. I am getting used to talking I think. I'm not gonna cry though!

T: That's fine. You don't need to cry, but you can if you feel like it. I just want you to be able to talk to me about how you feel and how you felt in the riot. And not just for the sake of being upset, but because in the very unusual context of PTSD therapy, this will help us put the trauma memories more into the past. Is that something you want to do?

N: God yes. That was the worst day of my life.

T: Yes, it sounded awful. Shall we try to talk about what happened again?

The work with Nelson on expressing emotions took several sessions, and he gradually became more able to access his feelings. The worst hotspot for Nelson was when he believed he was going to die and was begging for his life. This made him feel helpless, defeated, and ashamed. He and his therapist devised a survey that they distributed to men asking whether they thought Nelson's behaviour was acceptable. Most people responded that they would have done anything at all to escape from the situation and that appealing to the prisoner emotionally was a good strategy. One of the survey respondents gave a metaphor that Nelson liked: a rigid tree will fall over easily in a storm, but a tree that can bend and flex in the wind will not fall. Nelson began to see that the way he reacted to the prisoner did not mean that he wasn't strong, just that he had needed to do whatever he could to survive. This led to a change in Nelson's beliefs about himself.

Gradually, Nelson began to suppress the memories less and was able to 'turn up the volume' on the trauma memories, using imaginal reliving and introducing triggers. For example, Nelson was triggered by enclosed spaces, so they conducted a reliving session in a very small room. Nelson planned to return to work and arranged with his boss to carry out a site visit. On his first return to the prison, Nelson felt quite emotional but was welcomed back by his colleagues. Their positive reactions to him added more evidence to his new belief that he had behaved in a human way during the trauma, and that others did not see him as weak.

Recommended reading

Leahy, R. L. (2007). Emotional schemas and resistance to change in anxiety disorders. *Cognitive and Behavioral Practice*, 14(1), 36–45.

CHAPTER SIX
Dissociation

Laila had experienced a sexual assault and dissociated in therapy whenever the memories were triggered, losing awareness of her surroundings and becoming unable to move. Her therapist taught her strategies to manage the dissociation and used adapted reliving techniques to help her stay in the therapeutic window.

Dissociation is defined as a disruption, interruption, and/or discontinuity of the normal integration of behaviour, memory, identity, consciousness, emotion, perception, body representation, and motor control (APA, 2013). The term is used to refer both to the process of dissociation and the symptom or experience. There is a huge range of dissociative phenomena, from mild temporary dissociation, like depersonalisation (feeling detached from one's body, for example, when extremely tired) and alterations in time-sense, to complicated and enduring dissociative disorders. There remains much controversy about dissociative phenomena and how they arise (Loewenstein, 2018), but it appears that, as well as sitting on a continuum of severity, there are different categories of dissociative phenomena that are qualitatively distinct (Holmes et al., 2005).

Many people with PTSD experience dissociation, typically at a mild to moderate level. A flashback is a 'tuning in' dissociative experience, where people temporarily feel immersed in the trauma memory as if it is happening again, simultaneously losing touch with their present surroundings. Numbing, 'spacing out' and memory blanks, or 'tuning out' dissociation, are also common in PTSD. Tuning out may arise as a general mode (such as a pervasive sense of depersonalisation or derealisation) or only in response to triggers, such as trauma memories or anxiety.

Dissociation is often conceptualised as a way of escaping mentally and emotionally from a distressing experience. It is common, therefore, for people to dissociate peri-traumatically, which can affect how the trauma memories are stored. Dissociation may have been a pre-existing problem or tendency before the trauma. People may also dissociate when the traumatic memories are subsequently triggered and/or as a means of coping with PTSD symptoms. In this chapter, we will focus on these 'detachment' types of dissociation, as they commonly occur alongside PTSD. 'Compartmentalisation' types of dissociation, such as conversion disorders, dissociative fugues, and dissociative identity disorder may also be trauma-related but are much less common.

UNDERSTANDING DISSOCIATION

AN EVOLUTIONARY MODEL OF DISSOCIATION

There are various theoretical models of dissociation, but one that we find helpful to discuss with our clients is the 'defense cascade' (Schauer, & Elbert, 2010; Figure 6.1). This suggests that dissociation evolved in animals, including humans, as part of the various instinctive defence

DOI: 10.4324/9781003288329-8

tactics we use when placed in life-threatening situations. Confronted with sudden danger, we first freeze, and orient towards the threatening situation (the startle response). When the threat has been evaluated as real and imminent, 'fight or flight' is activated, firing up the sympathetic nervous system to prepare us to run away from the threat, or defend ourselves. However, if we cannot escape or fight back safely, we enter a 'fright' stage where we become immobilised, or 'scared stiff'. This response probably evolved as a way of 'playing dead' or appearing to submit, so the predator loosens its grip or ends the attack. It also minimises further harm if we are injured and, indeed, dissociation is common in penetrating traumas, for example being stabbed or raped. If this tactic doesn't work, the last survival options are to 'flag' or 'faint' to minimise harm. Instead of the rigid immobility and hyper-arousal of the 'fright' phase, we go floppy as our sympathetic nervous system shuts down and the parasympathetic system takes over. In these phases, our pulse and breathing slow, which may explain why we feel more distant and unreal, can have 'out of body' perceptions, and become numb to sensations including pain. At the 'faint' point, we may blank out altogether or lose consciousness.

The cascade outlined by Schauer and Elbert has not been empirically demonstrated in humans. However, we find it a useful heuristic for several reasons. Firstly, it provides a normalising explanation for some of the frightening dissociative symptoms that our clients experience during and after trauma, such feeling paralysed or unreal. By explaining dissociation as a 'hard-wired' survival response rather than a conscious choice, it also helps challenge self-attacking beliefs about not 'fighting back' during trauma. Secondly, the model explains why some people with PTSD dissociated during their traumas and some did not. In relatively short traumas, or where the individual has been able to escape or fight back, they may only reach the 'flight or fight' stage of activation. When re-experiencing trauma memories, they therefore feel a rush of adrenaline and intense fear, anger, or agitation. However, in more prolonged traumas, where people have been unable to escape or are immobilised, they move into the later stages of the 'defense cascade' and so, during flashbacks, feel helpless, defeated, drained, or numb. Lastly, the model explains why dissociation occurs during traumas, persists afterwards, and arises in

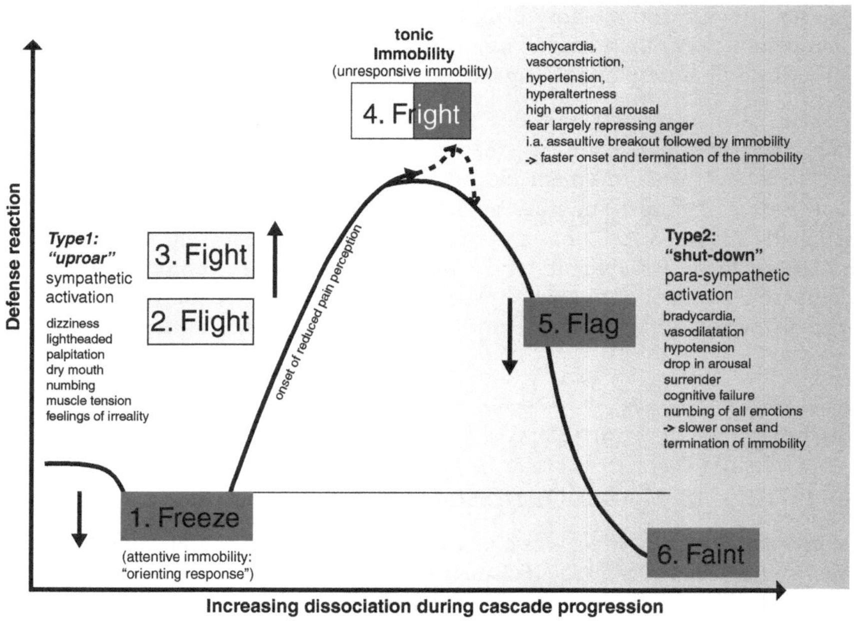

Figure 6.1 The defence cascade (Schauer & Elbert, 2010, used with permission from *Zeitschrift für Psychologie / Journal of Psychology* 2010; Vol. 218(2): 109–127)

therapy. Dissociating becomes a learnt behavioural response to stress that is reactivated when trauma memories are triggered. The more often this happens, the more quickly the cascade occurs, so people who have had repeated traumatic experiences can learn to dissociate very quickly. The response is also hypothesised to generalise over time to more and more triggers, making it more frequently activated.

LEARNT DISSOCIATION

For many people, dissociation is an automatic response outside of voluntary control. However, for others, it begins as a deliberate coping strategy for pain or distress. For example, some ex-military clients we have worked with learnt to deliberately dissociate as a way to deal with the physical rigours of military training such as long marches, and (usually later) to deal with the distressing situations they encountered. Other clients with abusive childhoods learnt to stare at a spot on the wall or repetitively self-soothe by rocking to take themselves away from pain. Later, these strategies become habitual ways of managing distress. For these clients, it is often important to examine beliefs about emotions (Chapter 5), as clients may believe they are unable to manage them in any other way, or that expressing them may place them at risk.

FLASHBACKS

Flashbacks are usually a sign that the memories are particularly poorly integrated and contextualised so, when triggered, are experienced in powerful somatic and sensory detail. Clients may re-experience the 'uproar' sympathetic nervous system activation illustrated by Schauer and Elbert, becoming highly distressed and aroused during a flashback. If the trauma was prolonged and/or inescapable, they may also re-experience 'shut down' dissociation during a flashback, appearing to 'tune out'.

Flashbacks normally diminish once the trauma memories have been fully processed, for example through imaginal reliving or writing a narrative. These activities can be challenging when they trigger flashbacks, which we want to avoid in sessions. As well as being very distressing, clients won't be able to access any contextualising information while they are having a flashback. However, alongside our client, we do need to take calculated risks of triggering flashbacks to progress with treatment. After all, evidence shows that trauma-focused treatments are still effective when a client experiences dissociation (Hoeboer, et al., 2020). This can be a delicate balancing act, so needs to be done collaboratively and from a 'no fail' perspective. If your client does have a flashback in session, you should rapidly and assertively support them in bringing it to an end, then try to derive some learning from the experience, to help you both refine your approach next time around. Occasionally, we learn something new about the trauma during a flashback that the client has been unable to otherwise remember or articulate, and this can be subsequently integrated into the trauma narrative.

THE EFFECT ON THE TRAUMA MEMORIES

Dissociating at the time of the trauma, and dissociation that persists afterwards, are thought to be risk factors for PTSD (Carlson et al., 2012). If our brains aren't processing information properly during the trauma, we don't form clear, continuous, and coherent memories. As we know, unclear and disjointed memories are harder for the autobiographical memory system to store, so they become easily triggered and intrusive. Clients may only recall fragments of memories, unisensory, emotional, or somatic memories that they struggle to place or make sense of. These can lead to 'affect without recollection' (Ehlers, & Clark, 2000). Furthermore, if it is hard to think about or talk about the trauma afterwards without dissociating, it can be hard to 'emotionally process', or make sense of the event and construct a conceptual memory representation that contextualises the sensory memories and puts them into the past.

EFFECTS ON APPRAISALS

As well as the impact on memory formation, dissociation is problematic because it contributes to beliefs like 'I'm weak', which lead to a sense of current threat. The relationship between peri-traumatic dissociation and PTSD is partially mediated by negative appraisals about the self (Thompson-Hollands et al., 2017). When we identify that a client may have dissociated during a trauma, we explore their beliefs, both in terms of their appraisal of their reaction at the time, e.g. 'I just lay there and let it happen', but also what it means to them about the future, e.g. 'I'll freeze again and be vulnerable', or more globally, e.g. 'I've lost my mind'. Furthermore, mental defeat (the sense of 'giving up' during a trauma, associated with loss of dignity, autonomy, and humanity) is a known predictor of PTSD (Kleim et al., 2007). Mental defeat is strongly associated with 'shut down' dissociative responses and may represent a cognitive counterpart to the later phases of the defence cascade (Wilker et al., 2017).

Hot cognitions

- Cutting off is my only way of coping
- Everything feels unreal
- I've lost control of my mind
- I feel like I'm watching from behind a pane of glass
- I need to do this to stop myself from feeling
- I lose track of time/time passes without me realising
- Not moving/fighting back in the trauma means I let it happen

MANAGING DISSOCIATION

PSYCHOEDUCATION

A good place to start is to help your client understand what causes their dissociation. Most people are familiar with the idea of 'fight or flight', but are less likely to know that other defensive reactions follow if they are unable to escape. We use the defence cascade model to normalise dissociation as an automatic, 'hard-wired' coping reaction which our brain uses to protect us and is typically the only coping resource we have in a 'no-win' situation. A normalising explanation is a hugely important intervention, that helps our clients make sense of what can be a disorientating and frightening experience, and tackles any beliefs about being crazy, weak, or untreatable. Short term, dissociation is designed to protect us from intense physical and psychological pain and potentially reduce injury. However, now that the danger has passed, dissociation is no longer helpful to survival and, longer term, may inhibit recovery from PTSD by interfering with emotional processing.

IDENTIFYING TRIGGERS

An important part of gaining control over dissociation is to identify triggers. These will usually be trauma reminders, like sensory details which were present at the time of the trauma, or internal experiences like pain or shame. For example, someone who has a domestic abuse history may be triggered by a raised voice, the smell of their ex-partner's aftershave, or an emotional experience like feeling criticised.

A good way to identify triggers is to keep a diary. Some triggers will be obvious, but others will be subtle and require some detective work to spot. Any experience of dissociation (whether 'tuning out' detachment or 'tuning in' flashbacks) provides an opportunity to recognise a trigger. The therapist can assist with this if the client dissociates in session, by 'tracking back' to the trigger.

GROUNDING

Grounding strategies are ways of bringing attention back into the here and now. To be effective, they should be easy to recall, accessible, and attention-grabbing as your client will need to use them quickly when they encounter a trigger.

Grounding strategies can be:

- Sensory, e.g. strong smells like smelling salts (these are more powerful than essential oils), tastes like strong-flavoured sweets or chewing gum, things to touch like ice cubes, stress balls, splashing or spraying cold water, a hairband around the wrist.
- Physical, e.g. moving around, stretching, shaking the legs and arms, using applied tension (especially for 'shut down' dissociation like fainting).
- Verbal, e.g. a certain phrase like 'I am safe' or 'I am at home'.
- Attentional, e.g. looking around the current environment and naming all the blue objects they can see, looking at photos or saved messages on their phone.

Some grounding strategies work better than others for different people, so your client can experiment to find their preferred technique. If you are working on 'tuning in' flashbacks, try using grounding strategies that match the modality of the trigger and/or memories. For example, if a particular smell is a trigger or forms part of triggered memories, using smelling salts or another powerful smell can be the most effective grounding technique. If they are re-experiencing the taste of blood, a strong mint may be better. If they are tuning in to an intense pain flashback in their hand, encourage them to softly massage it with hand cream. You can also combine techniques to target multiple senses. Grounding tools that represent a positive meaning or recent memories can also be particularly effective.

For people who experience frequent and severe dissociation, grounding techniques will need lots of practice. This includes deliberately introducing triggers and carrying out grounding techniques within sessions. A useful homework task is a grounding diary to record triggers, the grounding strategy used, and the intensity of the dissociative experience before and after grounding (see an example diary extract in Table 6.1). This will help identify which strategies are most effective for an individual.

Table 6.1 Example extract from a grounding diary

Trigger	Intrusion	Intensity (0–100)	Grounding method	Intensity (0–100)
Man who looks like ex	Him holding me down on floor	100	Looked around	90
Smell of aftershave	'Christmas incident'	90	Smelling salts	50
Anthony giving me a hug	Being held down on bed	100	Looked at Anthony Moved around	40
Headache	Being punched in head	70	Smelling salts Stroked hair	30

Incidentally, we see grounding as somewhat distinct from soothing or calming strategies. During dissociation, our priority is the reorientation of attention. However, there is also a place for emotion regulation strategies if a client is experiencing increasing arousal and is likely to dissociate soon, to bring them back into the therapeutic window.

STIMULUS DISCRIMINATION

Another important technique for dealing with triggers to dissociation is stimulus discrimination. As soon as the client has brought their attention into the here and now using a grounding technique, they can begin to notice differences between the trauma 'then' and the situation 'now'. The more often they can do this, the easier it should become, and the reminder should stop acting as a trigger to dissociation. Grounding can form part of stimulus discrimination, for example, naming and touching everything in the room that is different to at the time of the trauma, like the chair, carpet, wall, mug of tea etc. For people who dissociate rapidly, we practise noticing the 'now' firstly in the absence of triggers, to make this more accessible when needed. Saying them aloud and when moving can help.

ADAPTING MEMORY WORK

Memory work is still useful and effective if someone is prone to dissociation. But, if they dissociate when the trauma memories are activated, use the 'turning down the volume' techniques described in Chapter 4, namely written narratives, bird's eye view reliving, or decreasing the intensity of imaginal reliving, focusing on cognitions rather than emotions and sensations, and using distancing techniques. Have pre-practised grounding tools handy, systematically ask clients to rate how tuned in/out they feel, and to 'ground as they go', stopping every couple of minutes to use grounding and stimulus discrimination. As dissociation comes more under control, the intensity of memory work can be gradually increased.

Another adaptation that works well to prevent dissociation is continual movement while reliving. This can be walking on the spot, or in an outside environment, if possible. Passing a soft ball backwards and forwards with the therapist, or holding both ends of a rope and tugging it during reliving can be effective. The client can also use a fidget spinner, Rubik's cube, tear strips of paper, or squeeze a stress ball to keep them grounded. Having visual distractors where the client can see them is helpful for the person to focus on. Also, keeping whiteboards available and visible can help if the client loses the ability to speak.

Throughout any memory work, the therapist needs to keep a close eye on any signs of dissociation, such as long pauses, stuttering, slowed speech and movement, not responding to prompts, looking distant, or bowing their head. Check in regularly on how your client is feeling, and pause to reorient their attention to the here and now if they are dissociating. Staying in the therapeutic window can be a balancing act if someone is prone to dissociation, so you and your client need to work together to monitor and adjust their level of engagement with the trauma memories.

Plan for what they will do after the session, including how to get home if disorientated. Keep notes or audio recordings to remind clients what happened during a session, as dissociation can impair recall. In between sessions, clients can listen to session recordings providing they can keep themselves grounded, for example, by constant movement and keeping written updates to hand.

An alternative strategy is needed for people who have a constant general sense of being 'tuned out' or numb or those who are purposely using dissociation to cut off from strong feelings.

Here, we instead discuss gently 'turning up the volume' on the memories, bringing them back into the window of processing (Chapter 5).

FAQ: What are dissociative seizures?

Some people with PTSD experience dissociative (also known as functional, psychogenic, or non-epileptic) seizures, as well as other functional neurological symptoms such as weakness, fainting, and sensory disturbances (e.g. temporary loss of vision). These are usually considered 'compartmentalisation' rather than 'detachment' dissociation. Clients presenting with these symptoms should be assessed medically, but where an organic cause is not found, a psychological explanation and intervention may be most appropriate. Some functional symptoms may be transient forms of dissociation, like losing the sense of smell or hearing for a time. Others come and go with trauma-related and other stressors, or are present more or less all the time, like weakness in a limb. We recommend monitoring symptoms and trying to identify triggers. Where these are trauma-related, techniques such as stimulus discrimination and grounding can be taught. Recent models of dissociative seizures (e.g. Brown, & Reuber, 2016a) also emphasise expectancy processes, emotional repression, and emotional dysregulation, meaning that creating a normalising explanation for the experiences, identifying and addressing beliefs about symptoms, and managing the therapeutic window, as we've discussed in this chapter, should also help.

Not everyone with functional neurological symptoms (or, indeed, other forms of dissociation) has a trauma history (Brown, & Reuber, 2016b). Some clinicians assume that, if an organic cause has not been determined, they must be caused by 'repressed' trauma, but be wary of going on a fishing trip, as there may be another explanation.

PERI-TRAUMATIC DISSOCIATION: 'TUNING IN' TO 'TUNING OUT'

If someone dissociated during the trauma, there may be gaps in their recall and this may well reflect an accurate record of their experience at the time. Sometimes, as you work on such memories, other layers of emotion and meaning will emerge – thoughts and feelings that the peri-traumatic dissociation helped distance them from but which were nevertheless encoded in sensory memory. You can work on these hotspots as usual. If not, it is still worth trying to put words to as much of any dissociated memories as possible. You can help your client verbally 'code' the peri-traumatic dissociation, describing the feelings, perceptions, and sensations, updating them with 'what I know now is that I was dissociating as a way to cope with how horrible it is, which is why I feel nothing at this point' and using grounding alongside as physical updates, e.g. 'I had to dissociate then but now I can safely ground myself and feel real again'.

Where there are recall gaps due to dissociative amnesia, it may be helpful to 'map the gaps' with timelines and try to work out what likely happened, as a complete narrative will be easier to process (Chapter 8). Often very little happened during a gap, even if it lasted several hours or they travelled some distance, which can make for a reassuring update. By 'anchoring' the memories of being tuned out into the recollections before and after, it helps stop your client re-experiencing their peri-traumatic dissociation in the present. If only parts of the memory representation are recalled but others are missing, e.g. your client can recall a physical sensation but doesn't have visual memories, try to help them imagine what they would have experienced in their other senses. Make sure, however, that what your client adds in are 'best guesses' rather than 'worst cases'!

Kelly was throttled by her ex-partner, and only remembered the pressure around her neck and seeing black. She filled in the gaps in the representation by writing in her narrative 'I can feel his hands around my neck. I know now that I was terrified for my life and my brain froze up. This is called dissociation and it was a way of my mind protecting me from what happened. I couldn't speak or move. I don't remember it but I was pushed against the wall of the kitchen and I must have dropped my phone when he started to strangle me as I found it later on the floor. Freezing was probably the right thing for my body to do in that situation, as trying to fight back or run away would have just led to me being hurt further. I felt numb, but I was very scared underneath. Thinking about it now, I can allow myself to feel that because I know now that he didn't kill me, and that very soon after I managed to get away. I can also look around now and name all the objects I can see because I'm not dissociating anymore'.

Top tips: Think of the onion

Remember that dissociation is a coping strategy, and may be a long-held way for your client to protect themselves from painful emotions. It can feel exposing to remove this strategy and can bring to the surface some difficult emotions that your client has been trying to suppress. We think of dissociation as like the skin of an onion; a protective layer. When we peel that away, your client will encounter new layers of meanings and feelings that they haven't yet dealt with. One of our clients told us 'it felt like moving from a grey, blurry place to a land where everything was suddenly so much more bright, intense, and vivid, and I hadn't anticipated how exhausting that would be'. This is an important part of the process, so we support the client to gradually reduce dissociation, providing alternative ways of coping which promote acceptance and processing rather than avoidance. Further work will be needed to address the layers of the onion that lie beneath the skin. The onion metaphor can also help clients understand why they might experience the trauma more intensely when they have reduced their dissociation or why, as they resolve one bad feeling, it is replaced by another. Reminding them of the onion can help instil hope and reframe this as a sign of progress.

Notes from the therapy room: Laila

Laila came to treatment a year after she was raped by a man she had been dating. She had gone to his house to watch a football match. They began kissing but when the man tried to undress her, Laila resisted. He became more forceful and Laila became unable to move or speak. After he raped her, the man acted as if nothing was wrong and continued to ask Laila on dates, which she refused. She felt confused about what had happened and told her friends it was 'awkward sex' rather than rape. In childhood, Laila's stepfather had been physically and emotionally abusive, subjecting her and her sisters to punishments which she found terrifying. For example, they would be slapped or shut in the basement if they disobeyed his strict rules on modesty.

Laila developed a range of dissociative symptoms following the rape. She felt cut-off from her surroundings when she was out in public, especially in busy places. She experienced powerful dissociative flashbacks when she saw a man who looked like the perpetrator or when she was alone with a man. Before the rape, she had not experienced intrusive memories of the abuse from her stepfather; however, she now sometimes heard his voice in her head calling her a 'slut'. She began self-harming by hitting, burning, and pinching herself. In treatment, Laila dissociated whenever she talked about the trauma, becoming frozen and unable to move or talk.

In therapy, a model of dissociation as a coping strategy to deal with threat was discussed, and a shared formulation developed over several sessions (Figure 6.2). Laila had learned to dissociate during childhood, to 'disappear' mentally during abuse. During the trauma, when Laila felt under threat, this reaction was triggered, and Laila entered a 'fright' state where she

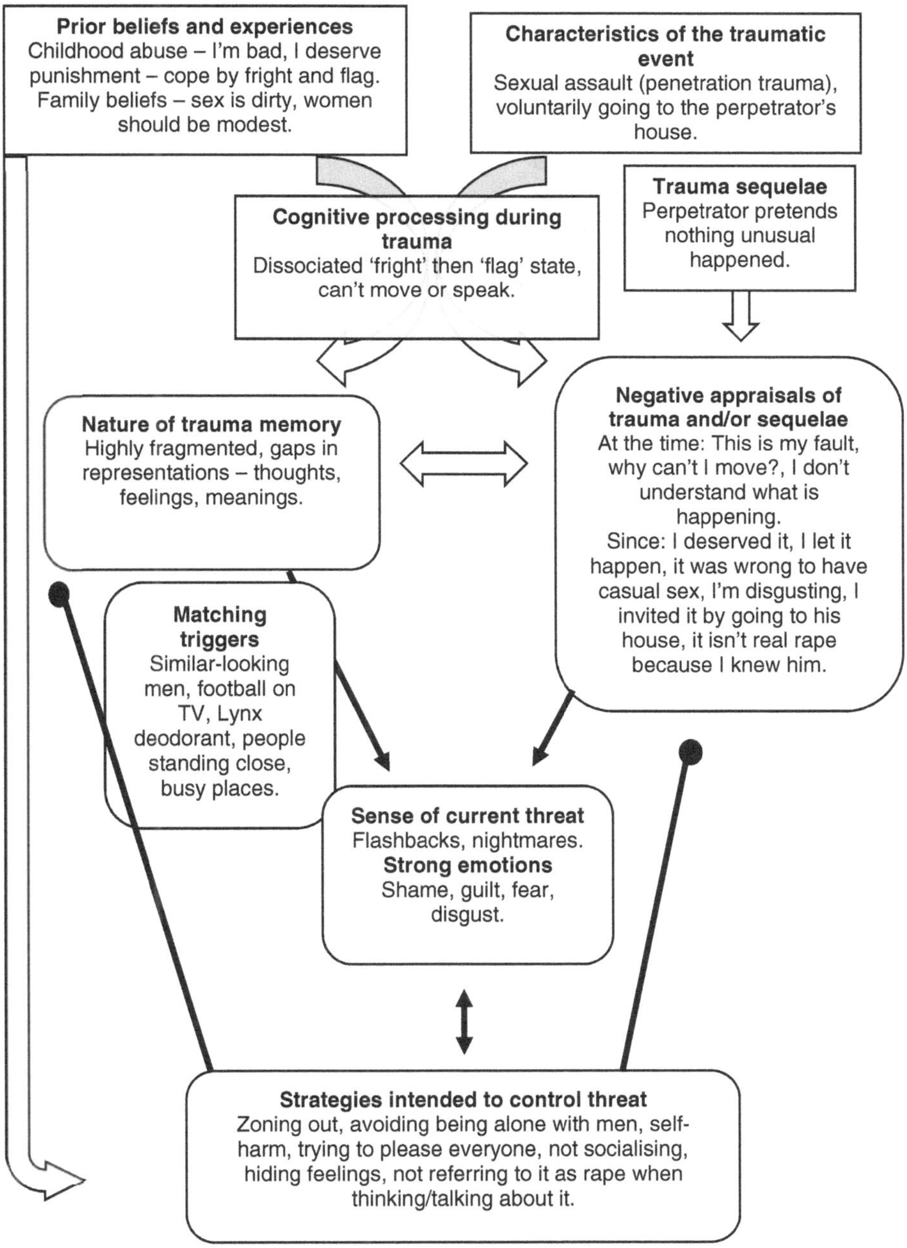

Figure 6.2 Laila's formulation

was terrified but unable to move. This reaction was retriggered when she accessed the trauma memories. Because she hadn't fought back, Laila had interpreted the rape as her fault and felt ashamed. Her stepfather, who was very religious and did not approve of pre-marital sex, had been strict with his daughters about how they dressed and acted. This had laid the foundation for Laila's beliefs that she had 'invited' the rape going to the man's house.

Laila began to monitor her dissociative symptoms. She identified multiple forms of dissociation which had different triggers and responses. Her therapist taught her various grounding techniques and stimulus discrimination, which were practised in session and as homework. As some of her intrusions were related to cognitions, Laila and her therapist also developed statements summarising the information Laila needed to remind herself of once she had grounded herself. They created a chart of her different types of dissociative symptoms, their triggers, early warning signs, and most effective responses (Table 6.2).

As Laila began to feel more control over her dissociation, some of the key appraisals associated with the trauma were identified. The main appraisal driving her sense of shame was that she had 'allowed' the rape to happen because she hadn't fought back and was, therefore, 'slutty' for having 'casual sex'. Her therapist encouraged her to review the evidence for and against this belief. Although Laila had not actively fought the man off, she had clearly said 'no' when he tried to undress her. Laila and her therapist researched definitions of sexual consent and together watched a video made by the Metropolitan Police about consent. They concluded that Laila's behaviour could not have been considered consent to sex, and it would have been clear from her total immobility that she did not want sex, nor was she enjoying it. Laila and her therapist developed a survey to gather opinions on her responsibility for what happened. Most

Table 6.2 Laila's dissociation chart

	Flashback – Dan	*Stepdad's voice*	*Feeling frozen*	*Self-harm*	*Spacing out*
Triggers	Being alone with a man Men who look like him Football on TV	Raised voices Footsteps Dressing in immodest clothes	Physical proximity Smell of aftershave	Male attention People commenting on my appearance Sexual feelings	Going out Busy places Meeting new people
Early warning signs	Images Heart rate increasing Getting numb	Listening for noises Not talking Strong urge to pinch myself	Hard to get words out Gripping arms Tense legs	Shame feeling Feeling sick	Feeling worried Time passing quickly Looking down
What I need to **do**	Show myself he isn't there Focus on their face 'then versus now' Move around	Look in mirror Look around at where I am – not in childhood home	Smelling salts Wriggle toes Hum Stress ball	Sit on hands Urge surf Read update flashcard	Look around Grounding – smelling salts, mints etc.
What I need to **know**	He's not here I'm not there I didn't deserve it	He isn't here I'm an adult now No-one is going to hit me	I can move This is only temporary I'm not in danger	I'm not a slut I'm not trying to draw attention to myself Sexual feelings are normal	I'm safer if I'm aware There's nothing to be scared of

people responded that Laila had not been responsible. Laila began to view what had happened as rape. Although she felt less guilty and ashamed, this shift in her appraisals made her feel more upset as she began to acknowledge that she had been violated by someone she thought she could trust.

Memory work was approached gradually using 'volume down' techniques. Laila agreed to try 'bird's eye view' reliving, using a fidget spinner to keep her hands moving so that she did not become immobile or hit herself. They initially relived only the first part of the evening, taking regular breaks to use grounding strategies. During the parts of the trauma where Laila had been unable to move, her therapist encouraged her to move around the therapy room as she talked. They incorporated updates within reliving immediately, including why she couldn't move or speak, that she was not responsible for what was happening, and that she was safe now. Gradually, Laila was able to add further details when reliving the memories and additional updating information.

Laila and her therapist planned a series of behavioural experiments to reduce her avoidance of triggers. She began by going to busier places while trying to keep her attention in the here and now. Laila felt more on edge when she was not dissociated, and realised she had been 'zoning out' to protect herself from those feelings. Although it was initially unsettling, being aware of what was going on around her enabled Laila to see that she was not in danger. Laila also experimented with deliberately dressing in less modest ways, like showing her arms, and reminded herself that she was an adult, and would not be punished as a result.

Becoming less avoidant helped Laila to engage in reclaiming your life assignments and she began to re-engage with friendships and social activities that she had stopped since the trauma. She did not feel able to date again yet, but practised being alone with men, starting with an old friend of hers, and went to a salsa class with a friend to test out being close to unfamiliar men. Although Laila continued to experience occasional episodes of dissociation as she encountered some of her trauma triggers, she was able to use her grounding strategies and stimulus discrimination to cope with these.

Recommended reading

Carlson, E. B., Dalenberg, C., & McDade-Montez, E. (2012). Dissociation in posttraumatic stress disorder part I: Definitions and review of research. *Psychological Trauma: Theory, Research, Practice, and Policy*, 4(5), 479–489.

Chessell, Z. J., Brady, F., Akbar, S., Stevens, A., & Young, K. (2019). A protocol for managing dissociative symptoms in refugee populations. *the Cognitive Behaviour Therapist*, 12(e27), 1–16.

Kennedy, F., Kennerley, H., & Pearson, D. (Eds.). (2013). *Cognitive behavioural approaches to the understanding and treatment of dissociation*. Routledge.

CHAPTER SEVEN

Multiple trauma memories

Jon experienced and witnessed hundreds of traumatic events during his career in the police, and had always thought he was unaffected. However, after a particularly upsetting incident, he began to re-experience many different trauma memories. His therapist found it hard to know which traumas to prioritise in treatment. They looked for commonalities in the intrusive memories and meanings driving his PTSD symptoms, hoping that by targeting memories that best represented the range of experiences, their work would generalise to other trauma memories.

Many people with PTSD have experienced more than one traumatic event. Some people experience several unconnected traumas, for example, two unrelated accidents at different times. Others have occupations that have led to repeated trauma exposure (such as military or first responder roles) or have experienced repeated traumas within a sustained period of threat, such as living through a war, an abusive relationship, or being detained and tortured in prison. Exposure to multiple traumatic events increases prevalence rates of PTSD in a dose-dependent manner (Wilker et al., 2017). In this chapter, we will discuss why this happens and address related issues in treatment, such as understanding how each trauma contributes to maladaptive beliefs and unhelpful coping strategies and deciding where to start.

The effect of multiple traumatic experiences

EFFECTS ON MEMORY PROCESSING

Repeated exposure to trauma has profound psychological and neurobiological effects, especially at younger ages while the brain is still developing (van der Kolk, 2003). When repeatedly exposed to danger, our brains become more threat-oriented, which affects how we process and respond to sensory information. In response to an ambiguous situation, someone who has been in a sustained high threat environment will perceive greater danger, activating a more powerful threat response in the brain and body. Furthermore, when the threat has passed, it will take their nervous system longer to return to a non-threat state.

This pattern of rapid reactivity and slow recovery affects how memories are laid down which, in turn, increases the risk of PTSD. Our immediate threat response, driven by the limbic system (especially the amygdala), bypasses cortical involvement – there is no time to think through information or integrate it with other memories when we are in danger, the priority is to react quickly. This leads to more 'data-driven' processing, with less conceptual and self-referent processing (making sense of and placing the event within the autobiographical memory system), which has been found to predict PTSD (Beierl et al., 2020), as has peri-traumatic dissociation, which also occurs more often with frequent trauma exposure. With an increased 'trauma load', potential triggers also multiply, as the fear network expands and the connections strengthen (Wilker et al., 2017).

DOI: 10.4324/9781003288329-9

Usually, conceptual processing continues once we are safe as we think through and make sense of what has happened, allowing a more elaborated version of the memories to be laid down. Being in a situation of continued threat prevents this from happening. Being around reminders of the threat, such as in the home with an abusive partner, can also mean the trauma memories, and associated fear network, are constantly activated and, if this includes dissociation or defeat as a response, then conceptual processing is further inhibited as the individual remains more shut down or persistently dissociated. Feeling powerless and dissociated also reinforces feelings of defeat, and resulting negative self-appraisals such as being weak or worthless.

Learning about the neurobiological changes that result from multiple trauma exposure can make us, and our clients, feel hopeless about the chances of recovery. However, we should remember that many people with extensive trauma histories do not develop significant mental health problems and, of those who do, many make full recoveries. Just as experiences of abuse and neglect cause neurobiological changes, so do experiences of safety and love. Helping our clients access and absorb those experiences often becomes part of treatment for people with chronic trauma histories.

EFFECTS ON APPRAISALS

Multiple traumatic experiences lead to layers of meaning building up over time. For example, after a single traumatic event, like an assault, someone may ascribe a neutral explanation, like they were in the wrong place at the wrong time, and what happened was a matter of unfortunate chance and unlikely to happen again. However, if they are assaulted again on another occasion, it may seem too much of a coincidence to be a matter of chance and, instead, the person may draw a different conclusion, such as that they look or act in a way that makes them vulnerable, or that there are far more potential attackers in the world than they had realised. This threatening set of appraisals becomes more central to their mental representation of themselves and others and may lead the person to start taking extra precautions to stay safe, beginning the cycles that perpetuate PTSD.

Early life trauma can have a profound impact on belief formation, as core beliefs about self, others, and the world may be distorted from a young age, with subsequent traumatic experiences seeming to confirm these beliefs, impacting personality and identity development. Clients tell us they 'don't know what normal looks like', as there is no baseline or 'good enough' foundation in safety and care. We'll cover how to work with more deeply ingrained appraisals which often develop as a result of multiple trauma in Chapter 12.

Hot cognitions

- There is something about me that attracts bad things
- Nobody can be trusted
- All men are potential abusers/rapists
- I can't cope with any more
- I'll never have a normal life/relationship

EFFECTS ON COPING

Just as beliefs can seem to be confirmed by multiple trauma exposure, coping strategies can be reinforced over time, and become less amenable to change. For example, if someone has coped with difficult experiences in the past by self-medicating with alcohol and has found some relief from negative emotions in this way, they are more likely to use this strategy again when faced with another traumatic event. Children, in particular, have few available coping strategies when exposed to trauma so those they develop, such as dissociation, may become more easily triggered and less under conscious control over repeated exposures to trauma.

Unfortunately, some ways of coping with PTSD symptoms can place people at risk of further trauma. Drugs and alcohol are one example, and have been found to partially mediate the relationship between childhood and adult trauma; survivors of childhood abuse are more likely to use substances, which in turn leaves them more at risk for further interpersonal abuse (Testa et al., 2010). Similarly, easily triggered anger and aggression as forms of self-protection can lead to further conflict. These are therefore important targets for treatment.

Even if coping strategies are not directly risky, for example brooding and isolating, they often form part of what maintains PTSD, so need to be identified and reduced or dropped. This can feel like an unsettling process. After all, coping strategies are generally your client's best effort at surviving and moving on. Simply pointing out that they are unhelpful and suggesting that your client drops them is unlikely to be an effective intervention. Instead, help your clients to first understand their coping strategies, work out their function and benefits, then evaluate their costs, both in the short-term (surviving) and the longer-term (recovering/thriving). In this way, you validate and normalise even their most extreme coping efforts while drawing their attention to the inadvertent costs of coping this way. This helps build both a rationale and motivation for reducing over-learnt coping strategies. You may also need to work on building up new, less costly, ways of coping to replace any unhelpful strategies. We cover this in more detail in Part 4.

Deciding where to start

One of the issues that therapists face when their client has experienced multiple traumas is choosing where to focus. Both the therapist and client can feel overwhelmed and it is easy to waste valuable session time simply 'talking through their life', trying to work out which memories to target. Here's how we decide where to start.

WORK OUT WHICH TRAUMAS THE PTSD RELATES TO

Experiencing multiple traumas is not the same as having PTSD symptoms from multiple traumas. Some people only re-experience one or two of their many traumas. Others re-experience many events, or a mixed-up 'blur' of memories, and find it hard to identify which symptoms relate to which traumas. Sometimes, events many years later trigger PTSD symptoms from earlier traumas, making it even harder to make sense of symptoms.

> Clive was a firefighter who had witnessed many deaths during his career but did not develop PTSD until he attended a fire in which a child died, who was a similar age to Clive's own daughter. He developed PTSD after this event and then began to have nightmares about other fires he had attended over the years, most of which he had not thought about since.

Assessment tools, such as structured PTSD clinical interviews and self-report measures, are often tricky to administer correctly when multiple traumas have occurred. To be helpful to treatment planning, they should be completed separately for each traumatic event. This can sometimes raise practical problems. For example, a client who had multiple traumatic events in childhood is unlikely to recall whether their insomnia started after the first trauma, the second, or the tenth. Questions about 'losing interest in previously enjoyed activities' are hard to answer for someone who has had PTSD for decades. However, PTSD re-experiencing symptoms can usually be linked in both their content and their onset to specific traumatic events, if not immediately then after some 'detective work'.

Traumatic events which are re-experienced are usually the best area to focus. However, other traumatic life events may still be highly relevant to understanding your client's PTSD and should be included in the formulation. This is where the box for 'previous experiences and beliefs' becomes useful.

> Stephanie had been bullied badly as a child for being tall and skinny. Although as an adult she had 'put it behind her', the experience meant she had come to view herself as an 'easy target', and she vowed never to let anyone get the better of her again. As an adult, Stephanie seemed outwardly confident but her underlying negative beliefs were reactivated when she was violently mugged and exerted a powerful influence on how she processed the trauma. Stephanie strongly believed the mugging was her fault because, in her words, she had 'failed to stand up' for herself 'as usual'. While not causing PTSD, the bullying had come to define her self-image and, in turn, this primed her to feel defeated during the mugging and to interpret it afterwards as confirming she was a 'failure'.

Where earlier traumas are not re-experienced, it isn't usually necessary to use techniques such as imaginal reliving to address them. Instead, it is usually the meaning of the earlier trauma which is important to understand and address in therapy, using cognitive techniques. In some cases, we also use imagery rescripting to work on these earlier memories and break the 'feed-in' from the past.

> Stephanie and her therapist agreed a verbal update for the adult assault memory, that it was not her fault and that she did not cause the assault by failing to stand up for herself. Since this meaning was being fuelled by her early bullying experiences, she also 'went back in time' to give this message to the younger Stephanie, by visiting her in imagination to comfort her and tell her the bullying was not her fault. Linking and rescripting those earlier memories helped Stephanie to feel that the adult trauma update was believable when she brought it into the memory of the mugging.

USING TIMELINES

Timelines are often the first memory-focused technique we use if we encounter some element of memory complexity. We use them to map out the details of specific traumas, as a structure for working with them, and to identify any gaps, fragmentation, or confusion in the order of the memories (Chapter 8). We also use timelines with multiple traumatic events, to map a time period or the client's whole life, then identify and select 'targets' for more detailed memory work. Here are ten reasons we like using timelines:

1. It is collaborative, creative, and can help overcome communication barriers.
2. It provides your client with a ready-made conceptual representation of their memories and engages their autobiographical memory system.
3. It puts everything into a coherent order, which aids the processing of memories.

4. It helps you to identify how re-experiencing symptoms may match to different traumatic events both by their content and onset.
5. It allows you to identify when particular beliefs, coping strategies, and feelings developed and how they have been affected by subsequent events.
6. It provides context for traumatic events, which can help when working on appraisals. For example, once they have an overview of all the preceding events, it might help your client make sense of decisions they made at points in their life, or understand why they responded in a certain way to later events.
7. It can be a less threatening way of working for self-conscious clients, as your and your client's attention are focused on the whiteboard, rather than each other.
8. Timelines can be built up gradually and in layers, allowing you to manage over-activation and dissociation, and incorporate information from multiple sources.
9. It hopefully gives your client a sense of order over what might be a jumbled collection of memories from across their life, although it can also be quite overwhelming for your client to see an extensive trauma history in its entirety. For this reason, we often include positive life events within the timeline.
10. Including positive life events can also help reduce the centrality of trauma memories in defining your client's life view.

There are various ways to construct a timeline. An example of a typical written timeline is shown in Figure 7.1. We tend to use a whiteboard where possible so that details can be added or changed as needed. Another way of organising a timeline is to add details in certain categories, such as Figure 7.2.

If a client does not speak English, we ask the interpreter to add a written translation underneath the timeline. Alternatively, a symbolic version can be used, similar to the 'lifeline' approach in narrative exposure therapy (NET; Schauer et al., 2011), using a rope (or ribbon, if ropes trigger trauma memories) laid on the floor of the therapy room. Objects such as rocks and flowers are placed on the lifeline to represent negative and positive life events respectively. This provides a useful way of mapping out the client's life story incorporating traumatic events within the narrative. In NET, the therapist and client then talk through each rock in detail (a process called exposition), usually only once rather than repeatedly. Unlike CT-PTSD, the key feelings and meanings are not discussed and updated. Timelines are also used extensively in EMDR to identify targets for memory processing (Lombardo, 2012).

INTRUSIONS DIARIES

If a client struggles to identify the traumatic events that most affect them, an intrusions diary (Figure 7.3) can help build a picture of which memories are re-experienced most often, and/or cause the most distress. This kind of 'live' data gathering is usually much more informative and accurate than asking clients about their symptoms retrospectively, and has the added advantage of prompting clients to note triggers to trauma memories.

This form is quite wordy, so we often construct an easier-to-use tick box version for clients. We list the traumas which have been identified from the timeline or through discussion, label them and ask the client to tick the box when they experience a related intrusion (Figure 7.4). Whichever form is used, it is important to clarify the difference between intrusive memories and rumination with your client (page 28), so that they only fill in the form in relation to re-experiencing symptoms.

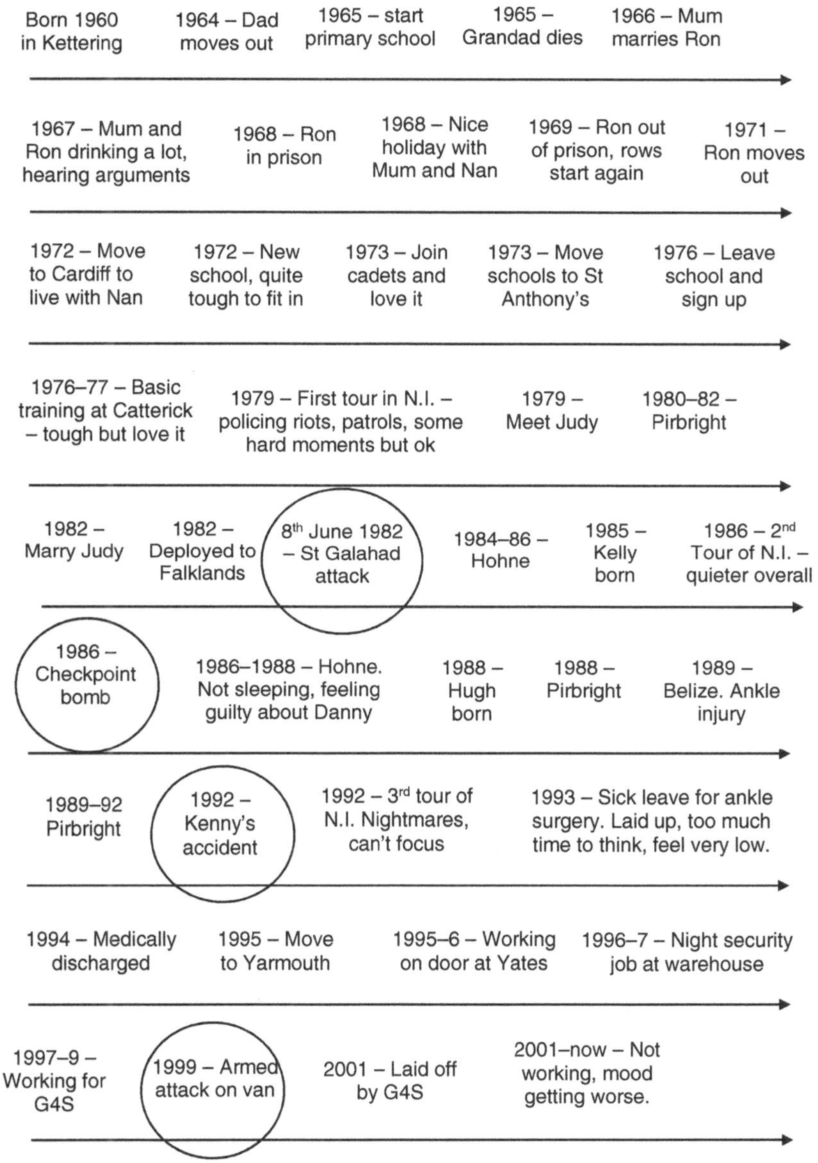

Figure 7.1 Example life timeline: Robert

PROS AND CONS OF WHERE TO START

Using timelines and intrusions diaries should identify the most problematic trauma memories. The next step is to decide which ones to work on in more detail. There are various options.

Starting with the worst

If possible, we encourage clients to start with the trauma memories which cause the most problems, as this should produce the most rapid symptom improvement, and hopefully instil

	1994 – 1999	2000	2001 – 2007
Living	Manchester, with mum, dad and Adam.	Taken into care.	Move back in with Mum.
Work/study		Start primary school	Primary school
Relationships	Close to Mum and Dad.	Miss family. Staff are kind.	Better with Mum, not seeing Dad.
Important events	Mum and Dad using drugs and fighting.	Moving into care. Court case over access.	Mum is clean, seems better. Like school.

Date	2007 – 2011	2011	2011 – 2013
Living	Sent to live with foster family.	Moved into a leaving care flat.	With Steve, at his flat.
Work/study	Start new secondary school.	At college.	Drop out of college.
Relationships	Not talking to family. Foster family are nice.	Start going out with Steve.	Only seeing Steve, losing friends.
Important events	Some bullying at new school. Start self-harming sometimes.	Treatment at CAMHS.	Steve getting more controlling, hits me sometimes.

Date	2013	2014	2014 – now
Living	With Steve	Move into hostel.	With Aunt Karen.
Work/study	Start at Boots, but lose job due to sick leave.	Not working.	Part-time at Karen's beauty salon.
Relationships	Fighting a lot with Steve. Isolated.	On/off with Steve. Back in touch with mum.	Not seeing Steve. Just seeing close family.
Important events	Steve pushes me down stairs and breaks my arm.	Hostel call Police when Steve breaks in. He is charged.	Steve given restraining order. Starting treatment.

Future plans:

Date	2020	2021 – onwards
Living	With Robbie	Get my own place
Work/study	Go back to college – marketing course	Get a job in marketing
Relationships	Build positive friendships	Consider a new (non-abusive) relationship
Important events	Do my PTSD treatment	Don't know yet!

Figure 7.2 Categorised life timeline: Jade

Date and time	Situation/trigger	What was the intrusion of?	How upsetting was the intrusion? (0–100)	How much did the memory feel like it was happening now? (0–100)

Figure 7.3 Example intrusions diary

	Monday	Tuesday	Wednesday	Thursday	Friday	Saturday	Sunday
St Galahad	✔✔	✔	✔✔	✔✔✔		✔✔	✔✔✔
Checkpoint	✔		✔✔		✔		
Kenny's accident		✔✔	✔	✔✔	✔	✔	✔
Van attack				✔			

Figure 7.4 Tick box intrusions diary for Robert

confidence in the rest of treatment. There is also a greater chance of a 'domino effect' of improvement whereby other memories become less intrusive as well.

Starting with the worst memories is preferential for a well-engaged, motivated client, who isn't having significant difficulty in talking about the memories, or therapeutic window issues, such as those described in Chapters 4 and 5.

Starting with a less distressing memory

If our client is unwilling to discuss their most distressing memories, engagement is poor, or we are concerned by an obstacle (e.g. dissociation, risk), another option is to start with less distressing memories. This has the advantage of providing an opportunity for the client to try out memory-focused techniques and hopefully experience success in reducing re-experiencing symptoms, which should build faith in the therapist and the therapy to tackle the most problematic memories.

The disadvantage of this approach is not targeting the heart of the problem, and therapeutic gains may be smaller than working on the most distressing memories. There is also a risk of colluding with avoidance. For therapists as well as clients, there can be an understandable temptation to avoid working on the most unpleasant memories, so we need to be sure that our reasons for choosing this option are sound.

Starting with 'easy win' memories

If we are concerned a client may drop out of treatment, we work first on 'easy win' memories if possible. We choose one which will hopefully update easily and quickly, providing our client with an experience of success. This can also be helpful where the client has strong negative beliefs about the consequences of memory work, for example, that they will become overwhelmed or risky; this can be set up as a behavioural experiment to test the feared consequence.

Memories that are quick to update usually have meanings that do not fit with pre-existing beliefs, and where key information has clearly not been integrated into the memories. For example, updating 'I'm going to die', with 'I didn't die, I survived' is much quicker and easier to add to trauma memories, than updating an appraisal like 'I deserved this because I am a worthless person', especially if this reflects a pre-existing core belief. In general, fear-based memories tend to resolve more easily than memories where the key emotions are shame, defeat, anger, or humiliation.

As above, we still prefer to target the most troubling memories first if possible, so only choose this option if there is a compelling reason to do so.

Start with the first

Another option is to approach the trauma history chronologically, starting with the earliest trauma to which the client has PTSD re-experiencing symptoms. This approach helps the client to build a coherent life narrative and to trace where certain beliefs originated. It also often helps clients appreciate the cumulative impact of the various traumatic events, and so normalise why they are struggling.

The risk of approaching a trauma history chronologically is running out of time to work on the most important traumas if they happened later in life, especially if we are working within limited session numbers. It can also be less efficient at decreasing symptoms quickly compared to working on the worst events first.

Choosing representative memories

Often a client will have experienced numerous traumas of the same type (for example, being tortured in a similar way repeatedly over some time, or assaulted numerous times by a partner). In these situations, it can be useful to choose 'representative' memories. This type of memory is a summary example, or representative simulation, of numerous experiences, that we construct together to include both the common features (e.g. how it tends to start) and key distressing thoughts, feelings, and sensations. The benefit of this approach is that it reduces the need for our client to describe every traumatic event in detail. If representative memories are effectively updated, it should mean that other memories which are very similar will also benefit. Working on representative memories can also be helpful when memories have become merged or unclear over time.

Maximising learning: the domino effect

When working with multiple trauma memories, we try to encourage generalisation of new learning from one set of trauma memories to others. In many cases, repeated trauma exposure is of a similar type (e.g. if someone has encountered traumas through their work, or through repeated abuse), which means that processing one set of trauma memories should help others to become contextualised as well. Even if traumatic events are not similar in concrete terms, the appraisals linked to them can be. For example, someone who is in an accident and feels helpless and trapped may be more likely to experience the same appraisals and emotions in a subsequent trauma, even if the events are unrelated.

After working on one set of memories, it is worth checking if re-experiencing of other memories has changed. This sometimes happens, probably due to updating of crossover meanings, changes to metacognitions, and a less avoidant coping style. If not, we encourage the 'domino effect' by identifying crossover meanings and prompting our clients to generalise their learning to other trauma memories.

Dalia was imprisoned and tortured due to her political activism in the Democratic Republic of Congo. After working on one of her trauma memories of being raped by a guard, her therapist encouraged her to consider what she had learnt in light of other trauma memories.

THERAPIST: It sounds like that memory has become a bit less intrusive now?
DALIA: Yes, it is different when I think of it. Not as real, not as clear.
T: That's really good. Are the feelings you have when you remember it any different?

D: Yes, I used to feel so dirty. Now I see that he was the dirty one. They were using it as a way to beat me down, you know, make me an animal. They wanted to silence me, but I know now I have a voice.
T: Good, that is a really important thing to remember. So, when we did your diaries, there were other memories that bother you a lot too, like the ones of being beaten?
D: Yes, they used to beat us with sticks and wire.
T: The way you felt when the guard raped you, dirty and like an animal, was that a similar feeling to the beatings or different?
D: The same really. Because they were doing the same thing, trying to make us feel small like we have no voice or power. Like animals.
T: That makes sense. So, do you think some of the things we have talked about with the rape memories, and some of the updates we did, might be relevant to the beatings memories too?
D: Yes, it's true. They wanted to silence me but I have a voice. They wanted to make me an animal, but I am still a woman. They are the ones who are animals.
T: Absolutely. So I wonder if it would help to do the same thing with the memories of the beatings as we did with the other memories. We could try bringing that same new information into the memory?
D: Yes, I think it would help.

Once one or two memories have been addressed and updated in session, clients are often able to follow the same process in between sessions with other memories. This should save session time, which can be used instead to review their trauma narratives, help with any tricky hotspot updates, and problem-solve unexpected obstacles.

Merged or very early memories

For some people, it is hard to isolate and prioritise trauma memories because they are very fragmented, lack any visual details, or have become coupled with other memories (where a fragment of memory triggers many others). Clients may also have 'fused' intrusions where, rather than being a recollection of a specific event, the perceptual and cognitive/emotional elements appear to relate to lots of similar events, and in this way are hard to pinpoint to a particular place and time. This is common in repeated and sustained 'captivity' traumas, and with very early memories because children's memory systems are not yet fully developed. For example, clients may have nightmares about someone being in their bed, or get a strong sense of fear when they experience certain physical sensations, but find it hard to link these intrusions to specific memories. This can make imaginal reliving or detailed narratives difficult to construct, and memories may be accessed only as a disjointed set of sensory memories without a clear context.

There are several options here. Where possible, we still seek to elaborate and contextualise the memories. If memories have become coupled, we make a timeline, to separate and articulate the memories individually. Where memories are very early or unclear, we try to access them through imaginal reliving and elaborate the narrative as much as possible. Some extra details may be accessible when the sensory memories are brought to mind and more complete, contextualised memories will be easier for the autobiographical memory system to store. For 'fused' memories which are difficult to separate, it is also possible to work on representative memories, to access the important meanings and update them. As already discussed, this should help to update other linked memories. Another option, where memories are difficult to separate and unclear, is to use imagery rescripting. The benefit of this approach is that full and clear memories are not needed;

if our clients only remember fragments, blurred details, or sensory memories, we can still create an imagined narrative. However, we still start the rescripting by helping our clients to access the emotions and meanings associated with the trauma, activating the parts of the memories they can recall, before making changes to the story.

To choose how to rescript the memories, we ask the client what they would like to change to feel different. The main goal is to meet the emotional needs the client had at the time. For example, if they felt scared and alone, the rescript should include a way for them to feel safe and cared for. How this is achieved is up to the client. For example, would they like someone (like a caregiver, superhero, the therapist) to come into the rescript to help them? Would they like a means of escape? Would they like to give themselves the ability to fight back or alter the outcome in some way? A popular rescript for childhood abuse is entering the scene as the adult self to stop the abuse, before comforting the child (Arntz, & Weertman, 1999). If the client struggles to think of ideas, we make suggestions for them to consider. Multiple rescripts can be tried to find the most helpful or to work through different layers of meaning and emotion.

Dalia rescripted a representative image of her torture memories. She had felt utterly helpless and defeated at the time, and felt angry now because she could never get justice. In the first rescript, she wanted to punish the guards by becoming enormously strong and battering them, so they knew how it felt to be hurt and humiliated. The rescripted image helped her feel powerful rather than helpless but made her uncomfortable as she was not a violent person. Her anger also persisted, alongside sadness at the inhumane conditions in her home country. In the second rescript, she instead imagined returning to the prison as a powerful angel, smashing through the walls, and freeing the political activists held there. Together they took the guards to the Hague and put them on trial, where she testified about what they did to her.

She imagined the guards being found guilty and then exiled to the desert, away from anyone they cared for, and unable to hurt anyone again. The first rescript helped reduce her feelings of powerlessness but did not fit with her values of non-aggression. The second version more effectively reduced both powerlessness and defeat, by enabling her to experience justice, and by restoring her sense of personhood through having her voice heard.

Top tips: Making an imagery rescript as effective as possible

We don't yet know how rescripting works, but there is emerging evidence that effective rescripts have the following features (Looney et al., 2021):

- *Believability*: This doesn't mean that the rescript is something that could have actually happened, and clients vary on whether they prefer fantastical imagery with magical powers, superheroes etc., or rescripts that are feasible in time and space. The important thing is that it feels emotionally believable and compelling.
- *Addresses the emotion in the memories*: Try to find rescripts that address the needs the client had at the time. If they felt dirty and contaminated, try rescripts to feel clean; if they felt scared, find a way to safety; if they felt helpless, give them power in the rescript. If there are multiple emotional needs, either introduce additional elements to your rescript or run multiple iterations for each need.

- *Vividness*: Try to ensure the rescripted memories are more strongly activated than the original memories by making the rescripted version as vivid and elaborated as possible.
- *Well-simulated*: Like directing a good movie, a good rescript flows logically, is detailed, and easy to imagine.
- *Matches the memory modality*: If you have highly sensory trauma memories, try to encourage a rescript that has lots of new perceptual information. If the client reports lots of cognitions in the memories, e.g. 'I keep thinking I am doing everything wrong', include more cognitive and verbal rescripts, like having someone there verbally reassuring them.
- *Consolidation*: New rescripts often need practice. We ask people to listen to recordings, write, draw, or make a collage of their rescript for homework.
- *Has a good balance of therapist guidance*: Clients may need help initially in activating a good rescript, but ideally become more autonomous as they progress.

Notes from the therapy room: Jon

Jon was in his early fifties when he came for treatment. He was a retired police officer with a long history of trauma. As a child, Jon was sexually abused by a priest over several years. The experience had left him with a strong drive to protect vulnerable people, which had been his primary motivation for joining the police. Jon worked for much of his career as an investigator of serious road accidents. As a result, he had attended numerous accidents, and seen many unpleasant sights.

Jon's PTSD was triggered when he was called to the scene of a suicide of one of his friends. He believed that if he had arrived sooner, he may have been able to save his friend's life. In the months that followed this incident, Jon began to experience nightmares where he was trying to save his friend but could not. He also began to re-experience scenes from the numerous accidents he had attended over the years, and occasionally of the childhood sexual abuse he had experienced. His formulation is in Figure 7.5.

Jon's therapist helped him construct a timeline of his experiences. The abuse memories were difficult to separate and articulate. Jon could remember the first incident fairly clearly, but subsequent abuse memories were confused and merged, and Jon could not remember dates or times. Similarly, his many road traffic accident memories were very difficult to separate or date. Jon recalled specific images of scenes but found it hard to put them in any order and there were lots of 'orphan' images that he couldn't match to a specific event.

Since the accident memories were the most frequent and distressing intrusions, Jon and his therapist agreed to work on these first. They chose an image that recurred frequently, of a partially clothed woman who had been thrown through a car windscreen. Jon identified his main feelings when re-experiencing this image were horror, helplessness, and guilt, linked to appraisals she had been dehumanised in this undignified state, and that he should have protected her from being seen and moved by strangers as they documented the scene for evidence. Reliving this moment, he recalled that her husband had arrived at the scene of the crash, but had been forcibly held back behind the police line. Jon was angry and upset at this and felt helpless to aid the man or his wife. He described an appraisal that he always arrived too late to help people and that he was like a 'vulture' who appeared after death.

Jon and his therapist discussed these appraisals. When Jon's therapist asked what his colleagues thought of the job that Jon did, he revealed that it was an unpopular role due to the constant exposure to death, bodies, and grieving families. Jon was respected amongst his colleagues for

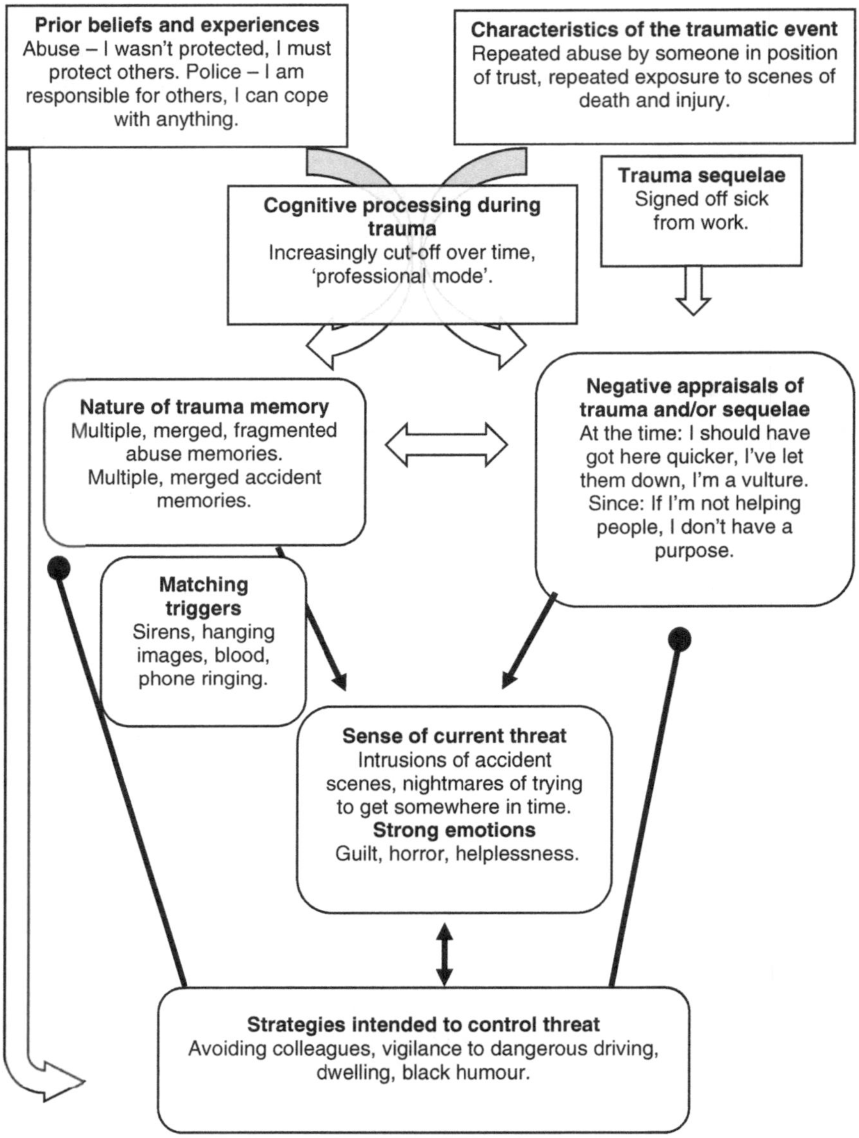

Figure 7.5 Jon's formulation

taking on such a role. When his therapist asked what was important to him about the job, Jon said that he wanted to ensure respect and dignity for those who had died, to protect their loved ones from finding their mutilated bodies, and to establish the causes of accidents to get justice and prevent future deaths. He used the phrase 'guardian of the dead'. Reviewing the evidence together, Jon agreed that this phrase better described his role than 'vulture'. He was able to acknowledge that it was a difficult job that he had done well.

Jon and his therapist rescripted the memories of the accident scene. He chose to clean and cover the woman's body, and remove her to a safe place, where she looked peaceful. He took her husband to a calmer environment, brought in his family to support him, and broke the news to him gently that his wife had passed away. He spent time with both of them and imagined the husband having the chance to say goodbye to his wife. He also imagined the scene of the accident now clean of any debris or blood, the road flowing normally again, with some flowers at the scene of the accident. The memories began to feel less painful to Jon, and he practised the imagery of the scene several times.

The therapist encouraged Jon to use a similar rescript every time that he experienced an intrusion to other accident scenes; 'cleaning' the scene, and protecting both the deceased and their loved ones from further pain. He also developed an image of himself receiving the support he needed for the difficult job he was doing, imagining speaking to a sympathetic colleague, and getting a hug from his wife. Gradually, the intrusions of accident scenes began to reduce.

Jon continued to feel guilty for not getting to his friend in time to prevent his suicide. However, when discussing the details of how his friend had died, Jon realised that he had carefully planned his suicide to make sure that he was not stopped. Jon concluded that his friend had wanted to die and that, even with his best efforts, no one could have saved him. Jon rescripted the scene of the trauma so that he calmly and carefully took care of his friend's body after finding it, and told him he was sorry for the pain he had been feeling.

Jon's therapist asked him if this new appraisal, that even with his best efforts he could not save everyone, was also relevant to his other traumas. Jon realised that he had felt guilty for not saving people who were in fatal accidents, even though he was only called to them afterwards. This need to save people stemmed from Jon's childhood experiences of abuse, and the desire to protect others from the pain he had felt. In an imagery rescript, he imagined entering one of his abuse memories, arresting the priest, and comforting his younger self.

Recommended reading

Stallworthy, P. (2009). Cognitive therapy for people with post-traumatic stress disorder to multiple events: Working out where to start. In N. Grey (Ed.). *A casebook of cognitive therapy for traumatic stress reactions* (pp. 194–212). Routledge.

Wheatley, J., & Hackmann, A. (2011). Using imagery rescripting to treat major depression: Theory and practice. *Cognitive and Behavioral Practice*, 18(4), 444–453.

CHAPTER EIGHT

Gaps in trauma memories

Eddie was assaulted by a gang in an apparent case of mistaken identity. He lost consciousness several times and, as a result, his memory for the assault was patchy, disjointed, and confused. He was frustrated that he couldn't remember more clearly. In therapy, he mapped the gaps in his memories to create a more coherent narrative. This also helped him to organise, 'join up', and process his fragmented intrusive recollections.

Many people with PTSD do not have a clear, coherent recall of their traumatic experiences. Memories can contain gaps, or be blurred, disorganised, and hazy. In some cases, very little of the trauma can be recalled, with fragmentary details only accessible when re-experienced in intrusions. Others may have brief intermittent periods of recall, like 'islands' of memory, alongside constructed images of what they think or fear happened.

Some clients have concerns about having memory gaps, for example, that it means they are brain-damaged or that something terrible happened during a gap that they cannot, or do not want to, recall. Gaps in trauma memories can impede some techniques, such as imaginal reliving. In this chapter, we consider how to use CT-PTSD with incomplete trauma memories.

WHAT CAUSES GAPS IN THE MEMORY?

There are various causes for memory gaps, usually affecting the encoding and storage of memories, or their subsequent recall. It can be helpful to try and work out the likely cause (or combination of causes), if it isn't immediately obvious, as it can help you decide what to do, and provides a normalising explanation for your client. Here are some common causes.

DRUGS AND/OR ALCOHOL

If someone is intoxicated at the time of the trauma (either voluntarily, through medication, or where the perpetrator has drugged them), this can affect memories. Different substances affect, in different ways, both the quality of the memory and the person's experience and behaviour when intoxicated. Often some visual memories will be intact, but images may be blurred or confused. For some people, the loss of explicit memory might be total, or there is only 'affect without recollection' reflecting implicit or somatic memories triggered by reminders. For example, people who have been drugged with substances like GHB or Rohypnol (usually to facilitate rape or robbery) may experience periods of total loss of awareness, as well as patchy, hazy memories, including of being physically paralysed (Gauntlett-Gilbert et al., 2004).

DOI: 10.4324/9781003288329-10

LOSS OF CONSCIOUSNESS

Traumas that involve physical injuries, particularly to the head, can lead to loss of consciousness peri-traumatically, which will naturally lead to memory gaps. Memories may exist for the moments before loss of consciousness and may be fragmentary or fleeting, such as a flash of something looming towards their head. People may drift in and out of consciousness during the trauma, leading to partial and disjointed memories. Traumatic brain injuries can also cause both retrograde and anterograde amnesia, including for periods where the person appeared awake and responsive at the time.

DISSOCIATION

If someone dissociates at the time of the trauma, they may not recall all of what happened. Memories may lack certain details or be distorted in perspective. For example, where someone has experienced an 'out of body' state during a trauma, they may have visual recollections recalled from an observer perspective, and may not be able to access sensory details like how their body felt.

In other cases, the trauma memories have been encoded and stored, but clients struggle to access them intentionally because they dissociate when the memory is triggered, or when certain hotspots are accessed. In these cases, the full memory is often present and recoverable, but memory work should be approached carefully, using the strategies described in Chapter 6. There can also be a complex interplay between the person dissociating when they recall the trauma and also vividly re-experiencing dissociation from during the trauma.

NORMAL FORGETTING

Forgetting and inaccuracies are normal features of memory, and people with PTSD sometimes overestimate how much they 'should' be able to remember about the trauma (Kopelman, 2002). There is some evidence that people with PTSD may struggle generally with recalling details of autobiographical memories (McNally et al., 1994). Additionally, there is evidence that trauma memories tend to be quite accurate as regards central details, but less so for peripheral details (Christianson, & Safer, 1996). This may lead to some gaps or inconsistencies in recalling certain details. It is also common for events leading up to a trauma to be forgotten, as at the time they would not have been significant and therefore were not stored in longer-term memory. Commonly this can include what the person did in the hours or days before, which may only feel important in hindsight, and in trying to work out how the trauma happened.

EARLY LIFE MEMORIES

Traumas that occurred early in life may not be recalled in the same way as memories from adulthood. Under the age of two years, most events are not stored as explicit verbal memories; although there is evidence that behavioural, or implicit ways of remembering start at a very young age (Cordon et al., 2004). Childhood memories may be blurry or fragmented, although no less disturbing for their lack of clarity. They may also consist of apparently unremarkable snapshots, but accompanied by a strong sense of something being wrong. Sometimes very clear memories exist, but lack context in terms of age or location. The sense children make of their traumatic experiences, and hence the qualities of their later recall, is affected by the child's age, gender, developmental stage, and their interactions with caregivers (Salmon, & Bryant, 2002).

Beliefs about gaps

Clients may have distressing beliefs about memory gaps, such as fears about what happened, or that gaps are a sign of brain damage, madness, repression, or unreliability. Beliefs about memories have been found to be more important in the maintenance of PTSD than the organisation of the trauma memories themselves (Bennett, & Wells, 2010), so addressing these beliefs can often relieve PTSD symptoms by reducing the centrality of meaning of the trauma and the behaviours such as rumination and avoidance which maintain PTSD.

Therefore, it is important to discuss with your client any concerns they have about the memory gaps and to address these before working on the trauma memories. Psychoeducation about the causes of memory gaps, such as the effects of certain drugs, injuries, or developmental stages, can help normalise gaps. Fears about what happened during the gaps, including imagined scenarios, can be gently explored and potential explanations and corroborative evidence considered. Many people assume something terrible happened during a memory gap. This is not usually the case, but there may be upsetting details which the client has not recalled, so the therapist should explore with their client the costs and benefits of learning more about what happened during memory gaps (see 'top tips' box).

Angelique had fragmented memories of her childhood, which had been characterised by physical and emotional abuse by her mother. There were various events that her sister remembered, which Angelique had no recollection of, including a time when they were both punished by being shut in a woodshed overnight. Angelique was concerned that she could not remember these events, and believed it was a sign that her brain was permanently damaged by the abuse, and that her memory system was unreliable.

Angelique's therapist helped her to consider different explanations for her memory gaps. They looked at information together about how memory worked, for example, that our brains do not record events precisely, like a video recorder, but are affected by lots of different factors, including age, our mood, and the meaning of the event. Angelique realised that there were events from childhood that she remembered and her sister did not, and others they did not agree about, suggesting that neither of them had a 100% accurate memory. Angelique's therapist also gave her information about dissociation, and Angelique recognised that this was something she had done ever since childhood, which might have affected her memories.

Angelique and her therapist also tested out whether her memory system was working currently, by checking recent examples. Although Angelique did not feel her memory system was perfect, she realised that her job at a nursery required her to remember many things, like the names of children and parents, food preferences and allergies, and the words of nursery rhymes and songs, all of which she remembered perfectly.

Hot cognitions

- Not being able to remember means I am repressing something awful/my brain is permanently damaged
- If I think or dwell on the memory long enough I will work out/remember what happened
- I am gullible for trusting the person who drugged me and for not watching my drink
- I am to blame/others blame me for becoming intoxicated
- If I can't remember everything I cannot recover from PTSD
- The gaps mean I can't be sure/others won't believe it happened

Memory work with gaps

Even without a clear or complete memory, it is possible to use many of the usual strategies for processing trauma memories, including timelines, imaginal reliving, hotspot updating, and stimulus discrimination. These techniques may need adaptation, depending on how much of the memory can be recalled.

MAP THE GAPS

First, we 'map the gaps' using a timeline or a written narrative of the trauma. The aim is to write out the details that your client can recall and identify the gaps or unclear memories. On timelines, we often draw a zig-zag to represent an unknown length of time, although the actual duration can sometimes be approximated.

Using 'map the gaps' helps organise memories that are fragmented or confused and to begin arranging them in order. On a practical note, we recommend using a whiteboard for a timeline, or an electronic document for a written narrative, to allow changes and details to be added. Figure 8.1 shows a timeline for Sam, mapping his recollections of a drug-facilitated rape, with the memory gaps marked.

FILL THE GAPS

The next step is to try and create as complete and coherent a narrative as possible for what happened. Fragmented, blurry memories are hard for our brains to make sense of. A more complete memory, even an unpleasant one, should be easier to process than a patchy and disjointed one, which should help reduce re-experiencing symptoms. However, before you start trying to fill the gaps, read the 'top tip' box below.

> **Top tips: Discuss whether your client wants to fill the gaps**
>
> A common fear about memory gaps is that something even more distressing occurred that hasn't been remembered. This is rarely the case but, occasionally, we do discover new, very upsetting information about the trauma when we work on the memories. This is especially likely if the reason for the gap is dissociation as, when this protective layer is peeled away (remember the onion on page 68!), further details may be recalled. Therefore, we need to have a conversation with our client about this possibility and check how they feel about potentially learning something new.
>
> Our clients often tell us that they want to know what happened, even if it is bad. This fits with our model of PTSD; we need to work through the meanings associated with a trauma, whatever they are, as continuing to avoid the memory and its implications maintains the problematic symptoms. However, we need to make sure that our clients feel safe and in control of the process of filling memory gaps, so we talk through the potential benefits and costs of the decision carefully. We also make a plan for how to manage if something upsetting does emerge.

If you have agreed that filling the gaps is likely to be helpful, start doing some 'detective work' to help your client figure out what really happened. This may produce several possibilities, which you and your client can then discuss, evaluate, and potentially test out. Here are some options.

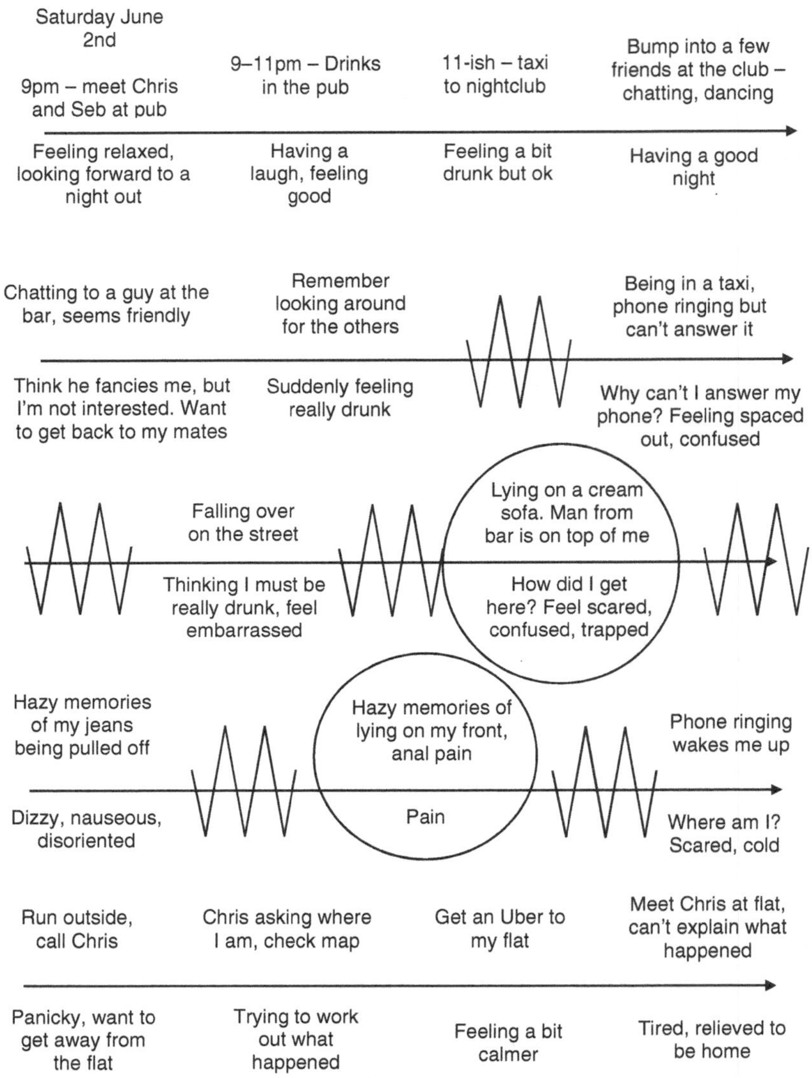

Figure 8.1 Sam's timeline

Imaginal reliving

Sometimes, more of the memories can be accessed through imaginal reliving. This is especially true when the cause of memory gaps is dissociation. Where someone has lost consciousness or been drugged, imaginal reliving will not lead to a full recovery of the memories, but some further details from before and after consciousness is lost may be accessed, which help make sense of the parts that are missing.

Revisit the scene of the trauma

Revisiting the scene of the trauma can often help fill memory gaps. The multiple strong cues present in the actual environment where the trauma occurred will potentially trigger parts of the memories that are difficult to access. We sometimes draw the analogy with clients of when the police use crime reconstructions to help jog the memory of witnesses. Where revisiting the scene of the trauma is not physically possible, using online resources such as Google Street View or looking at photographs of the location can help provide contextual details to access more of the memory.

Revisiting the scene of the trauma can also help to gather information to work out what probably happened, even if the memory cannot be accessed. For example, 'walking through' what is recalled of the trauma often provides information about the most likely locations or sequence of events and may reveal clues about how it happened.

Spatial maps

A similar way of mapping the trauma is to construct a spatial map of the trauma scene. This can be done by sketching the layout of the site as viewed from above and using 'bird's eye view reliving' to 'play out' what is remembered/known about events. You can also use pre-existing resources such as maps and police scene drawings. As with site visits, this may trigger recall of missing parts of the memories, or help work out the most likely sequence of events.

Other accounts of the trauma

Information about gaps can also be gathered from other sources. For example, other people who were present may be able to provide missing details. The client may have access to police witness statements or have known people who were there. Information may be available from elsewhere such as CCTV footage, media reports, and investigations. There may be discrepancies between different sources, and also with the client's recollections, so it is helpful to orient your client first to this possibility. You can give your client psychoeducation about the well-known problems with eye-witness evidence, to help them balance inconsistent accounts. Where the issue of difference is crucial to a key meaning, it is important to help your client weigh up both possibilities, and also what it means that they may never know for sure.

Logic

Where no additional information is available and your attempts to recall the missing parts of the memory are exhausted, we can use logic to consider the most likely course of events.

> Amal nearly drowned when he had an epileptic seizure while swimming in the sea. He remembered waking on the beach, having been rescued by another swimmer, and seeing the worried faces of his family but had no memory of the seizure or the rescue. This distressed Amal as he was worried about swimming again. As Amal wasn't able to trace the other swimmer, he couldn't get another account of the rescue, so he used detective work and logic to work out what happened. His family showed him the spot on the beach where he was pulled ashore so Amal could work out roughly where he had been swimming when he had the seizure. He had been wearing a smartwatch, so could see how long he had been swimming and when he had the seizure. He spoke to a lifeguard on the beach who told him that other swimmers that day had struggled with a strong current, which explained why Amal might have had a seizure, as they were usually triggered by stress. Reconstructing the trauma helped fill in some gaps in Amal's account of the trauma, although he was unable to recall the rest of the memories. It also reassured him that it was a very unusual event and likely safe for him to start swimming again in a pool.

Contextualise hazy and/or dissociated memories

If memories are vague, or lack some perceptual information (particularly a visual code), filling in more contextual details can make the memory feel more complete, and make it easier to process. For example, adding details about what most likely happened and any factual information such as the place, time, date, and presence of other people, can help hazy memories feel more concrete and understandable. Similarly, if the client dissociated during the trauma and can recall some aspects of the memory but not others, try filling in the gaps in the different levels of representation. For example, if physiological details are recalled, but not contextual or visual information, these can be added, and vice versa.

Top tips: Be careful of suggesting memories

As we'll discuss in Chapter 9, it is possible to inadvertently suggest false memories to our clients. So, when we are trying to help them understand a confusing part of the trauma, we need to avoid asking leading questions, making too many suggestions, or otherwise overtly influencing the content of memories. Instead, make it clear that further memories may or may not be recalled, and use the 'fill the gaps' techniques to try to activate existing memories, or to create evidence-based assessments (simulations) of probable scenarios. We avoid trying to fill the gaps for apparently new 'recovered' memories (Chapter 9) – it's better to let these emerge naturally.

Sometimes the problem is not that your client can't remember, but that they cannot put words to their experiences, or have fears around disclosing them. It is important therefore to check with them the 'quality' of the gaps – sometimes clients tell us that they can't or won't say what they recall. Again, be very cautious about 'fishing' or guessing in these circumstances, not least because, if you get it right, your client may become overwhelmed. Instead, try to support their natural process – like a midwife!

COMPLETE THE TIMELINE OR NARRATIVE

If additional information about memory gaps has emerged, this can be added to the timeline or written narrative in a different colour. You can also add levels of certainty into the timeline in this way: memories your client is sure happened, that others report seeing, that they recall only in intrusions or in nightmares, 'best guesses', 'worst case' constructed images, and also 'true' gaps. This allows your client to see and hold the trauma narrative in working memory in as complete a format as possible while maintaining a critical and accepting position to ambiguities and distressing intrusions. Reading it through in session or as homework and adding in further details can be useful exercises. It also helps open up a conversation about gaps that have not been filled and provides a 'scaffolding' structure for subsequent imaginal reliving.

RELIVE WHAT YOU CAN

If there are few gaps, we relive the whole trauma narrative, 'fast-forwarding' through the gaps.

Kevin was knocked off his bike while cycling home from work, and lost consciousness several times during the trauma. Here is an extract of part of a reliving session:

THERAPIST: Ok, so close your eyes and take yourself back in your mind's eye to that day. You've just left work and you're cycling along the main road. What can you see?

KEVIN: I'm on the main road. It's rush hour, it's quite busy, lots of cars and bikes.
T: How are you feeling in that moment?
K: A bit stressed with all the traffic. Hot, it's a hot day.
T: You're doing really well. What happens next?
K: I'm coming down to the junction with Morden Road and I hear a siren behind me.
T: What is going through your mind?
K: Just to stop, pull over. But before I can, this van suddenly pulls into the cycle lane. It's a split second I see it moving and I can't do anything about it.
T: How do you feel in that split second?
K: Scared. I know it's going to hit me. Then I'm in the air and then it's blank.
T: You are doing really well. How does that feel as you are in the air?
K: Horrible, out of control. It's going to hurt.
T: Do you remember landing?
K: No, nothing.
T: Ok, so just fast-forward the memory now. What is the next thing you remember?
K: Someone is crouched next to me, talking to me. I can hear voices. Someone says, 'don't move him'.
T: What can you see?
K: Nothing, just black.
T: Can you feel anything in your body?
K: I'm lying on my side. I can feel the hard pavement. There's pain in my shoulder and my head. I can't feel my legs.
T: Can you remember anything else in that moment?
K: No. It goes black again.
T: Ok, so fast forward again. What's the next thing you remember?

We can then add information to fill the gaps as part of reliving, shown here in a later session with Kevin.

K: I'm lifted up into the air. I feel scared and out of control. I know it's going to hurt when I land. Then it's just a blank.
T: What do we know now about that gap in your memory?
K: I was knocked out when I hit the pavement, probably for about 10 minutes. I must've landed on my elbow as it was broken. A pedestrian tried to help me and called an ambulance. The van stopped and so did the car behind. The van driver said I was in his blind spot. They waited with me until the ambulance came. Apparently I was moaning and they decided not to move me in case I had broken something.
T: Ok, good. What is the next thing you remember?

As well as adding in conceptual information (what they know now about the gap) you can also 'perceptually' reconstruct gaps in imagery. Some people will do this naturally if they have a powerful imagination. Kevin, for example, could be prompted to imagine (from a field perspective) the people around him, reassuring and protecting him while he is hurt, and update the gap with the meaning 'I can't remember, but people were there protecting me, I wasn't alone'.

Be aware that some gaps may become much more upsetting if you encourage your client to visualise what they know or suspect. You should discuss in advance the pros and cons of creating this more complete, albeit constructed, memory, and be ready to also bring in updates or rescripts of those new distressing images. For example, creating a perceptual reconstruction of what most likely occurred can be beneficial if it was positive (e.g. being rescued), or what the client is currently imagining is much worse. One option is to view more upsetting perceptual reconstructions from an observer perspective (e.g. bird's eye view) or 'fast-forward' through them to a safer point in the memory.

If there are many gaps and the memory is too fragmented to attempt to relive the whole event, an alternative option is just to relive the parts of the memory which are re-experienced, even if they are momentary. Elaborating even small fragments of memory with their key feelings, sensations, and meanings, then bringing in updated information (across multiple levels) can still help reduce re-experiencing symptoms for these moments.

FAQ: What if there is no memory to relive?

Occasionally, clients report PTSD symptoms while having no recollection at all of the trauma. This is rare because, to meet criteria for PTSD, they must be re-experiencing the trauma, so these symptoms need to be carefully assessed if someone reports no memory of the trauma. However, some people have nightmares about the moments before or after the trauma, or with thematically linked content, even if they do not recall what happened. Others will display physical and/or emotional reactivity alongside avoidance and vigilance to reminders of the event (it must be possible to specifically link the reminders and behaviours to the trauma to meet PTSD criteria), even without conscious recollection of it (McNeil, 1996).

Any re-experienced parts of the trauma, however fragmentary, can be elaborated, relived, and updated as we've described in this chapter. You can also work with representative or symbolic images that sum up the trauma and activate the key emotions and meanings. If the only re-experiencing symptoms reported are emotional or physiological reactivity to triggers, focus on identifying triggers and using imaginal/in vivo exposure and stimulus discrimination procedures to reduce reactivity. You can supercharge this by working with multiple triggers at the same time and across different contexts – so-called 'deepened extinction' (Craske et al., 2014). Additionally, problematic 'added meanings' associated with the trauma and threatening expectancies associated with encountering triggers can be addressed. Imagery rescripting can also be used to introduce new meanings and endings into thematic nightmares.

Lucia had no conscious recollection of an accident when she was seriously hurt after falling from a theme park ride. She developed strong physiological reactions in the form of shaking, pain in her legs and back, and nausea, intense distress when confronted with reminders of the accident, as well as nightmares about falling. With her therapist, Lucia worked on stimulus discrimination of her various triggers, such as watching rollercoaster rides on the internet, visiting high places, jumping on a trampoline, and ultimately visiting a theme park. They also used imagery rescripting on her nightmares of falling, changing the ending so that Lucia landed safely on a giant marshmallow, bouncing softly until she sank gently into it, then lying comfortably on her back, nibbling on little bits of marshmallow.

BRING IN NEW MEANINGS

As usual, after elaborating memories, we introduce new meanings to update problematic appraisals during imaginal reliving and through imagery rescripting.

Updating

The usual updating process can be followed. If a memory is very fragmented with long gaps, it may be easier to update one hotspot at a time rather than relive and update the whole memory.

After imaginal reliving and elaboration of the memory, Kevin continued to have intrusions of one moment in the trauma; the feeling of flying through the air. It was often triggered when he walked on a slippery surface and was associated with the belief that he would land painfully and seriously injure himself. After discussing new information about this belief, he updated the hotspot during reliving:

THERAPIST: Can you bring that moment to mind?
KEVIN: Yes.
T: What's happening?
K: He's hit me and I'm flying. It feels like the longest time I'm in the air. It feels horrible – I'm totally out of control and I know when I land it's going to really hurt.
T: What's the worst thing about that for you?
K: Anticipating the pain, knowing it's coming and not being able to stop it.
T: What do we know now about that moment?
K: It was probably only a second I was in the air, it just felt longer. I'm okay now. I broke my arm and I was briefly knocked out but I wasn't seriously hurt, my arm's fine now and I wasn't brain damaged.
T: Can you move around to show yourself that your body is fine now? Maybe touch your arm and your head and show yourself they aren't injured anymore. That's really good. How does it feel?
K: It feels okay. My arm is a bit tender but I can move it, it isn't broken.
T: Good. What do we know now about the pain when you land?
K: I don't actually remember the pain. I must have blacked out at that point.
T: Okay, so hold that moment in your mind, of flying through the air and anticipating the pain, and bring in that new information. There's no pain coming, you aren't going to feel it. How is that?
K: Strange, but it's good. There's no pain coming. I land, but I don't feel it. My arm hurts later on, and by then the paramedics are there to help me.
T: Now, hold on to that memory of flying through the air – can you jump up and down a few times? What do you notice?
K: I feel like I'm going to fall.
T: That's okay, you're doing great. Keep jumping, hop from one foot to the other, while you keep the memory of flying in your mind, like a short loop of video. How safely are you landing now?
K: I'm landing safely! I can feel the ground is solid.
T: Well done! How true does it feel now that your footing is sure?
K: Yes, I can feel it, my feet are landing flat, even as I'm remembering them being up in the air.

Imagery rescripting

Another way to introduce new meanings is via imagery rescripting. This can be especially useful when the memory is unclear, or when most of it is missing and therefore difficult to relive and update. Remember that imagery rescripting can be used in many different ways, and you can explore different options with your client. For example, bringing the adult self into childhood memories, changing the way a trauma memory ends, or enabling the client to do something that they wanted to do at the time but couldn't. Imagery rescripting can also be used to fill memory gaps in whatever way the client chooses.

Maura was held hostage by her neighbour during a psychotic episode where he believed Maura was the devil. He beat her badly and Maura lost consciousness. At the time, Maura thought she was going to die, and lacked any memories of being rescued, which seemed to contribute to her continued sense of unsafety. To bring in the meaning 'I was rescued and taken to a place of safety', Maura chose to imagine the memories she couldn't remember – the police breaking down the door of the flat, arresting her neighbour, and taking her to hospital. Her therapist encouraged her to focus on how it would have felt to be safe with the police and looked after by her husband, who came to the hospital. They also 'fast-forwarded' to a recent memory of Maura and her husband safe at home with their dog, and her neighbour receiving treatment in a secure psychiatric facility. The meaning of this new image was 'I'm safe now, my neighbour can't hurt me again. I am surrounded by love'.

Notes from the therapy room: Eddie

Eddie was assaulted by a gang in an apparent case of mistaken identity. He was dragged into a park, where he was beaten with baseball bats and stabbed. His memories of the assault were confused and contained gaps. His formulation is in Figure 8.2.

Eddie was bothered by the memory gaps as he believed that, if his memories were clearer, he could identify the men who assaulted him (who were never caught or charged) for the police and get justice for the attack. As the memory gaps were most likely caused by blows to the head, Eddie's therapist asked him how he would feel if the memories were never recovered. Eddie answered that he would accept this, as long he knew that he had done everything possible to try.

Eddie and his therapist wrote a narrative of the trauma to map the gaps, get the events in order, and identify any hotspots. Eddie took the narrative home to read himself a few times and add any further details he remembered. In the next session, he relived the trauma with his therapist, fast-forwarding through the memory gaps. This revealed some more sensory details, for example, Eddie remembered the smell of the earth as he lay on the ground.

Using Google Maps, Eddie and his therapist located where the attack took place. They returned to the park and re-traced Eddie's route on the night of his trauma, looking for further clues about what had happened during the memory gaps. The visit helped make sense of some fragments of memory that Eddie hadn't understood, including patterns of light and dark that seemed to have been caused by light from a nearby streetlamp coming through the trees above where Eddie was lying. This also helped explain why Eddie felt anxious since the assault when playing video games with flickering lights, and he was able to use stimulus discrimination to start to enjoy these again.

Eddie still couldn't access a clear image of his attackers' faces. On discussion, Eddie realised that it was probably because it had been dark, and his attackers had their hoods pulled on. He also realised that his attention had been on the baseball bats they were using. His therapist confirmed that 'weapon focus' was something psychologists had found in trauma research, and that it represented an adaptive survival strategy. Given that Eddie was 'blitz attacked' so suddenly, was out-numbered, and received many blows to the head, it made sense that he hadn't been able to get a good look at his attackers' faces. Eddie accepted this was the most logical explanation and that he would likely never be able to identify them. He also reasoned that, if they were in the habit of carrying weapons and attacking strangers, they would probably be caught eventually or would end up the victims of an assault themselves; this fitted with his pre-trauma view of the world as fair and that 'what goes around comes around'.

Eddie and his therapist added the information about what happened during the memory gaps to the written narrative in italics:

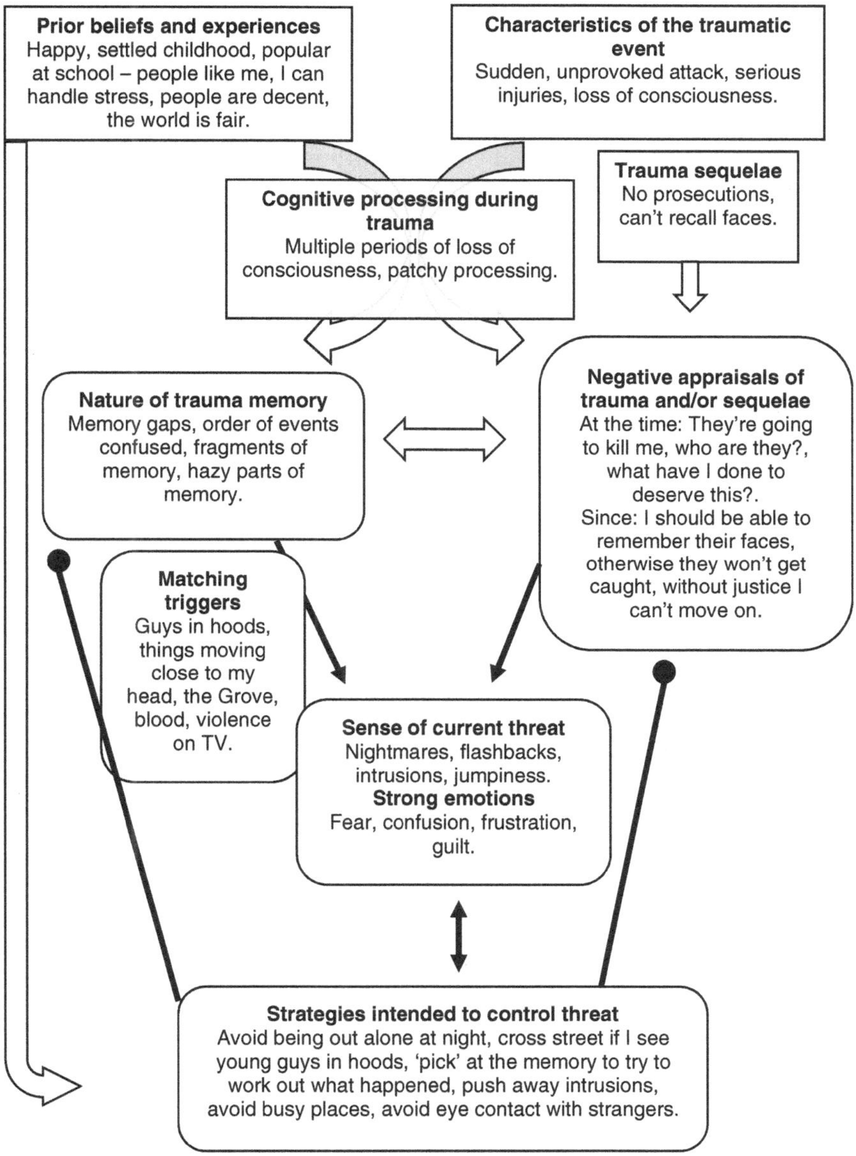

Figure 8.2 Eddie's formulation

'I'm on the train after a late shift. I'm feeling tired and want to get home and sleep. There's a guy on the train who keeps looking at me. I don't know him but I feel like he wants trouble. He keeps chatting on his phone and staring at me. I feel uneasy. I get off at Carshalton and start walking home. When I come past the pub on the corner, there are about six guys with hoods. At least two of them are holding bats. They grab me and start hitting me and then I'm on the floor. They drag me into The Grove. I'm so shocked, I've no idea what's going on – are they mugging me? But they don't ask for anything, they're just kicking and punching me. I see a boot coming at my face and then pain and then it's black. *I know now that I probably lost consciousness when I was kicked in the head. During the time I was unconscious, they must have dragged me from the bit of The Grove by the pub deeper into the park, to the area by the stream, probably because it was further from the road so they were less likely to be seen.*

I wake up to a guy shouting in my face something about "this is for Kenny" or "Kemi". I think "they're going to kill me" and I'm scared and sad that this is the way my life is ending, in the woods with some nutters. I must've blacked out again because I don't remember after that. I remember weird patterns of light above me, some shouting and laughing, and the smell of weed. *I know now that I most likely lost consciousness again, probably because of the blows to the head. My memory is quite confused – this is normal when someone has a head injury. I was probably in and out of consciousness. They seemed to be hanging around near me, talking and laughing, and smoking weed. The patterns of light were probably from the streetlight coming through the trees. I know that at some point I was stabbed twice in the stomach, although I don't remember it. They probably intended to kill me, thinking I was someone else, perhaps from a rival gang, but I survived.*

The next thing I remember I'm on my own. My stomach is wet and I realise it's blood. I think "I'm badly hurt, I can't move, I'm going to die here on my own". I feel really lonely and panicky. I manage to get my phone out of my pocket and I dial 999. I can hear the call operator but I can't speak, there's just weird gurgly noises coming out. I drag myself back to the main road. It's really painful and feels like I'm going to pass out. There's a lady on the road but she looks scared and walks away. I feel totally abandoned, and I'm sure I'm going to die. *I know now that I didn't die. I'm alive. The lady was scared but someone else helped me soon after.*

I see someone else walking down the road. I manage to put the phone on speaker and I hold it out to him. I'm lying on my front and I see blood spreading around me. That's the last thing I remember until I wake up in hospital and my mum is there and tells me I've had an operation but I'm going to be alright. *I know now that I passed out, probably because I had lost a lot of blood. I did the right thing by giving my phone to the man. He spoke to the 999 operator and got an ambulance. He used his jumper to try and stem the bleeding from my stomach and saved my life. They took me to hospital and I had emergency surgery. I survived to tell the tale.'*

After reliving the trauma with the information about the memory gaps included, Eddie found that he was getting fewer intrusive memories and nightmares. Several hotspots remained, including the moments when he believed he was going to die. He and his therapist added updates into the trauma memories before reliving it again.

Eddie continued to be very jumpy if something moved close to his head. This seemed to be linked to hotspots in the memories where he was kicked and struck around the head. They practised in session by first Eddie, and then his therapist, moving their hands near Eddie's head while using stimulus discrimination. Eddie also practised in real-life situations, including going to the barber.

The remaining therapy sessions included working on beliefs related to safety and addressing remaining triggers, such as going to the park, asking directions from men with their hoods up, and walking the streets at night.

Recommended reading

Ehlers, A. (2010). Understanding and treating unwanted trauma memories in posttraumatic stress disorder. *Zeitschrift für Psychologie/Journal of Psychology*, 218(2), 141–145.

Gauntlett-Gilbert, J., Keegan, A., & Petrak, J. (2004). Drug-facilitated sexual assault: Cognitive approaches to treating the trauma. *Behavioural and Cognitive Psychotherapy*, 32(2), 215–223.

CHAPTER NINE

Recovered memories

Sue became increasingly aware of 'recovered' memories of childhood abuse while she was receiving treatment for PTSD after a terrorist attack. Her therapist needed to formulate the role of both traumatic experiences and address Sue's symptoms of PTSD, without inadvertently influencing the emerging childhood trauma memories.

Memories of traumatic events can be forgotten and subsequently remembered, or 'recovered', later in life, often triggered by a particular event or reminder, and sometimes during therapy. Controversy has surrounded the accuracy of recovered memories, and the possibility for false memories to be recalled, with therapists sometimes blamed for inadvertently implanting or influencing memories of trauma. Understandably, these issues make clinicians cautious about working with recovered memories in therapy, raising the risk that PTSD symptoms are not addressed with evidence-based approaches.

Recovered memories can raise other issues in therapy, such as clients' concerns about what they do and don't remember, the impact of new memories on their relationships, and potential safeguarding and legal issues. In this chapter, we'll discuss these various issues and give some guidance on working with recovered memories.

THE RECOVERED MEMORY DEBATE

Freud first wrote about the concept of repression as a defence mechanism where, effortfully or otherwise, people banish trauma memories from their conscious awareness to protect themselves from overwhelming distress; but then experience them 'leaking through' in apparently unrelated emotional and behavioural problems. This idea underpinned forms of therapy aimed at retrieving the repressed memories thought to be the source of their psychological difficulties, such as through hypnosis, regression techniques, and drugs like sodium amytal; techniques which are now largely discredited. Concerns about this type of unsafe practice surfaced in some high-profile court cases, including one where the father of a patient successfully sued a therapist for implanting false memories of abuse (*Ramona vs. Isabella*; Mullins, 1996).

Adding to concerns was the publication of ground-breaking research into the fallibility and malleability of memories. Elizabeth Loftus famously showed that it was possible to implant false memories in lab studies (Loftus, & Pickrell, 1995) and argued that at least some recovered memories are probably false (Loftus, 1993). She, and others, raised concerns about self-help guides, particularly *The Courage to Heal: A guide for women survivors of child sexual abuse* (Bass, & Davis, 2002), which stated that if readers 'have a feeling that something abusive happened to you, it probably did' (p. 21); as well as survivors' groups and therapists who hold assumptions about the likelihood of abuse, even when a client does not recall it (Loftus, 1993).

DOI: 10.4324/9781003288329-11

Recovered memories have been a topic of intense and emotive debate over the years, and unanswered questions remain. Here is a brief overview of some of the key findings:

- Recovered memories, especially of childhood sexual abuse, appear to be quite common: A significant proportion of trauma survivors report periods of time when they have not remembered the trauma; around 16% in one study (Williams, 1995).
- Most childhood memories of trauma are accurate: Children over the age of two at the time of the trauma can recall accurate (although sometimes fragmentary) details later on (Terr, 1988) and, when researchers have sought corroboration for recovered memories of sexual abuse, it has been possible to verify the accounts in most or all cases (Coons, 1994).
- Memory is also subject to error and manipulation: Memories, including those of trauma, are often recalled differently over time (Southwick et al., 1997) and can be influenced by misinformation or suggestive questions (Weingardt et al., 1995).
- It is possible to implant false memories in some people, under certain conditions: Laboratory studies, such as Loftus's classic 'lost in the mall' paradigm (Loftus, & Pickrell, 1995), have shown it is possible to convince people that they remember events that did not happen. These studies may raise fears that therapists could implant false memories in their clients, although the therapy context is arguably quite different to these experimental conditions since therapists are unlikely to deliberately mislead their clients and trauma memories are presumably more salient.
- False memories are indistinguishable from real memories by content or quality: McNally et al. (2004) found that highly unlikely memories (of alien abduction) led to similar physiological states in clients with PTSD to verifiable traumatic experiences. It appears that 'false' memories can feel as real as 'true' memories.

Current guidelines

So where does this leave clinicians working with recovered memories? Several organisations published guidance on the topic in the 1990s, when the topic was being hotly debated. The Australian Psychological Society (1994), the American Psychological Association (Alpert et al., 1998), and the Royal College of Psychiatry (Brandon et al., 1998) all issued guidance warning their members to be careful of unintentionally implanting false memories in their clients.

The British Psychological Society (Frankland, & Cohen, 1999) produced guidance, much of which has stood up to subsequent research (see French, 2006, for an update), and which has been closely mirrored in more recent publications (e.g. Psychotherapy and Counselling Federation of Australia, 2017, which also provides a useful summary of other guidelines). Here are some key points for therapists:

- Be open to the emergence of memories of trauma that were not previously recalled.
- Take the recovery of memories seriously, accept this is the client's reality, and respect their feelings. But avoid drawing conclusions about the historical truth of recovered memories.
- Unusual, dramatic, powerful, and vivid memories or flashbacks of bodily sensations cannot be relied on as evidence of historical truth.
- Certain symptoms, e.g. eating problems, are not reliable evidence that abuse occurred.
- Tolerate, and help clients tolerate, uncertainty and ambiguity about early life events, as a factual truth may never be known.
- Recovered memories may be historically true, false, or partially true.

- Avoid imposing your own conclusions about what took place and avoid making suggestions.
- Avoid 'searching' for memories that have not arisen spontaneously and don't use techniques like hypnosis to reveal memories.
- Don't avoid working with recovered memories if they are important treatment targets.
- Be aware of the implications of recovered memories on wider family and social networks.
- Be aware of child safeguarding guidelines and when you might need to breach confidentiality.
- Remember guidelines for good practice, especially around note-taking and seeking appropriate supervision.

Understanding recovered memories

The mechanisms which cause memories to be forgotten and subsequently recalled have not been conclusively determined. The theory of repression remains contentious (e.g. Brewin, & Andrews, 2014; Patihis et al., 2014), and is based on the idea that memories are kept out of conscious awareness, perhaps initially deliberately and effortfully, and then unconsciously. Other possible mechanisms have been proposed, including dissociation, whereby memories weren't fully encoded or stored at the time of the trauma, avoidance (conscious suppression, minimisation and/or denial), 'simple' forgetting due to lack of retrieval cues and interference, lack of discussion (practice) due to shame, lack of state-dependent retrieval cues, 'enforced silence' due to threats of violence from perpetrators, or a combination of these (Smith, & Greaves, 2017).

It is possible that different mechanisms are at play, and that there are different types of recovered memories. Some of our clients report total amnesia for an event or time period, but others say that they always had a sense that something had happened but could not, or did not want to, recall details. Others had vague memories which become clearer over time or fragments of clear memory which had never been elaborated (by choice or otherwise) into a fuller picture. Some clients re-evaluate events that they have not thought about for a long time in light of later experiences. After all, abuse is not always experienced as terrifying peri-traumatically; sometimes an experience that only felt strange or confusing at the time is re-evaluated as horrifying or shameful later on.

Often there has been a trigger for memory recovery, such as an adult trauma that generates strong reminders through matching sensory, emotional, or cognitive features. Other triggers include having children, or when children reach the same age as the client was when they were abused, media reports of similar events, another victim of the same perpetrator reporting abuse, a sexual experience, or the onset of a new intimate relationship (Harvey, 1999). Undertaking trauma-focused therapy, which involves reducing avoidance of painful memories, thoughts, and feelings can also be a trigger.

Working clinically with recovered memories

Recovered memories can create anxiety for both clients and therapists. One potential risk is that therapists withhold evidence-based treatments that have the best likelihood of improving PTSD symptoms. Hence, our approach is to treat PTSD symptoms arising from recovered memories in the same way that we would treat PTSD from memories that have always been recalled, albeit with some adaptations.

TAKING MEMORIES SERIOUSLY

One of the more concerning consequences of the false memory debate is that people who have recovered memories of abuse may not be taken seriously or may have their experiences questioned. Whether or not memories are exactly factual, they are generally highly distressing. Memories of traumatic events are upsetting in themselves, added to which our clients will be grappling with the implications of realising later in life that they have suffered a trauma, not uncommonly abuse at the hands of caregivers. Our first goal, therefore, as with other trauma survivors, is to be respectful, empathic, validating, and supportive of our client's experience and how they have been impacted.

PSYCHOEDUCATION AND FORMULATION

Clients often have questions about why they have not recalled memories before, and why they have come back now. Some also have concerns about whether or not their memories are accurate, particularly as early memories can often be hazy and fragmented. We therefore often find it helpful to initiate a discussion, and offer psychoeducation, about the nature of recovered memories, why memories may be forgotten and subsequently recalled, and what might trigger delayed recall. Often the explanation for recovered memories that our clients relate to is simply that memories have been out of conscious awareness for a time, but that a strong enough reminder has brought the memories back, or a change has occurred whereby the memories have become newly meaningful in some way or that removed their usual capacity to keep the memories at bay.

We often explain briefly that there has been a debate in psychological research about whether recovered memories are always true, sometimes inaccurate, or a mixture of real events and imagined memories, but that research hasn't given us a clear answer about this. However, we do know that sometimes people have recovered memories that have been proven to be true. Other people have false memories, which feel as true and real as 'actual' memories. And, in many cases, we can never know for sure what exactly has happened. This topic is introduced to encourage a stance of curiosity and collaborative exploration, rather than to imply the client may be, intentionally or otherwise, 'making up' their memories.

In our experience, most clients accept that they may never know exactly what occurred and the conversation then moves towards living with that uncertainty. Some of our clients believe firmly that their memories are accurate and we do not try to dissuade them from this. Our job is not to be arbiters of truth, but to assist with distress.

FOCUS ON MEANINGS

Another priority is to understand the meanings our client gives to the memories and explore how these meanings contribute to distress. For example, sometimes the fact that the memories were not previously remembered is the main source of distress, and the therapist can help address related appraisals. Other times, the primary impact of recovering memories is the realisation that a trauma has occurred, and the implications of that, for example on family relationships.

Hot cognitions

- This means I am damaged
- There may be other bad things that I don't remember
- I can't trust my memory anymore
- I don't know what is a real memory and what isn't
- People who were supposed to care for me have hurt me, now I don't know who I can trust

Here, the meanings associated with the memories and their emergence become the main area for intervention, rather than the content of the memories themselves. As usual, the intervention depends on the formulation and the client's goals. In some cases, we have found that dealing with the implications of recovering memories is the only intervention required. Where the memories have become intrusive, and the client reports PTSD symptoms relating to the new memories, the usual trauma-focused approaches can then be used.

Piotr began to recover memories of childhood abuse after his wife gave birth to their first child. His wife noticed that Piotr was excessively anxious about the baby and never wanted anyone else to hold him. When she asked Piotr about this, he confessed that he had started having memories of being abused by a neighbour who had sometimes looked after him as a child. He felt very ashamed of the memories and also feared that he would not be a good parent if he did not deal with his past experiences.

In therapy, Piotr's psychologist explored the meaning of these new memories. They discussed possible explanations for why the memories were being recovered now when Piotr had not remembered the abuse for so long. They also addressed the shame that he felt about the abuse memories and his anxieties about being a good parent. Through guided discovery, Piotr began to accept that he was not to blame for the abuse and to realise that he could still be an excellent parent. The memories, although unpleasant, were not particularly intrusive except when he dwelled on them, and he did not re-experience them in nightmares or flashbacks. Piotr's goals of being less anxious about parenting his son, and of being able to accept his past, were therefore met without the need for a memory-focused intervention.

IMPACT ON RELATIONSHIPS

Recovering traumatic memories often has an impact on close relationships. For some people, this is the source of distress that brings them to therapy. The issue is particularly salient when the recovered memories are of abuse by a family member, where the client still has contact or a relationship with the perpetrator, or where a caregiver has failed to notice, believe, or protect the client from abuse.

Coming to terms with the relationship implications of recovering memories of early trauma can be a jarring and distressing process. We encourage our clients to take time to think through, and discuss in therapy, their thoughts and feelings about their new memories, before making decisions about if, or how, to disclose or address them with family members. An obvious exception is where they and/or you assess that there is current risk from the perpetrator (next section). The therapist's role is often to help the client to consider how to address the new memories within their close relationships and to support them in whatever they decide.

Samantha recovered memories of childhood abuse by her brother, triggered by a later sexual assault as a young adult. She had an ongoing relationship with her brother, seeing him several times a year at family events, although they were not close. Samantha also had reason to believe that her mother knew about the abuse; she recalled memories of her mother walking in on her brother abusing her and shouting at him to stop, but then never mentioning it again.

Samantha and her therapist discussed how she wanted to manage future interactions with her family. Samantha's mother was now unwell with dementia, and Samantha decided not to confront her about what had happened. However, she wrote a letter to her brother telling him that she recalled what he had done and wanted no further contact with him. She also decided to report him to the police, who questioned him but took no further action. Samantha decided not to attend family events where her brother would be present but chose to make separate arrangements to see members of her family with whom she wanted to maintain relationships.

Another area for clients to consider is to whom they will disclose their recovered memories; for example, whether to disclose their experiences to partners and family members. We help clients predict and prepare for a range of responses from others, from receiving support and corroboration from others to being dismissed or disbelieved, outright rejection, or even threats. The therapist can help by considering with the client what to say, and making a plan for each potential outcome of disclosure; to 'hope for the best, plan for the worst'. We sometimes ask clients if they would like to invite supportive family members to join a therapy session. This can provide them with a 'safe' environment to make their first disclosures, and/or enlist their support in making their disclosure plan.

SAFEGUARDING AND CONFIDENTIALITY

Where a client has recovered memories of abuse, and the perpetrator is still alive, we must always consider whether the perpetrator may still pose a risk to others. From the outset, be transparent with clients about your legal and professional responsibilities around disclosures, particularly where you believe someone may be at risk. Explain in advance how and where you will record clinical information, what you will do with it based on what they tell you, and who may then have access to it. In this way, everything you do should, as much as possible, be predictable and supportive of their choice-making and autonomy. You can help clients understand and weigh up the options for disclosing their recovered memories to social services or the police, and if they decide to, support them in the process. Equally, you may need to make a disclosure against their wishes, and balancing the interests and wishes of your client with your professional and legal responsibilities can be tricky. These issues are discussed in more detail in Chapter 23, and also in the British Psychological Society's guidance document on managing disclosures of non-recent (historic) child sexual abuse (BPS, 2016).

LEGAL ISSUES

Sometimes, recovering memories of earlier trauma may lead a client to pursue legal action against the perpetrator. Our role as therapists is to discuss the issues associated with undertaking legal action, but not to influence them, and to support our clients in the decisions they make. If they decide to contact the police, and you were the first person to whom they disclosed the trauma, you may be called on to give evidence, and your notes would be considered an important source of evidence (see Crime Prosecution Service (CPS) Guidance, 2020, draft version). Even if your client is not currently pursuing legal action, they may decide to in the future. All therapy records, including your clinical notes and any audio-visual materials, can be obtained retrospectively and, in this context, may become public, including to the perpetrator.

Part of the reason the recovered memory debate has been so controversial is that the reliability of memory plays a major role in determining the strength of evidence given by survivors of abuse in court cases. If your client does pursue legal action, there is a chance that their evidence will be challenged by suggesting that the therapy you delivered has influenced their recollections. This makes accurate note-keeping even more important than usual. You should also make use of supervision when making clinical decisions (and keep supervision records) and follow the guidelines in the following section around reducing the risk of inadvertently influencing memory recovery. However, as discussed in Chapter 22, CPS guidance (2020, draft version) is that therapy should not be delayed due to a legal case; the client's wellbeing is the priority.

FAQ: What do I do if memories are highly improbable?

In most cases, it is unhelpful and unnecessary to challenge the accuracy of our clients' memories. However, occasionally we have worked with people where their experiences seem highly improbable (see McNally, 2018, for possible indicators). We first remind ourselves that some events seem unbelievable simply because they are so extreme or unusual. More importantly, however 'true' they are, if we view these memories as distressing, meaningful mental representations, then they are still a valid target for intervention – we treat the intrusive memories as psychological symptoms, not historical records.

Very rarely, we have encountered situations where the traumatic events could not have occurred as described. One possible explanation is that a 'source monitoring failure' has occurred; for example, a hallucination, constructed memory, or dream has been recalled or appraised as a real event. In this situation, we may still use memory-focused techniques, focusing on their interpretations and experience of the memories (Chapters 10 and 11). Often highly improbable memories still have some emotional or representational truth; for example, they represent an experience of an emotionally neglectful childhood and the felt sense of being vulnerable and alone. However, we may try to raise the possibility that the event did not occur exactly as they experienced it, promoting a stance of curious uncertainty and helping clients to consider alternative explanations.

There are also rare cases where clients elaborate or fabricate trauma memories, to achieve some kind of 'secondary gain'. If we have strong evidence of fabrication, we attempt to understand and more adaptively address the need which is being met by this behaviour – to identify the 'primary loss' that motivates this 'secondary gain'. Where legal proceedings are involved, we attempt to separate the therapy intervention from the legal context, for example, by suggesting that therapy resumes after the case has concluded. Sometimes, the therapeutic relationship provides the 'secondary gain' in the form of validation, emotional support, and compassion, so an important therapeutic task would be to enable the client to meet those needs more sustainably, for example by developing their interpersonal support network. See Taylor et al. (2007) for further reading on malingering in PTSD.

Memories currently being recovered

Memories are sometimes recovered during therapy. New memories may arise from the same time period as the traumas being addressed in treatment; for example, new memories of experiences from a prolonged period of abuse. This can be a normal process of increasingly detailed remembering that occurs when people focus on memories, known as hypermnesia. At other times, completely unrelated traumatic memories may be recovered.

Abdullah was receiving treatment for PTSD following a train crash. One very distressing moment in the trauma was when Abdullah saw a look of terror and pain on the face of his 8-year-old son. When reliving this hotspot in therapy, Abdullah had a flashback to an earlier traumatic experience, of being beaten up by an older child when he was around 8 years old. Abdullah had not previously recalled this experience, but when his therapist encouraged him to focus on the look on his son's face during the trauma, the recovered memories were triggered.

When new memories are recovered during therapy, our initial priority is to support clients emotionally with the experience of retrieving new memories and understanding their implications. It won't be immediately clear whether they will develop PTSD symptoms from the new memories, so initially we employ a non-directive, supportive, and validating approach to help the client come to terms with their new memories.

The time period during which new memories are being recovered is when they are more vulnerable to being influenced by the therapist. It is therefore important to avoid any inadvertent suggestion. Here are some tips:

- *Check your assumptions*: One of the concerns raised about false recovered memories is that therapists have pre-existing assumptions that influence their responses to clients. These include always believing that certain symptoms (such as sexual problems, eating disorders, or borderline personality disorder) indicate that a client was abused, even if they do not remember it.
- *Explain your concerns*: As previously described, we explain briefly that there is a debate about emerging memories and concerns about therapists influencing them, so we want to avoid this. Being transparent means we can plan treatment collaboratively.
- *Use a non-directive questioning style*: Research has shown that witness statements can be influenced by certain questioning styles and we can draw the style of interviewing that the police use to minimise inadvertently suggesting responses to our clients. This includes avoiding forced-choice or leading questions, and just allowing our clients to give an uninterrupted 'free recall' version of events, prompted only with open-ended questions (e.g. 'what do you remember about that time in your life?') or specific-closed questions (e.g. 'where did that happen?').
- *Take detailed notes or record sessions*: If your client decides to take legal action against a perpetrator, and you are the first person to whom they disclose the memories, your notes could be a valuable source of evidence. For advice on what to note, see the CPS (2020) guidance.
- *Support natural processes but don't start fishing*: Don't try to prompt your client to remember more. For example, we wouldn't use the techniques in Chapter 8 for filling in gaps while memories are in the process of being recovered, nor would we use imaginal reliving or any other trauma-focused techniques to explore emerging memories. There isn't good evidence that these techniques do influence the recovery of memories, but it is better to err on the side of caution and let any memories emerge naturally. We may, however, encourage our clients to 'trust in their natural process', by which we mean neither to suppress or inhibit, nor focus or ruminate on new intrusive images. Rather, we suggest they keep a brief diary of anything that pops up, and not look over it between times.
- *Give memories time to settle before assessing for PTSD*: Not all our clients develop PTSD from recovered memories, and we wait until no further memories or details seem to be emerging before making that assessment. In the meantime, non-trauma-focused techniques can be used. If memories become and remain intrusive, other PTSD criteria are met, and the client wishes to, you can offer a course of PTSD treatment for the recovered memories.

Notes from the therapy room: Sue

Sue was in her mid-fifties when she started PTSD treatment after being injured in a terrorist bombing on a train. At assessment, she reported few memories of her childhood and no previous traumatic experiences. However, while working on the memories of the bombing, Sue began to recover memories of sexual abuse by babysitter when she was around six years old.

Following discussion with her therapist, Sue agreed to pause the intervention focused on her adult trauma, to allow the childhood memories to naturally emerge and settle down. They discussed why these memories might be emerging now, and Sue realised that she likely felt the same way as a child during the abuse as she had done during the terrorist bombing; helpless, alone, and dissociated. Her therapist explained that there was some debate about whether recovered memories were always accurate and that there was a risk they could be influenced by outside sources. They decided to discuss Sue's thoughts and feelings about the memories without discussing their content in detail or trying to remember more.

Sue reflected that the abuse memories made sense of some of her choices in life. For example, she had worked abroad most of her life and had very little contact with her family. She now remembered telling her mother that her babysitter had touched her vagina and being told that she was lying and should never speak of it again. This felt more like an old memory, that had always been there but she had not thought about since childhood. Sue figured this experience was why she had put the other memories out of her mind for so long. Sue had chosen never to have children and had never enjoyed sex, which she now believed was due to the abuse. They added this information to her formulation (Figure 9.1).

Sue and her therapist discussed how to deal with family members who would have known about the abuse. She had no current contact with her former babysitter, who was now in his sixties with adult children and grandchildren. Sue agreed for her therapist to report the abuse to social services. She did not want to pursue a prosecution against him but did want to make sure that he did not present a risk to his grandchildren. Social services recorded the report and confirmed there had been no other complaints made against him. Sue agreed that she would participate in an investigation if further evidence of abuse emerged. Sue decided not to confront her mother about her knowledge of the abuse. They had a difficult relationship while Sue was growing up, and Sue had chosen to distance herself from her mother as an adult, rarely visiting her family.

After several sessions, Sue reported no new memories were emerging. She continued to have intrusions of the terrorist attack and was also having occasional nightmares involving her babysitter. Sue agreed to continue the work on the adult trauma and monitor any PTSD symptoms relating to the recovered childhood memories, with the option of addressing them later on. Sue and her therapist returned to the task of reliving and updating her adult trauma memories. She also continued with work on reclaiming her life, focusing particularly on activities such as reading and seeing friends, which she had neglected since the bombing.

Sue reported no longer re-experiencing the terrorist attack but continued to have some nightmares of her babysitter. The memories to which they related were unclear, but Sue remembered feeling smothered by her babysitter as he lay on top of her and being frightened of suffocating. It was similar to a moment in the terrorist attack when Sue had been trapped under the body of another injured passenger, so Sue used the same updates as before: that no one was on top of her and she could now move and breathe freely. She used physical movements of spinning and jumping alongside these updates to help them feel more powerful. The nightmares became less frequent and less frightening.

As they approached the end of therapy, Sue's therapist helped her review her goals and areas for ongoing work. Sue felt glad that she had recovered the memories because they helped her make sense of some of the problems she had struggled with throughout her life. Sue planned ways of reclaiming aspects of her life that had been missing ever since childhood. For example, she made steps towards becoming more comfortable with her body by taking up a yoga class and having a sports massage. She tended to avoid talking about personal issues with her friends, instead taking the role of listener to the problems of others. She challenged herself to be more open about her own difficulties with a selected close friend.

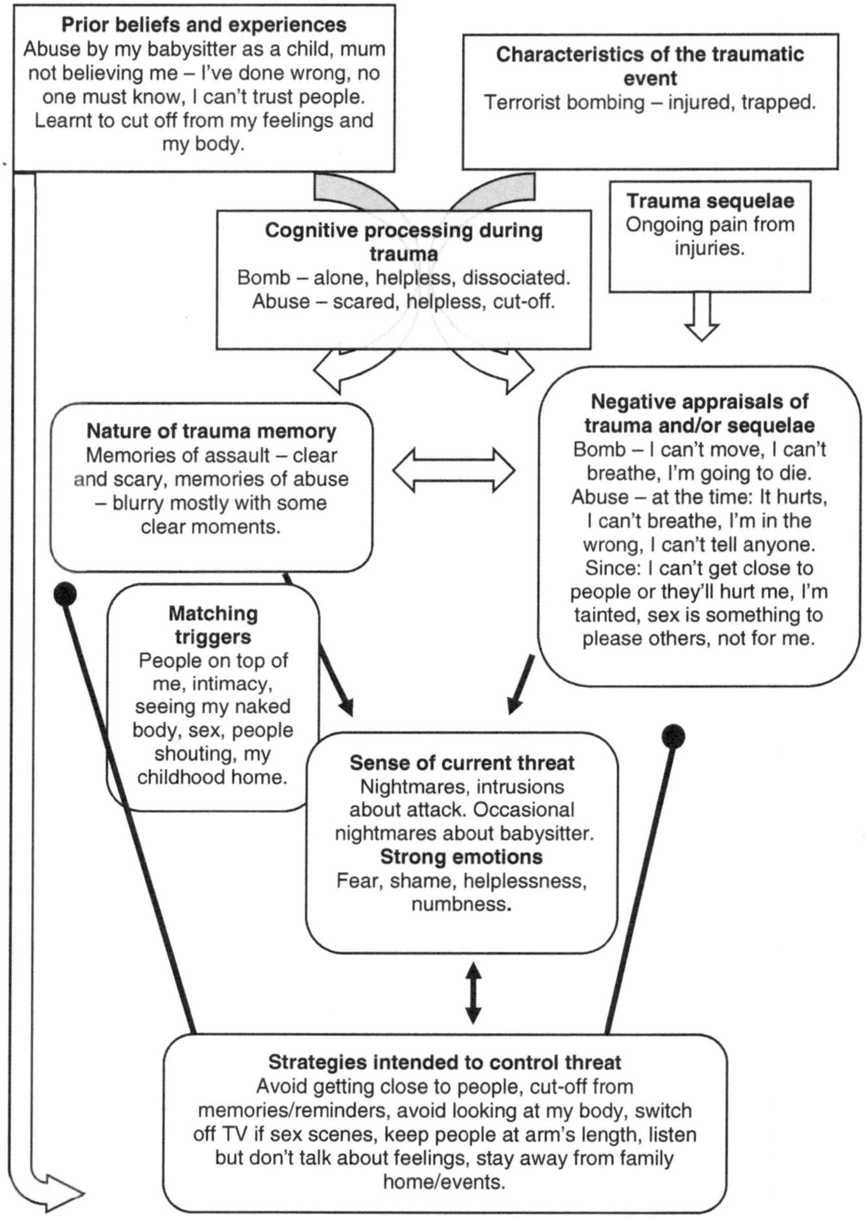

Figure 9.1 Sue's formulation

Recommended reading

McDonald, A. (2017). Occasional paper on recovered memory of childhood sexual abuse: An overview of research evidence and guidelines. Melbourne, Australia: PACFA. www.pacfa.org.au/

McNally, R. J. (2018). Recovered memories of childhood sexual abuse. In R. Rogers, & S. D. Bender (Eds.). *Clinical assessment of deception and malingering* (pp. 387–400). Guilford Press.

CHAPTER TEN
Constructed memories

Luisa's brother died by suicide. Afterwards, she found herself imagining his last moments, and these images started to recur as nightmares and intrusions. In therapy, she worked on both her 'true' memories of learning of his death, as well as these 'constructed' images which represented her worst fears of how he had died.

Constructed memories (also sometimes called 'elaborated memories' or 'non-memories') arise partially or completely from imagination, rather than through direct perception. These typically visual images may be formed at the time of the trauma, for example, a 'worst-case scenario' picture that pops into mind, or later on, for example, when finding out something new and distressing about an event. Constructed images commonly arise when someone hears about the death of a loved one and imagines their death vividly, or has been exposed to upsetting details of a traumatic event which they did not witness and spontaneously creates images of what happened. Sometimes their own similar experiences of trauma feed these images. Other times, the person was present at the trauma but witnessed only part of it, and their imagination has filled the gaps.

These mental constructions can be experienced similarly to 'true' memories, with a sense of reliving the event and of the self within it (Rubin, & Umanath, 2015). They typically differ from false memories, however, as the person is aware that they do not accurately represent their actual experience. Nonetheless, the person may believe they are possible or even probable simulations, and hence both feel 'true' and contribute to a sense of current threat.

Gunam fled Sri Lanka after he learned that the authorities planned to question him about his involvement with the Tamil resistance movement. One night, armed police came to Gunam's house and he escaped through a window. He fled to India, and eventually to the UK. Not long afterwards, Gunam found out that his brother had been arrested and the family had no news of his whereabouts. Gunam had heard many accounts of Tamil people being tortured and murdered by Sri Lankan authorities and had seen photos in Tamil newspapers of injuries they had suffered. He began having nightmares of his brother being tortured. He became increasingly distressed and struggled to sleep. Mixed in with the images of his brother were memories of the night he escaped from his home in Sri Lanka, and Gunam often had nightmares of being chased and tortured himself, even though it hadn't happened.

DOI: 10.4324/9781003288329-12

FAQ: Do constructed memories count as PTSD symptoms?

Diagnostic frameworks have historically assumed that PTSD re-experiencing symptoms are frightening 'replays' of a traumatic event the person directly experienced or witnessed. While often true, clinicians have gradually become aware that PTSD re-experiencing phenomena often go beyond 'replaying' actual memories, and that PTSD symptoms can arise from a traumatic event that is indirectly experienced, or internally generated (such as hallucinations – Chapter 11). DSM-5 was the first diagnostic framework to explicitly recognise that PTSD symptoms can arise following indirect exposure to trauma, specifying two instances that meet criterion A: learning that a close relative or friend was exposed to actual or threatened death through violence or an accident; or being repeatedly exposed to distressing details of a traumatic event (seeing pictures, videos, reading, or hearing narratives) in the course of one's work. In our experience, indirect exposure to traumatic events is commonly associated with distressing constructed memories, and these phenomena can be understood as PTSD re-experiencing symptoms.

Criterion A has been the subject of much debate over the years and has changed in each version of the DSM diagnosis. Indeed, ICD-11 has not specified the kinds of events that cause PTSD, instead stating that it 'follows exposure to an extremely threatening or horrific event or series of events'. This leaves the clinician to use their judgement as to what is extremely threatening, and so may encompass events that wouldn't meet the stricter DSM-5 criterion, such as protracted legal processes, discrimination, and bullying.

Understanding constructed memories

Contemporary accounts of autobiographical memories view them as dynamic mental constructions rather than static representations like photos or videos. Typically, they include mental images that represent aspects of actual experiences, but many of the details are filled in, missed out, inferred, or compressed; hence all memories are to some degree both inaccurate and constructed. This is because, rather than serving as accurate records of events, memories function as shortcuts to generating personal meanings that help us make sense of and navigate the world. Therefore, 'when people remember they imagine and when they imagine they use memory' (Conway, & Loveday, 2015). This idea helps us to understand how constructed memories in PTSD, viewed as meaningful mental representations, are really just a subset of normal memory processes. Indeed, constructed images, such as daydreaming future events, imagining 'near-misses', and seeing detached observer-perspective images of ourselves, are everyday experiences that are also common across emotional disorders.

There have been very few systematic studies of constructed memories in PTSD. Several have reported that a subset of people with PTSD experience intrusive imagery arising from 'elaborated cognitions' (Reynolds, & Brewin, 1998), or imagine additional distressing details of events (Oulton et al., 2018), often representing a 'worst-case scenario' version (Merckelbach et al., 1998). Both lab studies and studies of real events have shown that people will commonly and inadvertently 'fill the gaps' in parts of a scene that they did not witness using their imagination (Crombag et al., 1996; Strange, & Takarangi, 2012, 2015), and may report detailed images of traumatic events they did not see. Notably, these constructed memories are indistinguishable from 'real' memories across a range of characteristics including their vividness and associated distress and can become intrusive in the same way as other types of PTSD memories.

We've also observed the following:

- *They often occur in people with a high capacity for visual imagery*: People with powerful visual imaginations seem more likely to generate vivid, sensory, and emotional images of traumatic events they did not witness, and to be troubled by them afterwards. However, even people with a poor imagination may generate constructed images, and may indeed find them more meaningful and disturbing, in part because they are less familiar with experiencing powerful images (Grey, 2009).
- *They both represent, and maintain, key appraisals*: Constructed images tend to fit with the meanings our clients make of traumas. For example, if they believe that a loved one died in agony, this will be reflected in their images. The images may, in turn, strengthen the appraisal of how the death occurred, creating a maintenance cycle.
- *They are maintained by rehearsal, rumination, and a search for understanding*: People who are troubled by constructed images tend to be those who ruminate about the parts of the trauma they did not witness. The process of trying to make sense of what happened is natural and not in itself unhelpful, but people who become preoccupied with what might have been tend to construct more images, usually of worst-case scenarios, which then become a further target for dwelling.
- *Other memories or images can be incorporated into them*: Earlier experiences, information from other people, and media inputs can all influence imagery.

These processes are summarised in Figure 10.1.

TYPES OF CONSTRUCTED MEMORIES AND IMAGES

Grey (2009) highlights that intrusive imagery in PTSD can relate to 'veridical' ('true') memories, and/or 'non-veridical' (constructed) images, both of which may arise peri-traumatically (during the event itself) and/or secondarily (after the event). Indeed, people may report combinations of these types of memories, such as veridical peri-traumatic memories of the moments just before they lost consciousness, alongside non-veridical reconstructed images of what they feared happened while they were unconscious.

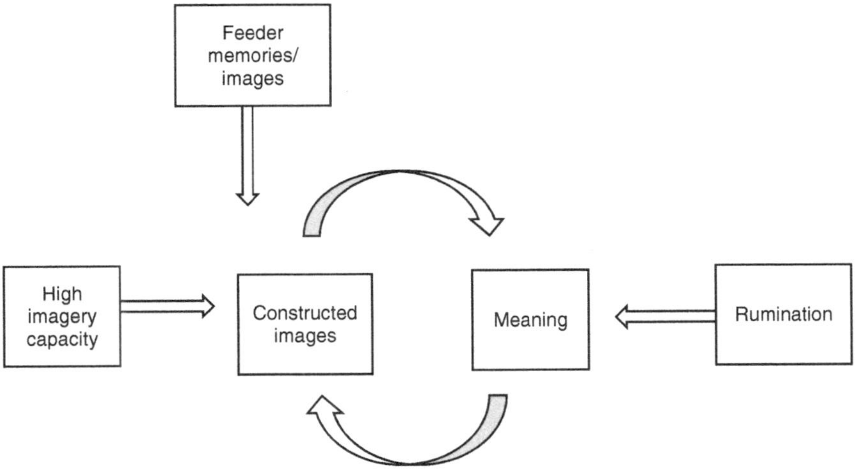

Figure 10.1 Visual representation of constructed image formation and maintenance

Peri-traumatic constructed images include those which are seen in the 'mind's eye' during a trauma or immediately on hearing about it. Examples include visualising worst-case scenarios of what might be about to happen, imagining upsetting details that are out of view, and dissociative phenomena such as seeing oneself from outside the body.

> Aurelie was an interpreter for the court service and worked on a trial of an organised crime network that had trafficked women into the UK for prostitution. As part of the case, Aurelie translated numerous testimonies of sexual and physical assault. As she did so, she imagined those things happening to the women giving evidence. The images were intensely distressing and she found herself re-experiencing them afterwards.

Secondary, or post-traumatic, imagery constructions are generated after the trauma, often fuelled by rumination or attempts to 'fill the gaps' and make sense of an aspect of the trauma which was not witnessed or remembered.

> Gunam did not experience any images when he first heard about his brother's disappearance. His initial reaction was shock and guilt that he had left his brother vulnerable by leaving the country. However, over the following days and weeks, he began to dwell on what might be happening to his brother. He read accounts online of others being tortured and imagined his brother in those scenarios. His nightmares began a month after he first learned his brother was missing.

Finally, some of our clients have described secondary constructed images that started some time after the trauma, triggered by exposure to new information.

> Elouise was a sex worker who was assaulted by one of her clients. A year later, she learnt that one of her friends had been murdered by the same client. Elouise realised that she had a lucky escape. She had heard details of the murder and repeatedly imagined what it would have been like if it had happened to her. She began to have intrusive images of both the actual assault she had experienced, as well as constructed images of the client murdering her.

Working with constructed memories

ASSESSMENT, PSYCHOEDUCATION, AND FORMULATION

When investigating our clients' re-experiencing symptoms, we always ask about disturbing images that may have arisen from imagination either at the time of the trauma or afterwards, and then explore their underlying meanings. As already discussed, some constructed images represent an important personal meaning associated with the trauma. Metacognitive beliefs about the images are also important to understand, e.g. 'because I can picture it, it must be true'. These types of appraisal can often be addressed through psychoeducation. We explain that constructed images and memories are common, especially if the person did not witness (or fully witness) the event, and can be as vivid and upsetting as 'real' memories.

It can be helpful to sketch out a simple maintenance cycle similar to that in Figure 10.1, showing how our beliefs about what happened can lead to the formation of images, which in turn make beliefs feel more true. This leads to interventions aimed at reducing rumination, addressing problematic meanings, reliving, and updating the trauma memories and, in some cases, the 'feeder' memories or images.

Hot cognitions

- If I can imagine it, it must be true
- I need to work out what really happened
- Imagining it brings me closer to the person who died/was hurt
- They died in terrible pain and distress

UNDERSTANDING AND ADDRESSING MEANINGS

Having explored the meaning of a constructed image, we can correct any distortions and help the client consider alternative meanings. A range of cognitive strategies might be appropriate, including guided discovery techniques to consider a full range of evidence, behavioural experiments, site visits, and so on. Here are some examples:

Jennifer developed PTSD after a traumatic childbirth. Her baby's heart rate was dropping and an emergency caesarean section was performed. Jennifer couldn't see what was happening, but she could feel pain and tugging sensations in her abdomen. She could see the faces of the medical staff and they seemed worried. Jennifer was terrified that her baby was dying. She had an image of her abdomen opened wide and people with their arms inside her. She imagined her baby was limp and lifeless.

After the birth, Jennifer kept re-experiencing the constructed images of her open abdomen and lifeless baby. In therapy, Jennifer and her therapist looked at the meaning of these images. The images represented her appraisals 'my tummy is wide open', 'I'm being gutted like a fish', and 'my baby is dead', linked to feelings of fear, helplessness, and detachment. Re-experiencing the images made the meanings feel stronger.

Jennifer and her therapist pieced together what had happened during the birth. Although her baby had been in distress, she was successfully delivered and was now healthy and happy. Together, Jennifer and her therapist watched online videos of caesarean sections to get an accurate image of what had happened outside of Jennifer's view. The images on the video were less horrific than in Jennifer's imagination. She realised that her abdomen would not have been wide open with people's arms inside, and this new information fitted with the size of her scar, which was only a few inches wide. In the videos, the baby was usually removed quickly and immediately moved around, which was different from her image of the doctor struggling to pull out a limp baby.

Farzeen's son died in a car accident and she had to identify his body, which was badly bruised and swollen. Farzeen believed that it had been damaged by being mishandled in the morgue. She developed images of him being mistreated, for example, his body being dropped on the floor, and the morgue workers handling him roughly. These images became intrusive and were intensely distressing.

To address her beliefs, Farzeen's therapist arranged for them to revisit the morgue and speak to the mortuary manager. He explained the process of how the bodies arrived at the morgue, how they were handled, and what tests were done. Farzeen was impressed by how seriously the mortuary staff took their responsibility to care for the deceased and how respectfully they spoke about them. When Farzeen asked about the damage to her son's body, the mortuary manager confirmed this had occurred during the car crash, and not at the morgue.

FAQ: What if the worst *did* happen?

Looking at meanings of images and trying to correct any misappraisals can help ameliorate strong negative beliefs about traumatic events. However, in many cases, something really awful did happen, and it would be inauthentic and unhelpful to pretend otherwise. As with other examples in this book, we cannot always update a trauma with 'the worst didn't happen', but we can look at the different layers of meaning associated with the event, and consider updates for the different meanings. For example, it was true that Farzeen's son had died. Yet, how he had been treated after his death was a major source of her distress and was linked to a misappraisal that we could tackle. If the distressing meaning associated with an image appears accurate, it's still always worth asking 'and what's the worst thing about that for you?' to explore any additional layers of meaning. And, in almost all cases, meanings can be updated by including the information that the trauma is now in the past, and the danger or suffering is over.

Sometimes, we need to help our clients accept the implications of a terrible event or the uncertainty of not knowing an outcome. In Gunam's example, he did not find out what had happened to his brother. The focus in treatment became how he could move forward with his life while living with this uncertainty. He found it helpful to put himself in his brother's shoes – if he was in prison or had been killed, what would he want for Gunam? He realised he would want him to take the opportunity of freedom to have a good life. We worked on the guilt that Gunam felt about leaving Sri Lanka, helped him to stop dwelling on what was happening to his brother (on the basis that it didn't help his brother, and only made Gunam feel worse), and supported him to build a life in the UK. We worked on the memories of his own escape, 'tagging' the constructed images of being tortured himself as having their source in his fears and things he'd seen in the news, updating them with the information that they hadn't happened to him, then using imagery manipulation techniques to 'shatter' the images into tiny pieces as a way of taking away their power.

RELIVING AND UPDATING MEMORIES

Images that occurred peri-traumatically are part of the trauma memories, so can be addressed through reliving and updating. Take, for example, this extract from Jennifer's session:

THERAPIST: Let's try bringing the new information back into the memories.

JENNIFER: Ok.

T: So, I want you to bring the memories to mind. They're starting the C-section, and you can't see what's going on.

J: Ok, they've put the sheet up and I can't see. I can feel them pulling at me. I can see their faces, and they look really serious. I'm so scared.

T: And what's going through your mind?

J: The baby, just the baby, that she's dead.

T: What's the picture in your mind?

J: She's grey and limp. They're trying to yank her out of me.

T: You're doing really well. What do you know now that's different?

J: She's fine. Ella's fine. She's 9 months old now and she's healthy. She was always healthy.

T: Can you look at a photo of her now?

J: Yes, on my phone. She's laughing.

T: What colour is she? Is her skin grey?

J: No, she's peaches and cream.

T: Good, just go back in your mind to the operating theatre. They are still working behind the sheet. How are you feeling?

J: I feel like a fish being gutted. It doesn't hurt exactly but I can feel tugging like they are rummaging around inside me.

T: What do you know now about what was happening?

J: They were doing an emergency C-section, they'd done it plenty of times before. They looked serious because they were concentrating. I wasn't wide open. The baby was right there. They just had to make a cut and get her out.

T: Can you picture the C-section from the video?

J: Yes.

T: How does that look?

J: Orderly, controlled. Not loads of blood and guts like I was picturing. Just a bit of blood and goo when they lift the baby out.

T: How big is the wound?

J: Just big enough to get the baby out. I wasn't cut side to side like in my imagination.

T: If you feel comfortable, can you just look down at your scar for me, maybe touch it?

J: Yes.

T: How big is it?

J: Not big. Four, five inches maybe.

T: That's really good, well done. How are you feeling?

J: Ok, better. It was just my mind working overtime. I was thinking the worst.

In this extract, the therapist threads together the memories, including the constructed images that the client describes, with the updated information, including the new images they have developed.

IMAGERY RESCRIPTING

Imagery rescripting is another option for working with constructed memories. As usual, imagery rescripting can introduce new meanings to memories, help an update to resonate emotionally, and do something in imagery that the client was unable to do in reality. Imagery rescripting may be a particularly useful intervention for constructed memories as we are already working in the realms of the imagination. Clients with a strong capacity for visualisation are likely to find new images easy to generate, which can then compete with the constructed image.

Marianne worked for the British Transport Police and was on duty during a terrorist attack on the London Underground. She was tasked with organising the passengers emerging from below one of the affected stations, many of whom were injured and terrified. Over her radio, Marianne heard details of the disaster unfolding, including the numerous fatalities.

From the people emerging from the station, the emergency services personnel, and the radio communications, Marianne painted a picture in her mind of hundreds of people trapped underground in the dark, in pain and dying.

Long after the bombings, Marianne continued to have images of the people underground. She had nightmares where people were trapped underground, unable to escape. Marianne also imagined ghosts haunting the underground network, trapped below. She was terrified to go back to work or to use the trains.

To address these distressing images, Marianne and her therapist used imagery rescripting to imagine opening the top of the tunnel at the station where Marianne had worked and putting in a golden escalator that came directly to the fresh air. Marianne stood next to it in her imagination, watching people emerge unharmed. The ghosts floated out of the tunnels and up into the sky, free. She imagined looking down into the station and the tunnel with an enormous searchlight that lit up the whole area to check that there was no one still trapped.

Another use for imagery rescripting is with recurrent nightmares. Nightmares sometimes persist even after clients report the memories feel less distressing and daytime intrusions have ceased. In this scenario, nightmares can be understood as constructed images, originating in the trauma but with such distressing content that they are themselves re-experienced even after the trauma memories are processed. In these cases, the nightmare itself can be directly rescripted (Krakow, & Zadra, 2010).

Jakob was working as a taxi driver when he was attacked by a drunk customer with a broken bottle and sustained very bad facial injuries. After his PTSD treatment had resolved most of the intrusions, he continued to have a recurring nightmare of a spinning metal ball with blades flying towards his face and would wake up as it was about to hit him. It reminded Jakob of an old horror film and, in therapy, they found it on the internet, which seemed to match and make sense of the origin of the image. However, the nightmares continued. Jakob and his therapist rescripted the dream by imagining the spinning ball transforming into a spinning windmill toy and seeing his son holding it while running on the beach. He rehearsed this new ending by reading it every night before bed and re-running it in his mind if he awoke after the nightmare.

WORKING WITH FEEDER MEMORIES OR IMAGES

As in Jakob's example, constructed memories have often been influenced by other memories, or images from elsewhere such as films or TV shows, or conversations with other people. Occasionally, earlier traumatic memories are triggered and re-experienced at the time of the trauma, leading to 'flashbacks of flashbacks'. It can be helpful to identify and process these other sources if they seem to be maintaining the constructed memories, by tagging them as mental events, e.g. 'this image comes from seeing news stories about other people being tortured' or 'this was an image that popped into my mind as he was talking, that came from my own experience of sexual assault'. If another source forms part of the content of the constructed memories or is re-experienced as well as the construction, it may need to be relived and updated separately. Other times, it is sufficient to identify and label it when updating the constructed image.

Gunam had watched videos online of torture techniques and was having nightmares about them. One particularly distressing video had shown someone being burnt alive and Gunam couldn't get it out of his mind. He imagined it happening to his brother, or himself, and had nightmares about being set on fire. Together with his therapist, Gunam did an imaginal reliving session of the video he had watched. He updated the memories with the information that it was not him or his brother being burnt, and the person in the video was no longer in pain.

Abbie's partner died from a heart attack while running a marathon. Abbie was watching the marathon but did not see her partner collapse. Afterwards, she experienced intrusive images of him clutching his chest, struggling for breath in extreme pain and fear. She realised that her images came from medical TV dramas and films, which may not be realistic depictions of heart attacks. To find more realistic information, Abbie found an account online of a runner who had experienced a heart attack during a marathon. She described feeling very hot and then suddenly collapsing but had no further memory. When Abbie worked on her constructed memories of her husband's death, she reminded herself that her image may be inaccurate, as it was from TV shows and films that were designed to be dramatic, and her husband's experience may not have been as painful or frightening as she imagined.

Notes from the therapy room: Luisa

Luisa grew up in Portugal with her parents and younger brother, Tomas. As a teenager, Tomas became depressed and made several suicide attempts. One day, when Luisa got home from work, she found a suicide note from Tomas in his bedroom. There was a train line near their house and Luisa realised he had gone there. When she arrived, she saw emergency services vehicles and a stopped train. She did not see Tomas's body but saw some blood.

In the weeks that followed, Luisa thought constantly about Tomas's death. She imagined him in distress, running to the train tracks. In her mind's eye, he felt alone and abandoned by his family. She pictured his body being shattered by the high-speed train and imagined the pain he had felt. She visualised his body parts strewn across the train and the embankment. The images were vivid and intensely distressing and came in nightmares and powerful daytime intrusions. She also imagined Tomas beyond the grave, disfigured and in pain, against a blank empty background. Luisa avoided reminders of the trauma, like going past the train line and going into Tomas's bedroom. Her parents had kept the suicide note, but Luisa could not bear to look at it. Her formulation is in Figure 10.2.

In therapy, Luisa and her therapist talked about her images. Luisa had a strong visual imagination and it made sense that her brain had come up with pictures of Tomas's death, although she could not know how accurate they were. They explored Luisa's appraisals of Tomas's death, that he had died alone and in pain, which were feeding the images, which in turn made the images feel even more real.

Next, they discussed rumination. Luisa thought constantly about Tomas's death. When her therapist asked her about the advantages and disadvantages of this, Luisa acknowledged that it made her feel sad and guilty, and stopped her from being able to access happy memories of Tomas. It also made her parents worry about Luisa, and interfered with her studies. However, Luisa felt that she needed to think about Tomas, otherwise she would be somehow letting him down, by forgetting about him. Her therapist asked if she would ever forget Tomas, even if she didn't think about him all day, and Luisa acknowledged that she couldn't forget him. She agreed

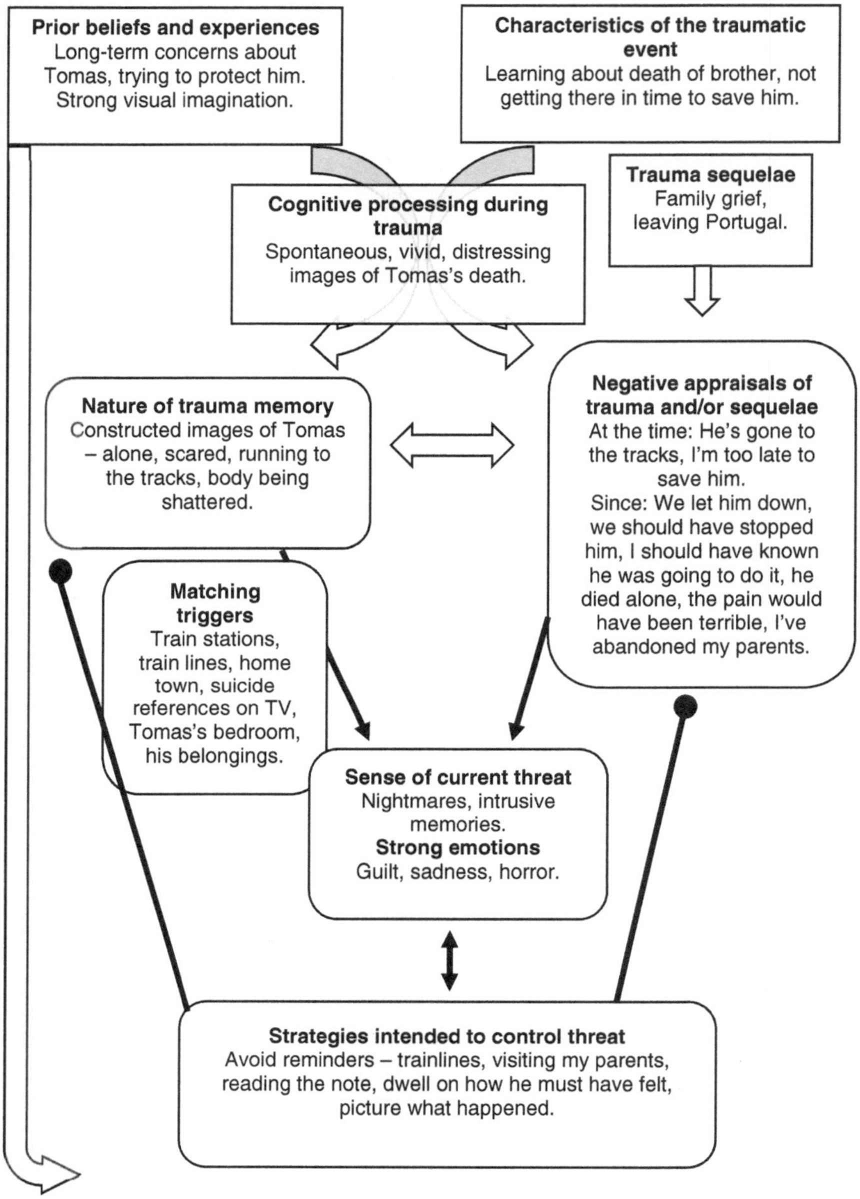

Figure 10.2 Luisa's formulation

to try an experiment – she dedicated an hour of her day to mourning Tomas, including looking at happy photos of them together and writing in her journal about him, and the rest of the day she tried not to dwell on his death, and put her attention into whatever she was doing, like cooking or studying. This was difficult at first, but Luisa found over time that she was able to engage in more of the activities she used to do, without forgetting Tomas.

Luisa and her therapist discussed the meaning of Luisa's images. Luisa felt guilty that Tomas had been alone on the day of his death, and believed this meant she had failed him as a sister. Luisa's therapist gently explored this belief with her. There was evidence that Tomas had planned his suicide for a day when he knew he would be alone, presumably so no one would stop him. He had tried to die before, and his family had intervened. They had also tried very hard to help him, including arranging professional help, staying with him as much as possible, and talking to him about his problems as much as he would allow. Luisa decided to read his suicide note again, and brought it to therapy. Tomas had written how much he loved his family and did not want them to blame themselves. He explained that he was in great emotional pain and could not bear it any longer. Luisa's belief that she had let her brother down began to change a little. Instead, she concluded that Tomas had been determined to die because his pain was so great, and she and her family had tried their best to help him. She still felt sad, but less guilty.

Luisa and her therapist also talked about physical pain. In Luisa's imagination, Tomas was in agony when he was hit by the train and could feel his body breaking apart. However, it had been a high-speed train and he had died on impact, suggesting his death would have been very quick and any pain would have been momentary. Luisa also reflected that Tomas was not in pain anymore.

Luisa did an imaginal reliving session where she brought this new information into her memories of the day of Tomas's death. She also brought new images into the constructed parts of the memories which reflected these meanings. Instead of picturing Tomas alone and in pain, she pictured him making a clear-headed decision that he wanted to end his life and writing a note to his family to tell them he loved them. She pictured his death as quick and painless and then imagined him ascending to heaven where he was pain-free and was reunited with their grandparents who would look after him in the afterlife. She practised this new image many times and gradually the nightmares began to fade.

Luisa and her therapist worked on her avoidance by visiting a local train station. When Luisa next went home to visit her parents, she laid flowers next to the tracks where Tomas had died. Her parents had not wanted to clear Tomas's room, and Luisa felt ready to go and look at some of his possessions. She found a picture in his drawer of the family all together and kept it as a reminder of how much they had loved each other. Luisa and her family agreed to always spend Tomas's birthday together at the beach, where he had loved swimming in the sea. Over time, Luisa realised she was able to think more about happy memories of Tomas and less about the day he had died.

Recommended reading

Grey, N. (2009). Imagery and psychological threat in PTSD. In L. Stopa (Ed.). *Imagery and the threatened self: Perspectives on mental imagery and the self in cognitive therapy* (pp. 137–165). Routledge.

Oulton, J. M., Strange, D., Nixon, R. D., & Takarangi, M. K. (2018). PTSD and the role of spontaneous elaborative "nonmemories". *Psychology of Consciousness: Theory, Research, and Practice*, 5(4), 398–413.

CHAPTER ELEVEN
Psychosis-related PTSD

Abdi had a psychotic episode during which he believed he would be arrested. Afterwards, he had nightmares about the visions and developed a fear of the police. His therapist helped him to make sense of what had happened and to process his memories of the experience.

Psychotic experiences are often terrifying. People can experience nightmarish hallucinations which they perceive as entirely real, or become convinced by delusions that their life is in imminent danger. Psychotic experiences arise for various reasons, including from drug use, medically related delirium, and as part of a psychotic disorder or severe mental illness. Those suffering from the most severe psychotic symptoms may also have aversive experiences associated with treatment (e.g. forced hospitalisations, restraint, and seclusion) or that result from disordered behaviour (e.g. reckless or suicidal acts). In some cases, psychotic symptoms and associated experiences can lead to PTSD, termed psychosis-related PTSD (PR-PTSD).

Whether psychotic experiences meet criterion A for a PTSD diagnosis according to DSM-5 has been debated. An objective threat of death or serious injury may not be present but nevertheless subjectively experienced. Certainly, a significant proportion of people who have experienced psychosis report PTSD symptoms afterwards (Buswell et al., 2021) so we tend to treat traumatic memories of psychotic experiences as we would other types of PTSD.

Although PR-PTSD is the main focus of this chapter, there are other ways in which psychosis and PTSD intersect (Morrison et al., 2003). Adverse and traumatic experiences, particularly in childhood, have been linked to psychosis (Bendall et al., 2008; Varese et al., 2012). Furthermore, many people with PTSD experience psychosis-like symptoms, generally audio-visual hallucinations linked to their trauma memories either directly, or indirectly as thematically linked content (Brewin, & Patel, 2010). Recently, a subtype of PTSD with secondary psychotic features has been proposed (PTSD-SP; Compean, & Hamner, 2019). Several similar mechanisms may underlie both psychosis and PTSD, probably including memory processes, negative beliefs, emotion regulation, dissociation, and attentional processes such as hypervigilance (Hardy et al., 2016).

Treating PTSD following psychotic experiences

CREATING A SHARED UNDERSTANDING

Normalisation, psychoeducation, and a shared formulation are particularly important with PR-PTSD, as clients may lack any understanding of what has happened, and potentially remain uncertain about what was, and wasn't, real.

A good starting point is to explore with your client the context of the psychotic experiences: where, when, and how they first happened, and their content: what was experienced (externally and internally) and how did the person understand what was going on? Depending on the

DOI: 10.4324/9781003288329-13

cause, this may involve joint research into how psychotic symptoms and experiences can arise, how common they are, and how they might have been triggered in a particular context. In many cases, the content of hallucinations and delusions has some relationship to stimuli or stressors present at the time, and/or to previous life experiences. Exploring these possible links can help your client to better understand the nature of their experiences and provide a normalising explanation for why they occurred.

Stephen was admitted into intensive care after a severe chest infection. He had multiple hallucinations while he was there, primarily involving groups of masked men hiding in the ward. At some points, he saw them gathering around his bed and believed they intended to kill him. Once, he experienced them trying to suffocate him. Stephen could do nothing to fight back and felt terrified and helpless.

In therapy, Stephen and his therapist tried to understand his experiences by searching for information online. They found a research paper showing that up to 80% of ICU patients experience delirium and that scary hallucinations and delusions are very common. They also read that the experiences don't usually recur after discharge from hospital, although some people do go on to develop PTSD. They discovered an online community supporting people who develop PTSD after intensive care. Stephen found this information reassuring, as he was worried he was losing his mind.

Stephen's therapist asked him if the groups of masked men reminded Stephen of anything he had seen or heard about it in the past. Stephen had grown up in Northern Ireland during the Troubles and remembered being frightened of paramilitary groups, who often wore masks. They wondered if these memories had fed into Stephen's hallucinations and delusions. They also considered the possibility that real events had triggered some of the strange experiences. For example, there would sometimes have been people gathered around Stephen's bed (such as during ward rounds). He had also been on a ventilator, so it seemed possible that the sensation of suffocating was related to a medical procedure like intubation.

FAQ: What do I do if it is unclear which memories are 'real'?

Therapists are sometimes concerned about using memory-focused techniques with psychotic experiences (or constructed memories; Chapter 10) in case they risk 'colluding' or strengthening memories of events that did not occur in 'reality'. Often clients with PR-PTSD are aware that their memories relate to events that did not, or could not happen. Others may be unsure or even convinced they did happen. Directly challenging your client's perceptions or beliefs too soon risks invalidating their experience and rupturing the therapeutic relationship. Instead, we gently explore whether the client has considered other explanations for their experience (for example, asking 'is there any possibility something else might have been going on?'), how well other explanations fit with their experiences, and whether those explanations are less distressing than their current understanding. If possible, it is preferable to develop a psychological explanation for their psychotic experiences, but this is not essential to treatment. Distressing memories, whether of real events or not, can still be addressed as trauma memories using the usual cognitive therapy techniques, so knowing the exact truth of a situation isn't essential. Although we use the term 'psychotic experience' throughout this chapter, we would not always use it with clients and are led by their way of describing their experience.

In some cases, it will be unclear what really happened. Trying to work this out can be a shared enterprise between the client and therapist, using information from any available source and applying logic, guesswork, and common sense. Sometimes this will be inconclusive, and the therapist and client may agree that they will never know for sure exactly what happened.

Li was drug-raped in Hong Kong by two men who told her they were members of a Triad, an organised crime network. She moved to the UK soon afterwards but remained convinced that the Triad was monitoring her constantly, and would find and kill her if she identified them. This fitted with threats that the men had made to her at the time of the trauma. Her therapist helped Li to distinguish what was true when she was still living in Hong Kong (where the men were very well-connected and could potentially have found her) versus what was currently true. They discussed a psychological explanation that PTSD leads to a sense of current threat, which may have been fuelling her current sense of unsafety. They then tested out whether the Triad was currently monitoring her, using a series of behavioural experiments. For example, Li believed that her phone was bugged, so made a phone call to her therapist in which she mentioned her rape experience and waited to see if there were any negative consequences. When nothing happened, Li decided to take the risk of writing down one of their names and pinning it to the clinic noticeboard. Li and her therapist couldn't know for sure if the Triad had ever had the power to find her, but, when nothing happened, Li concluded that she was likely not currently being monitored or followed.

BELIEFS ABOUT PSYCHOTIC EXPERIENCES

It is common for clients to hold distressing beliefs about what it means to have had a psychotic experience e.g., 'I've lost my mind and will never get it back'. Some fears have a basis in personal experiences or social contexts, such as having a parent who was hospitalised with a severe mental illness and fearing they have inherited it, or witnessing others in their community being rejected or ridiculed for mental ill-health. PR-PTSD symptoms can add to these fears as they can be bizarre and unpredictable, especially when re-experiencing symptoms make it feel as if the psychotic experiences are happening again. People may also worry that their psychotic experiences will return, and become vigilant for any warning signs such as perceptual distortions. Sometimes, psychoeducation about the cause of their psychotic experiences is sufficient to address these concerns, but additional cognitive work may also be needed, such as guided discovery, research, and behavioural experiments to test particular fears. For those with ongoing or recurrent psychotic symptoms, 'staying well' planning will also be an important intervention.

Amy had a series of distressing hallucinations after she took MDMA at a festival. She was in a crowd of people and believed they wanted to take her soul. Faces appeared distorted and threatening and Amy thought she was in hell with 'the living dead'. For months after the festival, Amy experienced nightmares about the experience and flashbacks where faces of people she knew appeared distorted. At times, she believed she must be dead and in hell.

Amy believed she had permanently damaged her mind by taking the drug and would end up in a psychiatric hospital.

Amy's therapist helped her to research her hallucinatory experiences. Amy had previously taken MDMA with no ill effects and realised the pill she had taken at the festival may have been laced with another substance, such as LSD or MDA, which would explain the vivid hallucinations. Her therapist also explained that the symptoms she was now having were typical of PTSD, and did not mean that her brain was permanently damaged. They researched reasons that people are admitted into psychiatric facilities and concluded that Amy's symptoms would not meet the criteria. They also discussed the possibility that Amy had died and was in hell. Amy reasoned she would only know this for sure if good things happened to her, so agreed to plan reclaiming your life activities as behavioural experiments, to see if she was capable of experiencing good feelings again.

Amy was taking various steps to 'control her mind'. She was not drinking alcohol or taking any drugs, including medication. She was meditating every day, avoiding crowds, and trying not to look at people's faces in case they distorted. Amy agreed to try some behavioural experiments to test whether these strategies were actually preventing her from losing her mind. She went with her therapist to a busy shopping centre. Although Amy felt anxious, she did not lose her mind. Her therapist taught her to use stimulus discrimination, and she practised this while looking at people's faces, which did not distort. Amy also agreed to try experiments including drinking a glass of wine, and another of taking a paracetamol tablet, neither of which led to her hallucinating again. She concluded that the symptoms she was experiencing were due to PTSD, rather than signs that she had permanently damaged her mind. As her symptoms improved, she also became sure that she had not died and gone to hell.

Hot cognitions

- People are out to get me
- I've lost my mind
- I don't know what is real and what is not
- My perpetrator can see inside my mind
- People think I am crazy

RELIVING AND UPDATING MEMORIES OF HALLUCINATIONS

Traumatic memories of psychotic experiences can be addressed using imaginal reliving, or a written narrative, and updating, in a similar way to memories of events that are externally, not internally, caused. If the client is aware that the experience was hallucinatory and/or delusional, it is often useful to update it with the information that the event did not occur in reality, and perhaps what stimuli were driving their misperception, if this can be established. Other updates can be included as required, for example, to include information about psychotic experiences and about current safety such as 'I'm not in danger now'.

Where memories are fragmentary or difficult to contextualise, the client and therapist can attempt to create a coherent narrative of what probably happened, where possible (Chapter 8). If it isn't possible to fill in the gaps, hotspots can be relived and updated individually.

Stephen, who experienced delirium in intensive care, completed a written narrative about his experiences. He reported multiple, disjointed memories, so he and his therapist selected a representative memory to write out, which included parts of the experience that Stephen had nightmares about. They added contextualising details where they could (in bold), from information in Stephen's hospital notes, and his wife's memories. They also gradually added hotspot updates (in capitals).

'I was admitted on February 22nd, with pneumonia. I'd been poorly for two weeks, but it just kept getting worse and eventually they decided I needed hospital treatment. On the ward, I was given antibiotics, fluids, and oxygen, but I was still feeling really unwell. **I don't remember it, but later that night they transferred me to ICU because I needed a ventilator**. On ICU, I started having really intense dreams. There were masked men on the ward, hiding under beds and behind curtains. I KNOW NOW THAT I WAS EXPERIENCING DELIRIUM, WHICH IS REALLY COMMON IN ICU BECAUSE OF ALL THE DRUGS I WAS BEING GIVEN. I KNOW THAT IT IS ONLY A TEMPORARY PROBLEM, AND I DON'T HAVE IT ANYMORE. THE MEN WEREN'T REALLY THERE, IT WAS PROBABLY SHADOWS OF PEOPLE MOVING AROUND THE WARD THAT I SAW AND THOUGHT WERE REAL PEOPLE.

In one memory, the men are gathered around my bed. They are wearing balaclavas. I KNOW NOW THAT PEOPLE WOULD HAVE SOMETIMES GATHERED AROUND MY BED, LIKE ON THE WARD ROUND, OR IF THEY WERE GIVING ME SOME KIND OF TREATMENT AND MY MIND MIGHT HAVE THOUGHT THEY WERE THREATENING. I MIGHT HAVE SEEN PEOPLE WEARING BALACLAVAS BECAUSE MY MEMORIES OF THE TROUBLES WERE GETTING MIXED INTO THE DREAMS. The men are covering my mouth to stop me shouting out. They put something in my mouth. I think they are trying to suffocate me, to kill me. I KNOW NOW THAT THIS MIGHT HAVE BEEN A MEDICAL PROCEDURE, LIKE WHEN THEY WERE VENTILATING ME, THAT MY MIND GOT CONFUSED WITH THE DREAMS. I AM STILL ALIVE. I KNOW THAT BECAUSE I CAN LOOK IN THE MIRROR AND SEE MYSELF. I CAN LOOK ON MY PHONE AND SEE PHOTOS OF ME AND THE GRANDCHILDREN. I CAN TAKE A DEEP BREATH TO SHOW MYSELF I CAN BREATHE OKAY NOW.

I had lots of different dreams like this, and it felt like it was going on forever. I know now that I was on ICU for three days. I'm not there anymore, I'm back home. The next clear memory I had was seeing my wife and her telling me I was going to be okay. **I got transferred back down to the ward when my oxygen levels had stabilised. My wife had visited lots while I was in ICU but I don't remember**. I felt really groggy, but it was reassuring to see Anne there beside me. I remember looking around to see if there were any masked men, and I couldn't see any. Over the next few days, my condition improved and I felt clearer in my head. I was discharged on March 6th and continued to recover at home.'

Working on trauma memories where the client has ongoing psychotic symptoms

For many people with PR-PTSD, the psychotic experiences have passed. However, some clients will continue to have psychotic symptoms, either due to a psychotic disorder or secondary to their PTSD. Issues of comorbidity are covered in Chapter 20 and involve careful assessment and joint decision making with the client about how to best address different disorders using evidence-based treatments. Current guidelines (NICE, 2014), and a growing body of evidence (de Bont et al., 2016; Keen et al., 2017; Paulik et al., 2019; van den Berg et al., 2015; Ward-Brown et al., 2018) have shown that treatment for PTSD in the context of psychosis is possible, effective, and safe. Van den Berg et al. (2020) describe a phased approach to working with PTSD within psychosis, involving a shared formulation and psychoeducation, trauma-focused work on memories, and work on related appraisals. These phases are flexible, and there is the option to include techniques drawn from CBT for psychosis as needed (e.g. Morrison, 2017).

FAQ: How do I know what is a flashback and what is a hallucination?

It can be challenging to disentangle re-experiencing symptoms from hallucinations because they have many similar qualities. Hallucinations often incorporate aspects of past experiences while feeling 'in the present' (Hardy et al., 2005); however, they may not be a direct replay of an experience, which is more typical of a flashback. For example, people may hear the voice of their attacker or abuser, or another persecutory voice, saying thematically similar things to the time of the trauma, but not exactly the same. This would tend to be considered a trauma-related hallucination. Flashbacks are when people experience a replica of the trauma happening again and afterwards recognise it as a memory.

Supporting your client to identify, label, and record their PTSD and hallucination symptoms can help build a sense of predictability and control over what they experience. Looking back at when and how different symptoms started can also help to make sense of how they are causally linked to specific events and each other.

All the strategies we have described in this chapter can be used with people who have ongoing psychotic symptoms, if PTSD is the priority and focus for treatment. Some additional considerations may be important.

TEACH COPING STRATEGIES TO MANAGE PSYCHOTIC SYMPTOMS

Helping your client to develop some control over their psychotic symptoms can be useful, especially if the client is feeling overwhelmed, and to help them approach associated trauma memories. Work on managing ongoing hallucinations may draw on techniques such as coping strategy enhancement (Tarrier et al., 1990), responding to command hallucinations through testing the power of voices (Birchwood et al., 2014), and other techniques derived from CBT for psychosis (Morrison, 2017).

CREATING A CONVINCING RATIONALE FOR MEMORY WORK

People with PTSD and psychosis will be troubled both by memories from the past, as well as current fears driven by hallucinations and/or delusional beliefs. In this case, the rationale for memory work may be that dealing with the troubling memories could help them to cope with their concerns in the here and now. Reducing the sense of current threat created by trauma memories may have a positive impact on some current psychotic symptoms (Brand et al., 2018).

PREPARE FOR TEMPORARY SYMPTOM EXACERBATION

Just as PTSD re-experiencing symptoms can temporarily increase following work on trauma memories, psychotic symptoms such as voices sometimes also become briefly more intense which, in some cases, can prompt disengagement from treatment (Brand et al., 2020). To mitigate this, we discuss the possibility with our clients before commencing the work and closely monitor their symptoms throughout treatment. Clients will generally be aware that certain forms of stress lead to an increase in symptoms, so a similar explanation for why symptoms may temporarily increase is usually understood.

PRIORITISE AND ADAPT FOR DISSOCIATION

Dissociation may be an important shared process in both PTSD and psychosis, so it is important to address this early in the treatment arc (Chapter 6). Paulik et al. (2020) provide a useful set of clinical recommendations for managing dissociation in voice-hearers they were treating using imagery rescripting. As well as techniques such as grounding strategies, they suggest slightly adjusting the process of rescripting, including agreeing details of the rescript before starting to reduce unpredictability and uncertainty, pacing the rescript as needed, for example by introducing the rescript earlier in the trauma memories to reduce the intensity of emotion, and the therapist taking a greater role in leading the rescript, as well as monitoring dissociation, reassuring, and grounding the client as required.

FORMULATING TREATMENT TARGETS

There are likely to be different pathways between traumatic experiences and psychotic symptoms (Hardy, 2017). As already mentioned, some hallucinations seem clearly linked to specific traumatic experiences, and may be explained as decontextualised trauma memories, much like those found in PTSD, but which are not experienced as memories, and are instead experienced as representing a current external threat (Steel et al., 2005). Imaginal reliving and updating may be most appropriate for these types of memories, which are relatively circumscribed, and show a direct relationship to the psychotic symptoms. A second pathway links voices not to particular trauma memories, but as auditory images which have been generated from beliefs influenced by trauma memories. For example, someone who has had an abusive relationship may experience auditory hallucinations of critical voices, including unknown people commenting on their appearance or threatening them. Imagery rescripting may be more helpful than reliving where the content of the hallucinations is indirectly or thematically related to traumatic experiences (see Paulik et al., 2019, for a case series and tips).

NOTES FROM THE THERAPY ROOM: ABDI

Abdi was born in Somalia and came to the UK with his family in his teens. Abdi initially found it difficult to adapt to life in the UK, struggling to keep up at his new school and missing his friends back home. His family experienced racial harassment from neighbours in the temporary accommodation where they first lived. By the time Abdi was 18 years old and had finished school they had a settled place to live, and Abdi made friends locally.

Abdi regularly smoked marijuana and sometimes chewed khat. He began to experience some paranoid symptoms, such as believing the police were following him and planning to arrest him to send him back to Somalia. One night, at a friend's house, Abdi began to hallucinate. He believed that his friends had reported him to the Somali authorities and that soldiers were coming to the estate to arrest him and his family. He had auditory and visual hallucinations of soldiers trying to break into his friend's house and hid in the bathroom. His family became concerned after they received numerous panicky phone calls and called an ambulance. Abdi spent a few days on a psychiatric ward, where he was assessed and prescribed medication. He was then referred to an early intervention for psychosis team.

Over the next few months, Abdi's mental state stabilised and he followed the advice of his medical team to stop using recreational drugs. He no longer had persecutory beliefs about being arrested, but he remained terrified of the police. He had no further hallucinations of soldiers but was re-experiencing memories of the night he had locked himself in the bathroom. He dreamt about soldiers coming to arrest him. Abdi felt nervous in small rooms and didn't like to lock the bathroom door. He felt anxious when he was outside, especially if he saw someone in uniform, and was avoiding seeing his friends. Abdi's therapist assessed him for PTSD and discussed the diagnosis with Abdi.

Together, Abdi and his therapist developed a shared understanding of what had happened that night. Abdi's therapist gave him information about the effects of marijuana and khat, including that they can both cause paranoia. Abdi had heard about people having bad reactions to drugs before but hadn't realised they might have been affecting his thinking processes. They also talked about the stress Abdi had been under in the lead-up to the episode. He had experienced several difficult life events, including the abuse from neighbours, and was feeling under pressure to get a job to support his family. They also drew links between the content of Abdi's persecutory beliefs and hallucinations and his experiences growing up in Somalia which, in Abdi's childhood, was an unstable and often frightening environment. His fears of being arrested also seemed linked to Abdi's experience of the protracted asylum process, during which he had constantly feared being deported. Abdi's formulation is in Figure 11.1.

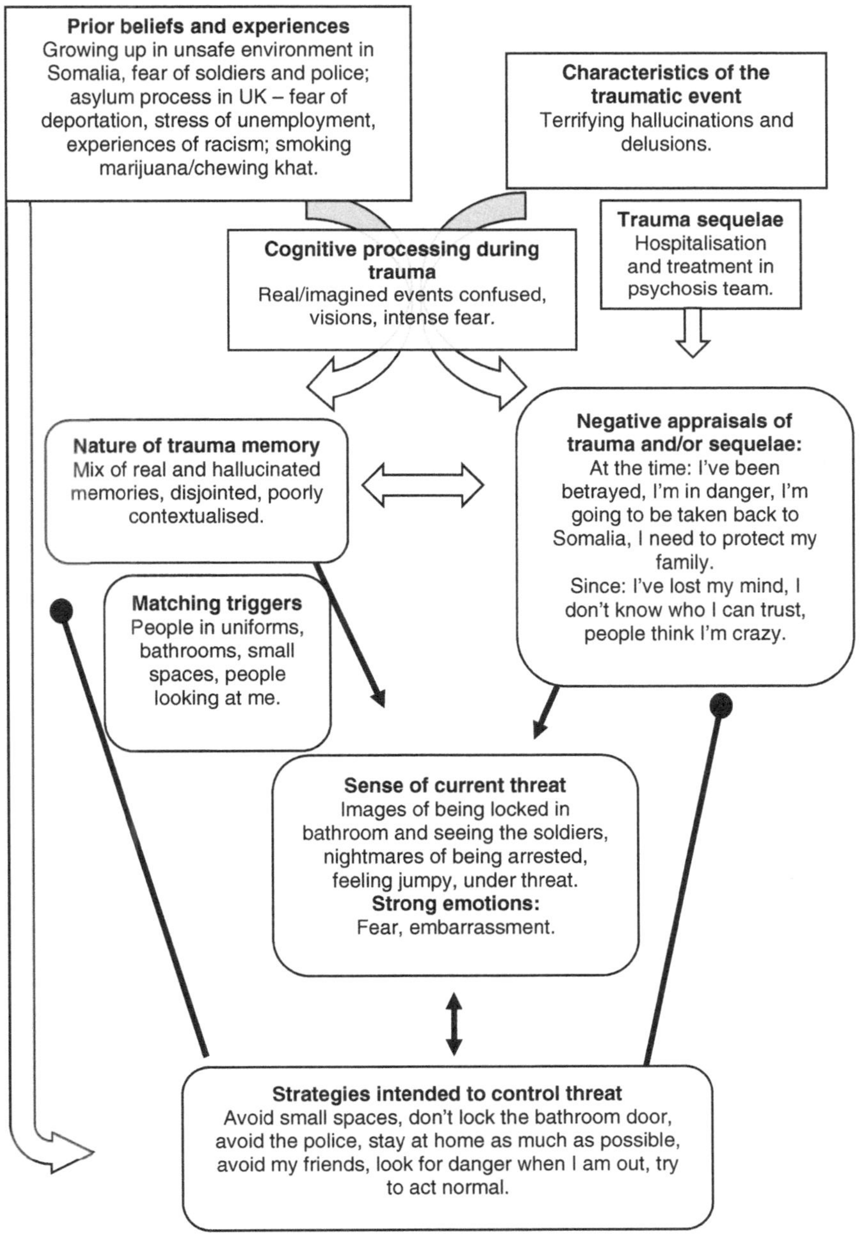

Figure 11.1 Abdi's formulation

This discussion helped to normalise Abdi's psychotic episode as an understandable reaction to stress. His therapist also explained about PTSD, using the metaphor of a linen cupboard to explain how Abdi's terrifying and confusing experience had not been properly put away into his memory system, so kept popping out in the form of images or nightmares. They decided to create a written narrative of the night when Abdi had believed he was going to be arrested, including updates of what he now knew to be true. Abdi found this process helpful, and read the narrative through several times with his therapist, clarifying details and discussing new updates. His re-experiencing symptoms reduced.

Abdi remained hypervigilant to people in uniform and was nervous of the police. His therapist taught Abdi to use stimulus discrimination and they practised looking at images of people in uniform online and noticing the differences between them and the Somali soldiers. They also discussed the differences between the UK police and the Somali authorities. Abdi had experienced some unpleasant interactions with the police in the UK but recognised that these were not as directly dangerous as his experiences with the military in Somalia had been. They also practised stimulus discrimination in small rooms, including the toilets at the clinic, and in his bathroom at home.

Focusing on these differences helped Abdi to gain the confidence to conduct some behavioural experiments. He first watched his therapist, then himself approached and asked a policeman for directions. He also went into a police station to request information about security marking his bicycle. Abdi found the police helpful in these experiments, which challenged his belief that he would be arrested.

In the final few sessions, Abdi and his therapist focused on relapse prevention. Abdi was concerned about having another psychotic episode, and the shame it would bring him and his family within the Somali community. They created a 'staying well' plan which incorporated the techniques which Abdi had found helpful in therapy, as well as general wellbeing strategies such as avoiding drugs, getting regular sleep, managing stressful situations, and how and when to seek further help if he needed it in future.

Recommended reading

Paulik, G., Steel, C., & Arntz, A. (2019). Imagery rescripting for the treatment of trauma in voice hearers: A case series. *Behavioural and Cognitive Psychotherapy*, 47(6), 709–725.

Stott, R. (2009). Tripping into trauma: Cognitive-behavioural treatment for a traumatic stress reaction following recreational drug use. In N. Grey (Ed.). *A casebook of cognitive therapy for traumatic stress reactions* (pp. 65–76). Routledge.

van den Berg, D., van de Giessen, I., & Hardy, A. (2020). Trauma therapies in psychosis. In J. C. Badcock & G. Paulik (Eds.). *A clinical introduction to psychosis: Foundations for clinical psychologists and neuropsychologists* (pp. 447–463). Elsevier Academic Press.

PART THREE

Complexity in cognitive work

CHAPTER TWELVE

Strongly held or long-standing beliefs

Beth was raped on holiday and described feeling guilty and stupid for having walked home alone. Her appraisals arose from long-held beliefs related to an earlier trauma, so were difficult to modify in therapy until earlier beliefs were also addressed.

Negative appraisals about the trauma and its aftermath often drive the sense of current threat that is central to the experience of PTSD. Working with these appraisals, and their underlying core beliefs, is a crucial element of CT-PTSD. Research suggests that changes in trauma-related appraisals during treatment predict subsequent reductions in PTSD symptoms (Kleim et al., 2013). As we'll explore in this chapter, strongly held negative appraisals, and long-standing core beliefs (grouped together, we often refer to these as 'meanings'), can be difficult to modify, so we draw on a wide range of cognitive and experiential techniques to address them.

Confirmation versus shattering of beliefs

We all hold fundamental assumptions, or core beliefs, about ourselves and the world, which are used to navigate daily life and generally go unquestioned. Most people who had a stable childhood with 'good enough' parenting hold relatively positive, optimistic beliefs. For example, they assume that the world and other people are benevolent, what happens in the world makes sense and is fair, and they themselves are generally decent, good, and worthy (Janoff-Bulman, 2010). By its nature, the experience of trauma strongly challenges these beliefs, and where they were overly positive or rigid, may even 'shatter' them (Janoff-Bulman, 1989), causing people to question everything they had assumed to be true.

> Richard had been a captain in the navy and was used to taking charge in highly stressful situations. He prided himself on being calm and decisive under pressure. After he retired, Richard was in a shop when an armed robbery took place. Richard panicked and froze. He stayed out of sight and did not intervene. Afterwards, Richard felt deeply ashamed that he had not tried to prevent the robbery. It shattered his view of himself as calm and brave, and left him believing he was now a failure and a coward. He began to doubt himself whenever he had to make a significant decision and feared that, if anything threatening happened again, he could not rely on himself to cope.

When people have experienced early life traumas, childhood adversity, abuse, or neglect, they may develop a much more negative view of themselves and the world. They may grow up believing there is something fundamentally wrong with them, that the world is unsafe and

DOI: 10.4324/9781003288329-15

unpredictable, and others will not protect them and will harm them. Subsequent negative life events may be appraised as further evidence for these beliefs, strengthening and confirming them. Events that do not fit with their beliefs (such as examples of people being kind or loving) are discounted or distorted to fit, for example, by labelling kind people as weak or stupid.

> Emma grew up in care because her parents were unable to look after her properly. She experienced numerous episodes of abuse as a child, including by older children in the care home and by staff. As a young adult, she met and married a much older man who was physically, emotionally, and sexually abusive. Emma described feeling that the abuse was normal and 'what she was used to'. She believed that she deserved to be mistreated, that it was 'all she was good for' because she was 'unlovable'; beliefs she had held since childhood. Her husband was repeatedly unfaithful and eventually left her for another woman, which devastated Emma despite meaning she escaped his abuse. She saw it as further evidence that others always betrayed her because she was worthless. Later, whenever her new partner was kind to her, she would become suspicious that he was covering up infidelity, angrily confront him, and call him weak when he wouldn't argue back.

Whether we are addressing 'shattered' or 'confirmed' beliefs in therapy, our goal is to help our clients to build flexible beliefs which can accommodate and adapt to a broad range of experiences including traumas. For example, that they are 'good enough', i.e. capable but imperfect, as susceptible as all humans to errors of judgement, but fundamentally decent with strengths and positive qualities, as well as flaws. Similarly, that the world is generally safe, predictable, and fair, but with occasional, sometimes entirely undeserved and random exceptions, both positive and negative, and that most people are good most of the time, but that rarely they may encounter very bad people. Building these beliefs can be particularly challenging for people who have held excessively negative, or rigidly positive, beliefs for a long time. However, it is still possible. Long-standing beliefs do not always require different cognitive strategies to those we typically use in CT-PTSD, but we may also need to add experiential techniques and take steps to address potential obstacles to belief change.

Discovering cognitions

Although there may be common themes, appraisals are highly idiosyncratic, so it is important to avoid making assumptions about the meanings people attach to their traumatic experiences. It is also important to closely attend to, and reflect back, our client's own words when talking about their appraisals, rather than our version of them. Some people can easily access and describe their appraisals, but others will struggle to put their thoughts and feelings into words. Here are our top tips for discovering them:

- *Ask*: Simple questions like 'what sense did you make of that?' and 'what went through your mind at the time?' will hopefully reveal appraisals, which we can further explore using 'downward arrowing' questions such as: '… and what did that mean to you?' or 'what was/is the worst thing about that for you?'. To check whether beliefs have been confirmed or shattered by the trauma, explore pre-existing beliefs and how they have changed, for example: 'is that something you've always believed?', 'has the trauma changed the way you think about that?', or 'what would you have said about that before the trauma?'.
- *Activate the traumatic memories*: Peri-traumatic appraisals might only be accessible when trauma memories are activated. When talking through memories, especially in imaginal reliving,

we ask our clients about what they were thinking at the time. This is especially relevant for hotspots, so, if your client is feeling emotional, it is a good opportunity to learn about 'hot' cognitions (alongside offering empathy and validation). You can do this during memory work or afterwards, e.g. asking 'you looked quite upset when you talked about that moment, what was going through your mind at that point?'.

- *Use a measure*: The Post-Traumatic Cognitions Inventory (PTCI; Foa et al., 1999) lists 36 common trauma-related cognitions (a 20-item version is also available) and is a useful tool, particularly if someone struggles to identify cognitions, as well as for monitoring how cognitions change during treatment. Another option is the Post-Traumatic Maladaptive Beliefs Scale (Vogt et al., 2012) which can be used similarly. Reviewing the results together, and discussing the most strongly endorsed themes, can help the client put their own exact words to each appraisal.
- *Follow the emotion*: Use your client's emotions to guide you in discovering appraisals. For example, fear is linked to appraisals about threat, guilt to appraisals of responsibility, anger to appraisals about unfairness, and hopelessness to appraisals of permanent change. Sometimes our clients describe emotions such as guilt, but the only appraisals they report are threat-related. This provides a clue that we have missed something and prompts further discovery.

Hot cognitions

- The trauma shows I am not the person I thought I was
- The world is more dangerous than I realised
- The trauma is just another example of how people always betray me
- My reactions during the trauma just prove again that I'm a useless person
- It's my fault that the trauma happened, and others think so too
- Life is pain, and it always will be

A HIERARCHY OF COGNITIVE TECHNIQUES

Once we have a good idea of our client's main appraisals, we can start addressing them in turn, starting with the ones most strongly linked with distress. All of the cognitive change techniques used in CBT are potentially relevant (for a recap, we recommend Westbrook et al., 2011). We use a hierarchical strategy to select a technique (Figure 12.1). By this, we mean starting with guided discovery techniques, which are relevant to everyone and highly effective for many, even those with long-standing beliefs. The next step, which is necessary for most people, is to actively seek evidence to challenge negative beliefs or strengthen new beliefs. If beliefs have not been successfully addressed by these two steps, we try to identify and address obstacles to change. All these steps may happen within a single session as we identify, modify, and test beliefs and, as new perspectives emerge, reintegrate them into the traumatic memories via updating techniques.

Working on appraisals and beliefs should never feel as if we are telling someone they are mistaken or irrational, and that we know what's right. Instead, we take an approach of collaborative empiricism, working together to understand the appraisals and their origins, consider alternatives, discover new evidence to test them, and weigh up the costs and benefits of holding on to them. Although we use the more common term 'thinking errors' here, we prefer to talk about 'thinking patterns' with our clients.

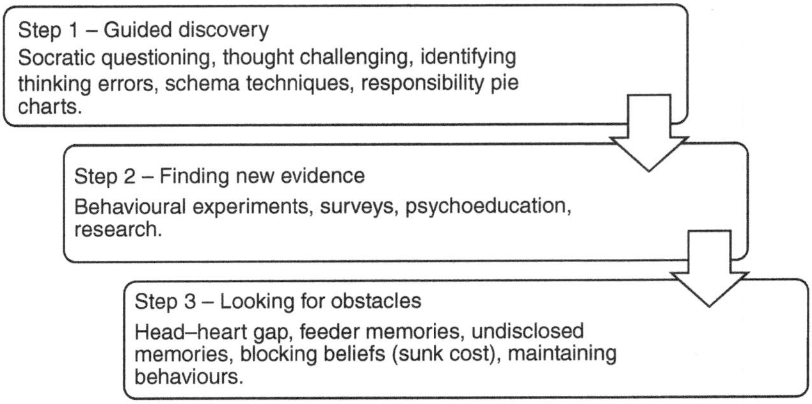

Figure 12.1 Hierarchical model of cognitive methods

STEP 1: GUIDED DISCOVERY

Socratic questioning

Guided discovery aims to bring our client's attention to information they already know, but haven't considered, or have discounted. Techniques such as Socratic questioning are fundamental to this process. As Padesky (1993) elegantly summarises, the aim of Socratic questioning is not to guide our clients to a conclusion that we have already made, but a genuinely curious approach to understanding our client's appraisals, and helping them reflect on them. The therapist asks exploratory/informational questions to learn more about a belief, listens carefully, summarises, and then uses analytical or synthesising questions to help the client examine how the information fits with their belief.

Richard's therapist explored his beliefs about his actions during the armed robbery.

THERAPIST: Has the trauma changed the way you think about yourself at all?
RICHARD: Yes, it's just made me feel ... you never know how you would respond in a situation like that, but I always thought I would be the kind of person who would step up, you know? Not someone cowering in the background. I'm so embarrassed.
T: So the way you responded didn't fit with the kind of person you thought you were? Can you tell me more about how you saw yourself before this happened?
R: I'm a navy man as you know. So there's that pride in facing up to danger, being brave, being disciplined. You're trained to turn towards danger, not away from it.
T: And I know you moved to quite a high rank during your career.
R: Yes, I was often in command of a ship and quite a lot of people. I had a lot of responsibility.
T: Do you think those experiences shaped how you saw yourself?
R: Yes, and I've always been quite sure of myself, quite decisive. And now I can't decide what to buy in the supermarket, it's so embarrassing.
T: You've mentioned being embarrassed before – is that a feeling you've had a lot recently?
R: Yes, I feel like I've let myself down, I suppose, and I feel like others can see that in me and they can't respect me.
T: Ok, so let me check I'm understanding. It sounds like you've always seen yourself as a responsible person, someone who faced up to danger and was respected by others. But how you responded in the robbery wasn't what you expected of yourself and it made you question that?

R: Yes, I suppose so. It was so sudden, the robbery. And not being at work maybe threw me off guard. I wasn't expecting it.
T: It sounds very sudden and unexpected. Did that affect your reaction?
R: Yes, I think so. In the navy, things were planned and there were systems in place, and other people there. You knew how to deal with situations that arose.
T: I see. So even though you were facing danger at times, you had systems in place to deal with it. But the robbery was different.
R: Yes ... my defences were down, I was just popping to the shop, it was so normal, you don't expect something like that.
T: No, of course not. And it makes sense that your defences were down, it was just an ordinary day. Looking back, what is it you could have done differently?
R: I don't know. This is what I go over and over in my mind. I could have tried to disarm him, but I wasn't in a good position, and it would have been risky for the shopkeeper. I could have tried to de-escalate it, talk to him.
T: Do you think that would have worked?
R: Well, the shopkeeper tried to reason with him, and he wasn't in the mood to listen. He was fired up. I think he was on drugs. I really thought he might use the weapon.
T: Could it have made it worse if you tried to intervene?
R: Possibly. Yes, I think it could have.
T: It sounds like there isn't anything obvious that you could have done differently? And acting might have in fact have made it worse?
R: I know. I just feel like I should have done something. I was the one with all the training, I know about firearms. If someone should have done something, it was me.
T: Yes, I see that. And I guess that fits with your view of the self before the trauma. That you would be someone who would face up to danger. But it sounds like this situation was different in some ways. You weren't at work, the situation was unexpected, and there wasn't an obvious beneficial course of action to take. How does that fit with your belief that you should have responded differently?
R: I guess it's just my pride talking. Maybe I need to accept that I couldn't have stopped it.

In this example, the therapist asks exploratory questions to help the client think through their belief, where it comes from, and how it fits with their trauma experience. They are led by the client's responses, rather than directing the discussion in a particular way, and use regular summaries. Ultimately, they bring the discussion back to the client's belief.

Thought challenging

More structured techniques to address negative thoughts can be used. Useful strategies include reviewing evidence for and against both the negative belief and an alternative belief, using the 'theory A/theory B' approach.

Rahul was a junior doctor covering a night shift when a patient under his care became seriously unwell and died. Rahul blamed himself for the death and stopped trusting himself to work with patients alone anymore. He was considering changing his career.

In therapy, Rahul's therapist explored his belief that he was to blame. Rahul thought he was not good enough to be a responsible doctor, and gave other examples of this, such as other mistakes he had made, and exams he had failed during his training. When his therapist asked how he had seen himself before the trauma, Rahul said that he had always been hard on himself, and had felt like he was under-achieving throughout his life.

Rahul's therapist helped him to consider an alternative theory, that everyone made mistakes sometimes, and that he was a good enough doctor. They looked for evidence for this theory and found plenty – Rahul had been considered good enough to pass his course so far, including positive feedback on his placements, a review into the patient's death had not found Rahul to be to blame, and there were many examples of him doing his job well.

Thinking errors

Thinking errors and distortions are common when people attempt to make sense of a trauma. For example, hindsight bias often exacerbates trauma-related guilt, where people believe they could have prevented the trauma if they had acted differently. Typically, this thinking error arises from people using what they know now (hindsight) to judge the outcome of their decisions and actions then. Working with this kind of appraisal involves helping the client to focus only on the things they could have known at the time of the trauma, as well as the context for making their decisions (e.g. events unfolding very quickly, effects of shock). Other common thinking errors in PTSD include over-generalisation (e.g. 'a group of youths attacked me, therefore all youths are dangerous'), all-or-nothing thinking (e.g. 'you are either good or bad, so I am bad'), and emotional reasoning (e.g. 'I feel guilty therefore I must have done something to cause this'). For a reminder of common thinking errors, read Burns (2008).

Emma was in an abusive relationship for 20 years. One of her appraisals was that she 'let it happen' because she had not left her husband when he started abusing her. Emma's therapist helped her to review this appraisal by looking at her timeline. The first time he had been violent was when Emma became pregnant with their first child, six months into the relationship. Emma's therapist encouraged her to cover the rest of the timeline and think about what she had known at the time and her reasons for not leaving her husband. Then, Emma was homeless, having recently left care, and did not have any close friends or family to support her. She was financially dependent on her husband and newly pregnant. Emma's husband had been apologetic after the first assault and promised it would not happen again. Emma loved him. It was her first serious relationship, and Emma had little experience of positive interpersonal relationships in general. In short, at the time, Emma was in a precarious social situation, with little experience or support to help her understand her husband's behaviour. She had no way of knowing that the assault was the start of a pattern of behaviour, and believed it was a one-off.

Reviewing her history in this way helped Emma to see that she had good reasons for staying with her husband at the time of the first assault and that choosing to leave would also have carried lots of risks. This helped reduce her hindsight bias and lessened her belief that she had 'let it happen' by not leaving her husband sooner.

Schema techniques

Long-standing and strongly held beliefs rarely change smoothly, nor suddenly with an 'aha!' moment. Instead, belief change is more a process of slowly 'chipping away', with evidence systematically being gathered and reappraised. Strong beliefs are hard to change because the experience of cognitive dissonance (evidence not fitting with an already held belief) is aversive. Instead, new evidence can be assimilated in a way that preserves the old belief, by categorising it as an exception, or with a 'yes, but …'. However, by gradually accumulating evidence that doesn't fit with the old belief, a 'tipping point' is often reached where it can no longer resist the weight of evidence. Schema change methods such as those described by Padesky (1994) can be useful here, particularly the continua methods and positive data logs.

Agneta was neglected by her parents throughout her childhood. As an adult, she worked as a carer and experienced an accident at work which left her with chronic back pain. Her employer was unsympathetic and Agneta lost her job. Agneta believed 100% that she was worthless, a belief that she had held throughout her life, but was further confirmed by her experience of the accident and its aftermath.

In therapy, Agneta's therapist used continua techniques to address the belief that Agneta was worthless. They identified an alternative belief: 'I am as worthwhile as other people'. Agneta's therapist asked her to define what qualities made someone worthwhile, and Agneta identified these as helpful to others, kind, caring, and loved by others. When Agneta rated herself on each of these attributes, she was able to see that she was a person who always tried to help others, was kind and caring to the people she had looked after at work, and was loved by her daughter and an elderly neighbour. Her belief that she was worthwhile increased from 0% to 20%. Her therapist also asked her to keep a positive data log to gather evidence that she was as worthwhile as other people by noting times when other people treated her with care, kindness, or respect.

Responsibility pie charts

People with PTSD often overestimate their responsibility for a trauma, so a useful intervention when working with guilt is to construct a responsibility pie chart. The therapist helps the client to list any people or situational factors which contributed to the traumatic event and/or their actions, with themself at the bottom of the list. A proportion of the responsibility is allocated to each person or factor and the pie chart is then drawn. In general, the client's 'slice of the pie' is then much smaller as it is shared with others.

Matt was based in Iraq with the British Army. One day, his unit was fired on while on patrol. Matt returned fire and killed one of the gunmen. Later, they came across the body alongside pictures of the gunman's family. Matt felt very guilty because he had 'taken away a little boy's father'. He rated himself as 100% responsible for the man's death

In therapy, Matt listed all the factors which contributed to the gunman's death. He included the man who had died, as he had made the choice to take up arms, and had also fired first. He also included his commanding officer who had ordered the return of fire. Matt's therapist encouraged him to think about factors that had led to him being in Iraq. Matt listed his stepfather who had been the reason Matt had joined the army, as well as Tony Blair and George Bush who had instigated the Iraq War. When he allocated slices of the pie to all these factors, Matt left himself with 20% of the responsibility for the man's death.

STEP 2: FINDING EVIDENCE

The techniques described so far often lead to changes in appraisals. However, very often these changes require consolidation, or further testing, through experiential techniques. Additionally, Step 1 techniques rely on a client already having access to the necessary information that challenges their beliefs. Sometimes, people do not have experiences or knowledge to draw on, so more investigation is required.

Behavioural experiments

Behavioural experiments are a core technique in CT-PTSD. They can be used to test a huge range of trauma-related beliefs and to collect evidence for new beliefs. Experiments can be spontaneous and carried out during therapy sessions; others will require more planning, or need to be done between sessions. Behavioural experiments are powerful, and often the most memorable sessions for our clients so we encourage you to do lots of in-session behavioural experiments, getting out of the office if you can. Read Murray and El-Leithy (2021) for more about behavioural experiments in PTSD.

Mukisa was beaten and tortured in his native country of Uganda when he was discovered having a same-sex relationship. In the UK, he was scared to go out in public, and particularly to be around African people, as he believed they would realise he was gay and attack him. Although Mukisa and his therapist had discussed different attitudes towards gay people in the UK compared to Uganda, Mukisa still felt very unsafe. His therapist helped Mukisa devise some behavioural experiments to test his belief. They walked together down a busy high street, and then Mukisa walked some distance on his own. He was not abused or attacked, and people did not seem to be staring. They also went together to an African restaurant and ordered a cup of coffee. Mukisa was not treated differently from other customers. Mukisa concluded that it was not apparent to others that he was gay or, if they had realised, he had not been mistreated as a result.

Top tips: How to design an effective behavioural experiment

We want our behavioural experiments to be as impactful as possible. Here's how:

- *Make it specific*: Try to make your experiment a true test of an appraisal. Remember these are idiosyncratic, so your experiment will be too.
- *Be spontaneous*: Many appraisals can be tested on the spot. You don't always need to complete a record form – check the belief rating and then go for it!
- *Make it memorable*: We want our clients to remember our experiments, and this sometimes means going outside their (and potentially your) comfort zone. Do something quirky or playful as part of your experiments.
- *Model it first*: In some experiments, you will need to model the behaviour first. Ask your client to observe and try it after you.
- *Take photos*: Ask your client to take a photo on their phone which captures the moment a belief is disconfirmed.
- *Watch out for safety-seeking behaviours*: Doing experiments together helps us spot subtle safety-seeking behaviours. If your client is doing something to guard against the feared outcome, try the experiment again without the behaviour.
- *Use momentum*: Often when a behavioural experiment has been successful, you can move immediately onto another. We may spend several sessions out of the office, doing multiple experiments.
- *Use the therapeutic relationship*: Your client is likely to be anxious, so you will need a strong therapeutic relationship. Stay warm, collaborative, and supportive throughout, use humour as appropriate, and respect your client's limits.

Surveys

A great way to get more data about a belief is to conduct a survey. This is particularly important if the belief concerns others' opinions. Free online survey tools make it easy to set up and conduct surveys anonymously and to collate the data. We recommend using a mix of quantitative and qualitative questions and discussing with your client who to circulate it to (page 148–9).

> Emma believed that other people thought she was weak and pathetic for not leaving her husband when he started abusing her. With the help of her therapist, she devised a survey which her therapist circulated amongst friends and colleagues. The survey briefly described the scenario Emma had found herself in and then asked:
>
> - What do you think about the woman in this scenario?
> - What do you think about her husband?
> - To what extent do you think this woman was weak and pathetic for staying in the relationship for so long? (0–100%)
>
> Please explain your answer
>
> - To what extent do you think the woman was responsible for the abuse happening because she didn't leave? (0–100%)
> - To what extent do you think her husband was responsible for the abuse? (0–100%)
>
> Please explain your answer
>
> - If you knew this woman, what would you want to say to her when you heard about her experiences?
>
> To Emma's surprise, none of the respondents thought she was weak or pathetic or responsible for the abuse. In their comments, they expressed sympathy and concern for her.

Psychoeducation and research

Another way to gather information about beliefs is via psychoeducation (if the therapist has access to relevant information) and/or research. It may be useful to speak to an expert in a particular area.

> Andrej was a security guard in a museum who tried to resuscitate a man who had a heart attack. Andrej had done first aid training and used the defibrillator that the museum kept, but the man died before the paramedics arrived. Andrej was devastated and believed he must have done something wrong during the resuscitation.
>
> Andrej's therapist helped him to research his belief. From an internet search, they learnt that less than 10% of people survive when resuscitation is attempted outside hospital, and only slightly more in hospital. Andrej's therapist also arranged for him to speak to a first aid trainer. Andrej explained what he had done and the trainer gave him feedback that he had acted correctly and had done everything he could to save the man's life. Andrej began to accept an alternative belief that 'I did everything right, but he was too unwell to survive, no matter what I or anyone else did'.

STEP 3: LOOKING FOR OBSTACLES

Head–heart gap

Head–heart gap describes the experience of believing something cognitively, but not feeling it emotionally. In our experience, it is one of the most common blocks in cognitive work, so much so that we have devoted a whole chapter to it, so see Chapter 14 for more.

Feeder memories

Another common block is when other memories which we have not addressed are 'feeding' the negative belief. These memories (even if they are not trauma memories) may require work in therapy, such as identifying and restructuring key meaning(s), updating and/or rescripting.

> Anthony was emotionally and physically abused by his wife for several years. He believed that he was weak for allowing the abuse to happen, and that other people would think the same. His therapist helped him to consider the evidence for and against this belief, conduct a survey, and complete behavioural experiments in disclosing the abuse to others. Although these interventions helped a little, Anthony continued to feel ashamed.
>
> When his therapist explored the origins of his belief further, Anthony mentioned the court case where his wife stood trial for assaulting Anthony. During the trial, his wife's lawyer had been scathing about Anthony's claims, suggesting that his wife (who was petite) could not have possibly assaulted Anthony, who was physically stronger. At the time, Anthony felt deeply shamed and believed everyone in the courtroom thought he was pathetic and a liar. When the case was dismissed due to lack of evidence, he felt even worse.
>
> Anthony's therapist thought these memories were supporting his beliefs about being weak. They rescripted the memories to allow Anthony to respond to the lawyer. In the new image, Anthony explained to the lawyer that he would never have fought back or harmed his wife, as it went against his morals. In the rescripted image, Anthony had irrefutable video evidence that the assault had taken place, which he showed to the courtroom, to vindicate himself, and convict his wife. The rescript made Anthony feel more powerful and less ashamed, which in turn helped address his belief that he had been weak for not preventing the abuse.

Undisclosed memories

Another block we sometimes encounter is when undisclosed memories relate to a particular belief. We access these using 'affect bridge' questions (Watkins, 1971) such as 'is there a time in the past when you felt this way?' or 'when was the first time that you believed that about yourself?'. These may elicit memories that the client has not previously thought to be important, or has deliberately not disclosed, perhaps due to shame or anxiety about possible negative consequences. Sometimes the client becomes more comfortable talking about these memories later in therapy when they have built sufficient trust in the therapist. If we suspect important undisclosed memories, we wonder aloud with our client whether we may be missing something important. This helps support our clients' autonomy and control over what they choose to disclose, rather than 'going digging' into their past. We also remind clients about confidentiality, reassure them that we are used to hearing about unpleasant traumatic experiences, and that, whatever they tell us, we will hold them in positive regard.

MAINTAINING BEHAVIOURS AND BELIEFS

Our work on appraisals is interwoven with identifying behavioural and cognitive strategies which maintain them. In turn, these may be driven by beliefs about appraisals, such as their uncontrollability or feared costs associated with challenging them. Addressing these is implicit in many techniques, such as surveys to overcome avoidance of talking about experiences with other people, and behavioural experiments in dropping safety-seeking behaviours. When beliefs do not appear to be changing, we review any further strategies which may be maintaining them, such as rumination or avoidance. It can also be helpful to explicitly discuss obstacles to change, such as 'sunk cost'. This arises where clients fear that costs of change – for example, letting go of blaming themselves after so long – means accepting having lost years of their life to unwarranted self-blame. You can find lots of helpful techniques for addressing these 'meta-beliefs' in Leahy (2003).

THE ONION

On page 68, we introduced the idea of trauma-related beliefs and emotions being like an onion. Once the outer skin of avoidance and other coping strategies is peeled away, we often find many layers of emotions and meanings underneath. We mention it again here as a reminder that cognitive work is often iterative, as we work through different layers of meaning. Don't be disheartened if you do some work on a particular belief and the client comes to your next session troubled by another belief or emotional reaction. This is perfectly normal. We don't usually have only one thought or feel only one emotion during traumatic events, and especially following multiple traumas. Keep working gradually and patiently through the different beliefs as they are revealed.

INTEGRATION WITH MEMORY WORK

Some trauma-related appraisals have arisen since the trauma, while others have their origin peri-traumatically, i.e. at the time of the trauma. For these types of appraisals, we include updates into the narrative or through imaginal reliving.

In some cases, updates will be very quick and easy and can be done in a single session. For example, if someone thought they were going to die in a traumatic incident, it is self-evident that they survived and we can immediately include that updated information when we work on the trauma memories. Other types of beliefs will require considerable work outside of the trauma memories. For example, if someone thought peri-traumatically 'I deserve this because I am a terrible person', and has a long-standing belief that they are a bad person which the trauma only seems to confirm, we may need several sessions of work on that belief to generate a meaningful update. There is little point in trying to update trauma memories with a new perspective that the client doesn't agree or emotionally connect with. Instead, we work outside the memories on addressing the underlying beliefs which are associated with key hotspots, and then we bring that information back to the trauma memories often in multiple 'layers' of update.

NOTES FROM THE THERAPY ROOM: BETH

Beth sought PTSD treatment after she was raped by a stranger while on holiday. She had left a night out with friends early as she was feeling unwell and was walking back to their apartment along a beach when a man approached her, engaged her in conversation, and then suddenly threatened her with a knife. He led her to a disused changing room where he assaulted her. Beth didn't report the rape or tell her friends. However, after a few weeks, she started experiencing gynaecological problems, and tests revealed she had contracted a sexually transmitted infection. Beth broke down in front of her doctor and revealed she had been raped.

In therapy, Beth was reluctant to talk about the rape and described feelings of guilt and fear when she thought about it. Beth completed the PTCI, and scored highly on items such as 'the event happened because of the way I acted' and 'the event happened to me because of the sort of person I am'. When they discussed these cognitions, Beth revealed that she felt stupid for having walked home alone and for having talked to him, and that she was an 'easy target'. Her therapist helped her to review the evidence for and against these beliefs but Beth struggled to think of any evidence against the belief and disclosed that she had always thought of herself as stupid, after struggling at school with learning and being picked on by bullies.

Beth's therapist decided to help her gather more evidence to address her beliefs. They conducted a survey about the attack, asking people whether they thought Beth was 'stupid' or an 'easy target' for having walked home alone. Most people disagreed with these statements and thought the rapist was to blame for the attack, not Beth. They also completed a responsibility pie chart, but Beth wanted to give herself at least 50% responsibility for the assault, even when other factors were taken into account. Her belief ratings remained at 90%.

In session six, Beth revealed that she was raped by her first boyfriend when she was 16 years old. Beth had never told anyone and tried to forget it, but was finding it impossible since the second rape. Beth's therapist commended her courage for disclosing the earlier trauma, and they added it to her formulation (Figure 12.2). Beth had not experienced PTSD after the first rape, but it had fuelled her belief that she was an easy target.

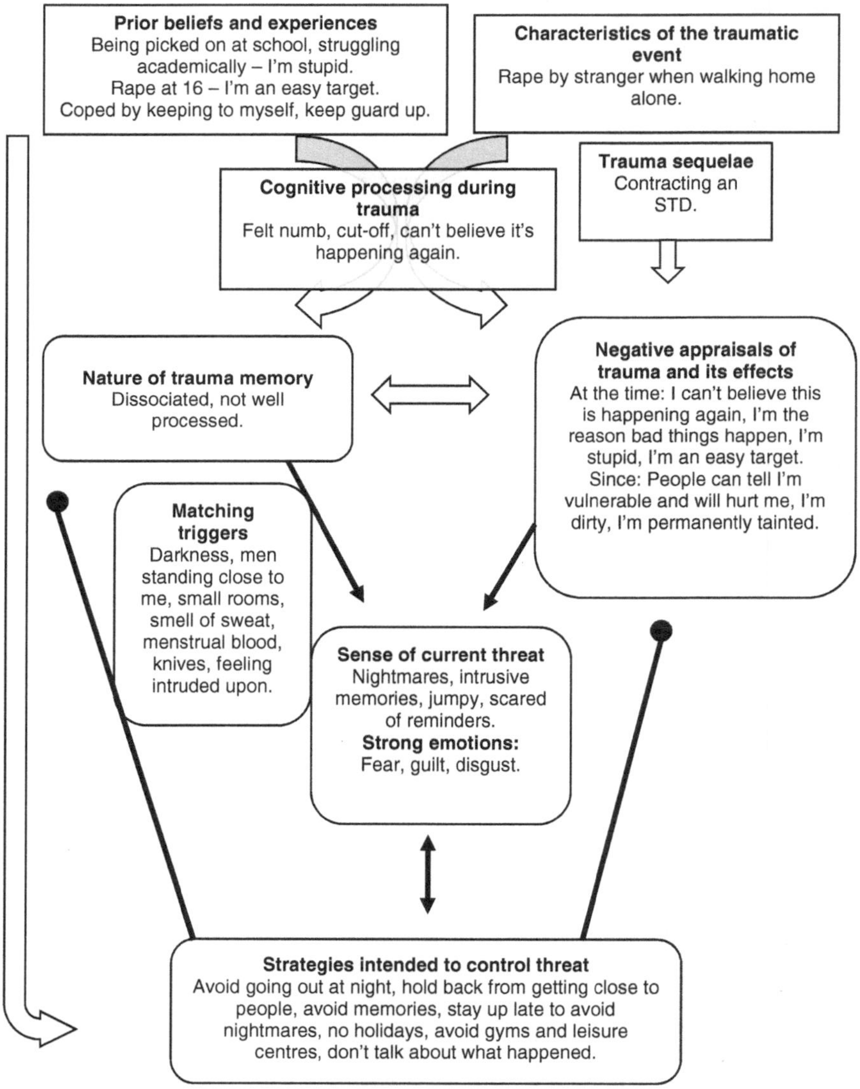

Figure 12.2 Beth's formulation

Gradually, Beth was able to give more details about the first rape. Her boyfriend had told his friends that Beth was 'easy' afterwards, and Beth felt humiliated. She believed he had targeted her because she had few friends and wasn't confident enough to stand up for herself. However, when they examined the evidence for this belief, Beth acknowledged that she had refused to have sex with him several times before the rape, and had broken up with him afterwards, both signs of standing up for herself. They did an imagery rescripting session where Beth told all of his friends that he was a rapist, and they were disgusted with him and threw him out into the street. She also imagined her older sister, who Beth was close to, comforting her 16-year old self and reassuring her that she was not stupid or an easy target.

Beth's belief ratings in being 'stupid' and an 'easy target' reduced to 70%. Beth reviewed the survey and the evidence chart again, trying to imagine she was reading about a stranger rather than herself. She agreed with most of the survey respondents and was able to identify more evidence against the belief. Beth acknowledged that she was harder on herself than she would be on someone else.

Beth's therapist helped her plan some behavioural experiments to gather further evidence. She practised disclosing information that made her feel vulnerable to her friends, to test if they then mocked or took advantage of her. She tried going out after dark, first with her sister, and then alone, to test whether she was attacked again. She also visited a gym with her sister, taking the risk to use a changing room on her own. Beth was working as a receptionist at a doctor's surgery and asked her boss for a review of her progress. Beth's boss gave her positive feedback which boosted her confidence. She also told one of her colleagues that she sometimes worried about making mistakes and often felt stupid. Her colleague was surprised, and told Beth she saw her as smart and reliable. Beth's therapist set her the task of noting down any examples of times when she did something which wasn't stupid. Over several weeks, Beth's belief ratings dropped to 30%, and the strength in her new beliefs (that she was of normal intelligence and had been unlucky rather than an easy target) rose to 70%.

These updated beliefs, together with the evidence Beth had gathered for them, were added into the trauma narrative at related hotspots. After reading this several times, Beth described increased confidence in the new beliefs and said the memories were feeling less powerful.

Recommended reading

Murray, H., & El-Leithy, S. (2021). Behavioural experiments in cognitive therapy for Posttraumatic Stress Disorder: Why, when, and how?. *Verhaltenstherapie*, 31(1), 50–60.

Padesky, C. A. (1993). Socratic questioning: Changing minds or guiding discovery. *A keynote address delivered at the European Congress of Behavioural and Cognitive Therapies, London* (Vol. 24).

Padesky, C. A. (1994). Schema change processes in cognitive therapy. *Clinical Psychology & Psychotherapy*, 1(5), 267–278.

CHAPTER THIRTEEN
Self-attacking beliefs and emotions

Yusra was imprisoned for eight months in prison in Sudan and subjected to humiliating and degrading sexual torture. Her PTSD symptoms included a continuing felt-sense of being 'dirty' and she was highly self-critical about feeling defeated during the torture. Her therapist used a combination of cognitive and imagery techniques to address her beliefs and update the trauma memories.

Self-attacking beliefs are extremely common after traumatic events, linked to feelings of guilt, shame, contamination, self-disgust, and humiliation. These beliefs and associated emotions may arise peri-traumatically and are therefore re-experienced when the trauma memories are triggered, or may arise after the trauma. Either way, they represent an important target in therapy. Not only are they highly distressing, but self-attacking beliefs also maintain PTSD by creating a sense of internal threat and driving strategies that prevent recovery such as withdrawal from others. Secondary problems such as depression may also develop, and guilt and shame have been linked to self-harm and suicide (Chapter 23).

The cognitive, experiential, and memory-focused techniques described in Chapters 12 and 14 are highly relevant; in this chapter, we focus on how to implement them effectively to target self-attacking beliefs and related emotions.

Understanding self-attack

People internalise social norms and expectations, leading to the development of core beliefs against which we compare our experiences and behaviours (Cunningham, 2020). When we fail to meet our internal standards, negative self-beliefs arise and lead to emotions such as guilt and shame. These commonly co-occur and overlap conceptually. Guilt after trauma usually relates to perceived responsibility, for example for failing to prevent the trauma, acting in a way that contributed to a worse outcome, or failing to recover afterwards. Shame usually follows a more global negative judgement of the self and is associated with feeling small and inferior, with an urge to hide, whereas guilt is more commonly associated with an urge to make amends. Guilt and shame may have been experienced peri-traumatically, or later on when looking back on the trauma, and can be internal (beliefs about the self) or external (beliefs that others will blame/shame them) (Lee et al., 2001).

Humiliation is a slightly different emotion from guilt or shame, as it is usually inflicted on one person by another. We may have felt humiliated during a trauma, but not feel ashamed or guilty about it. Humiliation is often linked to powerlessness, and consequently to anger, and the frustrated urge for revenge. Anger may have been felt peri-traumatically, or develop when viewing the trauma in retrospect, and is often maintained through rumination. Prolonged traumas such as torture often result in an experience of mental defeat, where an individual loses

DOI: 10.4324/9781003288329-16

a sense of their own identity and autonomy, feeling they are an object rather than a person, and no longer caring whether they live or die (Ehlers et al., 2000). Some clients feel embarrassed or ashamed that they experienced mental defeat.

Disgust is a common peri-traumatic emotion, particularly during traumas involving contact with dead bodies, bodily fluids, some forms of torture, as well as sexual assaults, and can lead to an ongoing sense of mental contamination (Fairbrother, & Rachman, 2004). Beliefs related to being 'tainted' or 'polluted' are reinforced by re-experiencing symptoms that bring back the peri-traumatic sense of being dirty, infected, or contaminated. A sense of 'moral disgust' is also common after traumas that violate an individual's personal standards (Chapter 15). Attempts to wash the feeling away, or neutralise it, are generally unsuccessful, reinforcing the belief of permanent change. Mental contamination is a common experience for many OCD sufferers (Coughtrey et al., 2012), and some people with PTSD develop similar compulsive washing behaviours.

Tanaka was a military nurse who assisted with clearing a mass grave while he was based in Bosnia. Tanaka had seen dead bodies and bad wounds before, but handling the partially decomposed bodies in the grave, some of which had been mutilated, made Tanaka feel disgusted and disturbed. Tanaka had always been someone with high personal standards of cleanliness, but after clearing the grave he began to wash excessively, cleaning his hands many times a day in response to a feeling of contamination.

Hot cognitions

- If I hadn't done x or y, the trauma would not have happened
- I should have seen it coming and prevented it
- The trauma happened because of the kind of person I am
- The trauma shows I am pathetic/worthless/unlovable
- The perpetrator wanted to degrade me
- I gave up, I wanted to die
- I'm dirty, I'm permanently tainted, 'damaged goods'

How to help

Although we have listed our interventions here depending on the primary emotional response, typically clients experience multiple emotions, and there may be various layers of meaning within a particular hotspot that need to be addressed, some of which will only become apparent as you progress (peeling the layers of the onion, page 68). Furthermore, some important appraisals may not have been present peri-traumatically, but arise later. The techniques in this section can be used for either type of appraisal. In general, those which arose and were present peri-traumatically need to be updated during imaginal reliving of the associated hotspot, as they tend to be impervious to change without activation of the memory itself. However, it can still be helpful to update post-traumatic appraisals while reliving aspects of the traumatic memory that might feed into them, as a way of enhancing the reappraisal and/or bridging head–heart gap.

Michelle was sexually assaulted by her boyfriend's housemate. During the assault, he forced her to perform oral sex and Michelle's most distressing re-experiencing symptom was the taste and smell of semen which engendered a strong feeling of disgust and revulsion. After working on this hotspot in therapy, it became less intense and Michelle became aware of other emotions and meanings about the assault. Another hotspot emerged of the man telling Michelle 'she wanted it'. Although, at the time of the assault, Michelle was certain that she did not 'want it', afterwards it made her wonder if she had somehow behaved in a way that had encouraged the assault, which made her feel ashamed. Addressing this in therapy, Michelle and her therapist talked about sexual consent and Michelle recognised that she had never given consent or encouraged the assault. They updated the trauma memory with this information, and Michelle imagined telling the perpetrator that he was lying and deserved to be in prison. Michelle felt less ashamed and instead began to feel very angry with the perpetrator of the assault, and with her boyfriend who had initially refused to believe Michelle. She decided to report the attack to the police.

DISGUST, HORROR, AND CONTAMINATION

Formulation and normalising

As usual, helping clients to better understand their symptoms is a good starting point. A feeling of dirtiness in the absence of an actual contaminant is distressing and can be confusing, so normalising the experience is helpful. We usually sketch a simple formulation to explain how the unprocessed memories of the trauma are bringing back the feelings of contamination experienced peri-traumatically, emphasising that trauma memories aren't re-experienced just in our minds, but also in our bodies.

This can also help explain why attempts to wash away the feelings tend not be effective, as the sense of dirtiness is created by internal processes such as images, memories, and thoughts, not by any external physical changes. We can demonstrate this quickly using an in-session behavioural experiment, by picturing with our client something unpleasant (but not linked to the trauma) like biting into an apple and finding half a maggot, or putting our hands in a jar of soiled nappies, or by accessing another unpleasant memory, like the last time we vomited, and noticing what feelings this provokes.

Psychoeducation

It can help clients to know that disgust and horror are natural responses to potential contaminants, and most likely evolved to protect us from infection and disease. Therefore, it is completely normal to experience feelings of disgust and physiological reactions around certain stimuli. We include this information to help people understand their feelings and reactions, and to reduce any self-blame.

Steve was a police officer who was called to the home of a man who had died some weeks ago. The smell was very bad and the body looked disfigured because it had been partly eaten by the man's pet dog. Steve experienced an immediate disgust reaction, retching and leaving the house to get fresh air. He felt embarrassed by his response and believed his colleagues would have handled the situation better. His therapist explained that disgust was an automatic response, with an urge to vomit an evolutionary strategy to protect against contamination. They conducted a survey that showed that most people believed they would respond similarly in such a situation and did not judge Steve's reaction negatively.

Separating self-disgust from other-disgust

A common thinking error occurs when people conflate disgust at others and their actions (often towards them) with self-disgust. It can be helpful to discuss this and to make the difference clear. Important updates often include 'he is the disgusting one, not me' or 'it was disgusting, but I am not'.

Cell renewal update

A useful strategy developed by Jung and Steil (2012, 2013) includes asking clients to research how often their cells renew (about every 4–6 weeks for skin cells, more frequently for mucous membranes), and then to calculate how many times they have renewed since the last contact with the contaminant (they developed it for survivors of sexual abuse, but we have found this works well with other types of contamination trauma too). This is followed by an imagery exercise (see later), which clients are encouraged to access when the feeling of contamination is triggered. We also find the exercise leads to useful updates which can be reintegrated into the trauma memories, e.g. 'my skin cells have renewed 92 times since he last touched me. Not an atom of him is left on me anymore'.

Other 'clean' updates

Similar updates can be created through Socratic questioning, to demonstrate that the client is no longer physically contaminated (e.g. counting how many times they have washed since the trauma, evidence that other people do not perceive them to be dirty etc.). Updates need to encompass the full range of perceptual and sensory details as well as cognitive and verbal information (see also page 160) and frequent interweaving between cognitive work and memory work will be needed to fully integrate new information. For example, when using a verbal update like 'I'm clean now, there's nothing on me', the client could look at and touch their skin to show it is clean, apply hand cream and smell their hands to show that they smell pleasant.

Imagery rescripting

Updates can also be introduced through imagery rescripting. Jung and Steil (2012) recommend helping the client to develop an idiosyncratic image to represent the concept of skin renewal and give examples such as imagining the old skin as a suit which they can unzip and step out of, or can shed like a snakeskin. We have sometimes used the image of a speeded-up film of cells renewing, like those on nature documentaries.

As well as skin renewal, we have found other imagery rescripts helpful to support updates like 'I am clean now', such as a beam of light passing over the body or a 'magic waterfall' which washes away any contamination. We may use a 'body scan' exercise to identify where the sense of contamination is felt and then help the client to develop an idiosyncratic image of it being washed away, elaborating it with sensory details including smell and taste.

Behavioural experiments

Many people with mental contamination avoid looking at and touching their own bodies because it feels dirty to them. This maintains the belief, and prevents the memory being updated. We use behavioural experiments to test the effects of interacting more with their body. Such experiments can also incorporate elements of compassion through self-care, such as rubbing moisturiser into parts of the body that are normally avoided, and viewing the body with kindness rather than disgust. Later behavioural experiments may include allowing others to touch the body, for example having a manicure, haircut, or foot massage.

For clients who are washing excessively, or using other behaviours compulsively to feel clean, behavioural experiments focus on testing the effects of reducing and, ultimately, dropping the behaviours. We find these experiments tend to be best attempted after some memory work, as the physiological sensations generated by re-experiencing symptoms can otherwise overpower cognitive learning. It can be helpful to encourage clients to respond to the urge to clean by using their 'mental cleaning' imagery, perhaps augmented by a 'clean' smell, such as sniffing a tissue with a drop of very diluted antiseptic.

Resuming intimacy

Resuming or establishing intimacy after a sexual assault or abuse is a treatment goal for many of our clients. If the client has a partner, we ideally involve them in therapy, to develop a plan everyone is happy with. Often sex has become a source of anxiety and tension so we advocate initially 'banning' sex, and first focusing on building up intimacy without the expectation it will end in sex. A graded hierarchy can be established, for example starting with hugs, holding hands, or wherever the client feels comfortable, and gradually increasing the level of physical intimacy at a pace determined by the client. Using stimulus discrimination helps when aspects of sexual contact are triggers to memories and, if possible, we teach the partner how to prompt discrimination.

For clients who aren't in a relationship, an intimacy hierarchy can still be created, with tasks such as hugging friends, going to a salsa class, or having a massage to become more comfortable with physical contact, and items like telling a trusted friend something personal as exercises in increasing emotional openness.

GUILT

Responsibility pie charts

As discussed in Chapter 12, a pie chart can be used to illustrate the degree of responsibility held by the different people and situational factors contributing to the occurrence of the trauma. In general, on reflection, the client will see that they have been allocating too much of the blame to themselves. Young et al. (2021) recommend doing this exercise with objects rather than simply drawing a pie chart, for example making piles of buttons, rice, or clay to represent portions of responsibility. Norman et al. (2019) recommend another visual tactic: making a row of dominoes to represent the different factors that led to the trauma occurring. The message is that, even if the client represents one of the dominoes, the action that makes the dominoes fall, and all of the other dominoes, also contribute to the outcome.

Surveys

Surveys are a useful way of assessing a range of opinions on someone's responsibility for a trauma, especially when they are struggling to see it from a different perspective (example in Chapter 12).

Top tips: How to get the most out of a survey

Surveys can be a powerful intervention for guilt and shame. Here's how to make the most of them:

- *Design it together*: Ask your client what questions they would like answered by the survey and offer suggestions if they get stuck.

- *Target the appraisals:* The most effective surveys target the client's idiosyncratic appraisals, so try to choose questions that will address these.
- *Choose your audience*: Check with your client whose opinions they would like to gather. It may be a general range, in which case you can circulate the survey amongst your own friends and colleagues, or a specific group you need to target, e.g. new mothers.
- *Use a mixture of quantitative and qualitative items*: Quantitative items allow a neat presentation of statistics and graphs, e.g. 'how much do you believe the woman in this scenario was responsible for the attack? (0–100%)' while qualitative items often provide useful detail e.g. 'what would you want to say to this person if you knew her?'.
- *Use software*: Online survey tools make it easy to circulate, anonymously collect, and collate responses.
- *Check predictions*: Before discussing the results, ask your client for their predictions or ask them to fill in the survey themselves.
- *Generalise meanings*: After looking through the results, review the implications for the target appraisals, e.g. 'what does this tell us about your belief that you are 100% to blame for the attack?'.
- *Check for 'yes, but ...*: Check for any thoughts that might minimise the findings. e.g. 'they are just being nice' and address them. If needed, do another survey with a different group or different questions.

Bird's eye view or different perspective reliving

Another good way to access a different perspective on responsibility is to ask the client to relive the trauma from a different angle, such as from above, or imagining they are a neutral bystander observing the trauma. This encourages a more objective standpoint on responsibility and can encourage self-compassion.

Aalia was sexually abused by her uncle in childhood. She felt very guilty when she remembered the abuse as she had felt very close to her uncle as a young child and believed she had invited the abuse by wanting to cuddle him and sit on his knee. Aalia's therapist asked her to imagine watching one abuse memory from above as if it was someone else. Aalia saw that the little girl just wanted attention and did not invite or want sexual contact. She felt sad for her younger self and more self-compassionate.

Busting rape myths

Beliefs about sexual assault are often influenced by so-called 'rape myths'. For example, that sexual assaults by strangers are 'worse' than those by partners, friends, or colleagues, leading many survivors feeling that their experience isn't 'real rape' or is somehow less traumatic if it didn't involve being snatched off the street. 'Perfect victim' myths include ways that people behave before, during, or after a sexual assault; for example, if they had previously been friendly towards their attacker then they have 'invited' it, or that failing to report an attack immediately makes it less credible.

Consent is an issue that often needs discussion, as many sexual assault survivors feel they somehow consented to sexual activity if they did not fight their attacker. More commonly, people freeze up, are too drunk or drugged to fight back, or comply with the assault for fear of being killed. Coercion into sexual activity is also common, whether it is a result of grooming, an abusive relationship, or a power imbalance. We find resources such as the 'Tea and Consent' video made by the Thames Valley Police and a useful worksheet designed by the NHS entitled 'What is consent?' (both available online) provide a good starting point to establish whether the client gave consent or not. It can also be useful to discuss the possible consequences of fighting back as, often, this would have led to greater physical harm. Education about the freeze response as a natural instinct to avoid further injury can be useful (Chapter 6).

Other thinking errors

As described in Chapter 12, several common thinking errors are linked to guilt. Kubany and Manke (1995) suggest that guilt is usually linked to appraisals about perceived wrongdoing, acceptance of responsibility, perceived lack of justification, and false beliefs about pre-outcome knowledge caused by hindsight bias. We also commonly encounter emotional reasoning ('I feel guilty, so I must have done something wrong').

SHAME

Silencing the inner critic

Many clients with high levels of shame report an inner voice that criticises them continually. Noticing, labelling, and externalising this 'inner critic' is the first step to reducing its impact. Some clients will recognise the voice from earlier experiences, such as a critical caregiver in childhood.

The 'teacher A/teacher B' metaphor is a useful exercise to recognise the detrimental impact of the inner critic (Stott et al., 2010). Clients are asked what the impact would be of a teacher who consistently criticises and puts down a child (teacher A) versus a teacher who encourages and supports a child, even if they don't get everything right (teacher B). Clients usually recognise that teacher A would cause a child to be demotivated and more likely to underperform compared to teacher B. Parallels can then be drawn to the effect of negative self-talk.

Clients are encouraged to practise speaking to themselves with kindness. Exercises such as imagining they are speaking to someone they care about who is feeling hurt and upset, or writing a compassionate letter to themselves, are useful ways of familiarising clients with this skill. Self-compassion may take some time and practice to embed, especially if someone has a long history of self-criticism.

The perfect nurturer

Another useful technique, developed by Deborah Lee (2005) is to imagine a perfect nurturer, an idealised caregiving figure who encompasses the qualities of compassion, to provide a cognitive and emotional reframe to self-criticism, helping clients to access feelings of self-compassion.

> Darrell had been continually criticised as a child, as his father believed it would 'build his character'. When Darrell sought treatment for PTSD following an abusive relationship, he realised that his inner voice was highly critical, constantly telling him that he had deserved the abuse. Initially, Darrell found it very difficult to speak to himself with kindness. With the help of his therapist, Darrell learnt to recognise when his 'inner bully' was talking and to instead consult his perfect nurturer (an elderly man with the kindness of Darrell's grandmother, and the reassuring voice of David Attenborough).

Addressing earlier beliefs

Many people who report high shame during or after a trauma have pre-existing beliefs which have left them vulnerable to self-critical interpretations of events. Where high shame is present, we ask clients if they already held similar beliefs before the trauma, or felt that way at other times in their life. Adding earlier experiences and beliefs to the formulation and drawing links to their current appraisals can be helpful. Long-standing core beliefs can be addressed using schema techniques such as continua methods and positive data logs (page 136–7). 'Feeder memories' may need to be addressed (page 140) through reliving or rescripting.

Surveys

Surveys are useful tools, especially for external shame, where the client has negative beliefs about how others will view them. Collecting responses anonymously allows the client to experiment with disclosure, and can form a first step to disclosing the trauma to others.

HUMILIATION, MENTAL DEFEAT, AND ANGER

Getting on side

Normalising and empathising with these types of emotions is important, rather than seeking to immediately relieve them, as clients often need to vent their feelings and have them acknowledged before they can move forward. These traumas can be difficult to disclose and can trigger anxiety about being judged by the therapist, so we make it very clear that we are on the client's side.

Psychoeducation

We normalise the client's emotional response as completely appropriate given their experiences and provide psychoeducation if necessary about their peri-traumatic behaviours and emotions. For example, we would explain the concept of mental defeat, and how it is an appropriate reaction to an inescapable situation, referencing research into learned helplessness and the '6 Fs' model of dissociation (Chapter 6).

Another useful area of psychoeducation can be understanding the motives and techniques of perpetrators. For example, the intent of torture is generally to mentally destroy an individual rather than to extract information, and/or to spread fear in a community. Interpersonal abuse often includes stages of grooming or 'love bombing' to gain an individual's trust, followed by strategies to control and silence them. Understanding such tactics can reduce self-blame by helping clients reattribute their responses to the perpetrators' strategy and intentions, not their own personal qualities.

Updates differentiating then from now

Other important updating information includes making a clear distinction between the situation the client was in at the time of the trauma, and the situation now. This is important because clients may have generalised the meaning of what they did or felt at the time of the trauma.

> Carmen was abducted and tortured by FARC rebels in her native Colombia. Amongst other punishments, she was forced to strip naked and repeat 'I am a cowardly Colombian woman' in front of her guards and other prisoners. Carmen felt deeply humiliated at the time, and felt angry and dirty when she remembered this part of the trauma.
>
> Carmen believed 'because I did and said those things, it means I am a coward'. She updated the memory with 'I did and said those things because they made me – it does not mean they are true. Then I had no choice, but now I have the power to decide what I do and say.'

Restoring identity, dignity, and connections

'Reclaiming your life' tasks when the main peri-traumatic emotion has been humiliation or mental defeat should include those which restore or reinforce a sense of identity, dignity, and autonomy. These types of traumas also often lead people to withdraw from social contact, as they fear judgement and their trust in others may have been damaged, so reclaiming connections with other people is also important (Ehlers et al., 2000).

> Lucy was groomed and abused by a sex abuse ring as a teenager. The abuse continued over several years, and Lucy described a sense of losing any self-respect and feeling she was a 'toy' to be passed around and used by men. Her reclaiming life tasks were chosen to help restore Lucy's sense of identity and autonomy. She began to choose clothes and make-up which she liked, rather than those she had been told to wear. She signed up to an adult education college and frequently looked at her ID card from the college to remind herself of the person she now was. Her therapist encouraged her to mix with other students at college, and slowly open up to new friendships based on mutual respect and trust.

Imagery rescripting

As usual in imagery rescripting, we discuss with the client what they would like to happen in a memory for it to feel better. Where the peri-traumatic emotion is humiliation, mental defeat, or anger, rescripts will often include an element of mastery such as gaining strength to overpower the attacker, and sometimes to shame or humiliate them. The aim here is to regain a sense of control, rather than to fuel revenge fantasies or rumination (page 186), so we monitor the effect of rescripting on these emotions, and shift tactics if they are not resolving. Other options include imagery rescripts involving mastery without revenge (such as imagining scenarios in which the client feels strong, loved, and not preoccupied with the perpetrator) and interventions to reduce rumination.

Notes from the therapy room: Yusra

Yusra was arrested for protesting against the government in Sudan. In prison, she was tortured and raped over an eight-month period before she was freed and fled to the UK. Yusra described nightmares and flashbacks of the torture, and a continual sense of being dirty and 'ruined'. She had developed behaviours such as washing herself with bleach to try and feel clean, and had been for numerous HIV tests but did not feel reassured by the negative results. Her formulation is in Figure 13.1.

Yusra's therapist helped her complete a timeline of her experiences and fill in an intrusions diary so they could identify the most distressing events. They agreed to work first on a torture memory during which Yusra had been sexually assaulted and urinated on by one of the guards. The memory was strongly linked to Yusra's feelings of contamination. Talking about it made Yusra feel nauseous and have a strong urge to wash, so they agreed to work on some 'clean' updates before reliving the memory. Yusra found the skin renewal update helpful and practised an associated image which she generated of peeling off her old skin as if it was a layer of glue, to reveal her clean, fresh skin underneath. They updated the memory with this new information and image, and also used an imagery rescript where Yusra overpowered the guards, tied them up, and freed herself and the other prisoners. Yusra began to feel less contaminated and was able to engage in

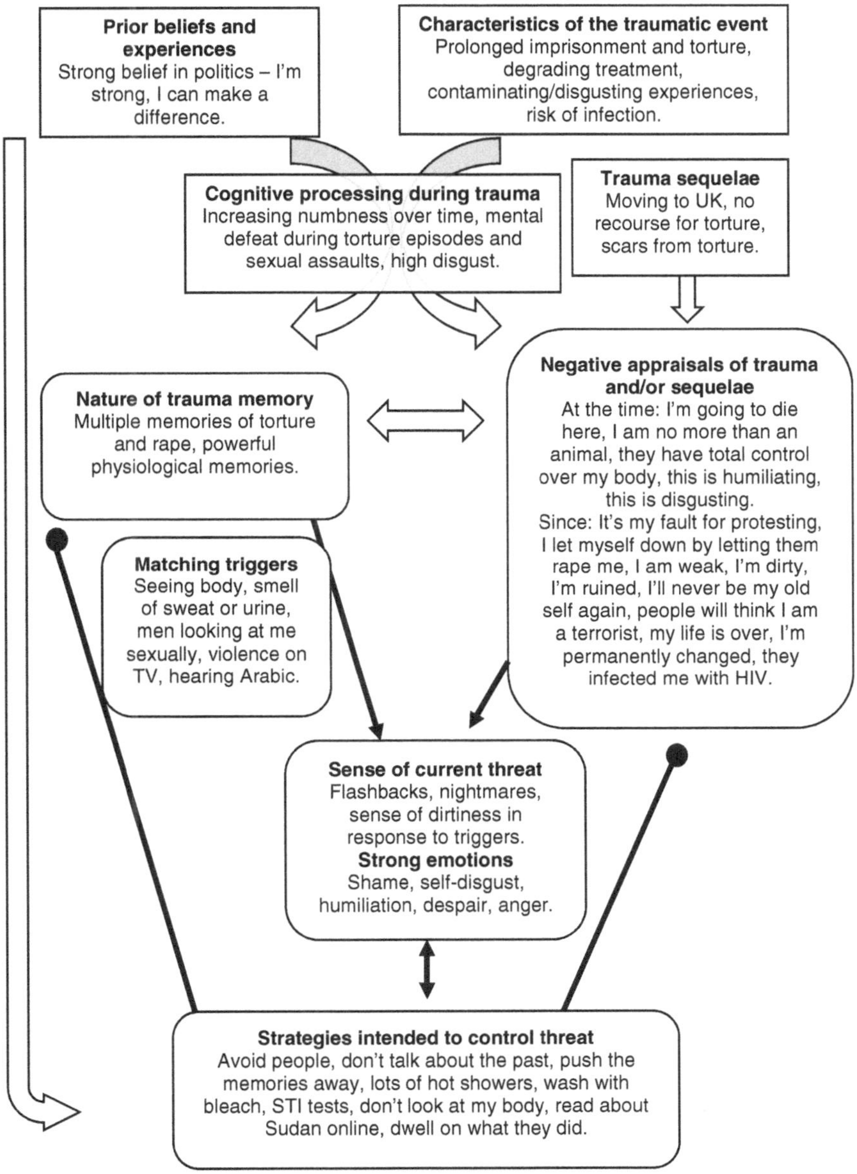

Figure 13.1 Yusra's formulation

behavioural experiments in dropping her excessive washing, and viewing and touching her own body again.

Another major cognitive theme was guilt associated with the sense of mental defeat Yusra had experienced during her imprisonment. Here, her therapist tries to better understand her beliefs and provides some psychoeducation about learned helplessness. The information forms the basis for a more compassionate reframe of Yusra's experiences.

THERAPIST: Tell me more about this belief that what happened was your fault?

YUSRA: I helped organise the protest, I made that decision.

T: Does that mean you deserved what happened later?

Y: No, I didn't deserve it. But, what hurts me most is that I stopped fighting it.

T: What do you mean?

Y: By the end, I was so weak. I was tired, I was hungry, I was sick. I stopped caring, I just wanted to die. I let them do whatever they wanted.

T: So, you stopped caring, and you stopped fighting, that makes you think it was your fault?

Y: Not so much my fault, it just pains me that I was so weak.

T: What do you think would have happened if you did fight back?

Y: I tried at the start, but it didn't help.

T: I see. Can I tell you about something you might find interesting? There's something called 'learned helplessness'. It's when we learn that we can't do anything about a situation and we stop trying. Years ago, there were some famous psychological experiments conducted with dogs and cats. They had them in a box and they gave them electric shocks. Some of them could escape and some couldn't. When they couldn't escape, they stopped trying after a while. And then, when they were later in a situation where they could escape, they didn't try. They lay down and accepted the shocks.

Y: That's so sad.

T: It is. Why do you think I am telling you about this?

Y: Because I am like the cats. I couldn't get out, so I just accepted what they did to me. It makes me sad, thinking about those cats.

T: What do you think those cats needed after the experiment?

Y: They need someone to hold them and care for them and show them it is over now.

T: I know cats can't understand, but what would you want to say to them?

Y: I talk to my cat! I think she can't understand, but she knows my voice.

T: How would your voice be if you were speaking to the cats?

Y: Calm, nice. I would tell them they are good cats, it isn't their fault, they were in the cruel experiment. It is over now.

T: Do you think they would believe right away that they are free?

Y: No, maybe they need to run around a while, see they aren't in the cage anymore.

T: So the cats need someone to speak to them kindly, to hold them and care for them, to show them they are free. Is that what you need too?

Y: Yes, I suppose I do.

T: What you said to the cats, what would it be like to say that to yourself?

Y: That I'm a good cat?

T: Ha, yes, exactly. Or you are a good person, and it wasn't your fault what happened, and it is over and you are free now.

Y: These are things I need to say to myself, but it's hard.

Yusra's therapist asked her to keep a photo of some cats on her phone, with a note about what she wanted to say to them. She practised this every day, and said the same words to herself as well. The information formed the basis for a more compassionate update which her therapist helped her to bring into the trauma memories.

Recommended reading

Jones, A. C., Brake, C. A., & Badour, C. L. (2020). Disgust in PTSD. In M. Tull & N. Kimbrel (Eds.). *Emotion in Posttraumatic Stress Disorder* (pp. 117–143). Academic Press.

Jung, K., & Steil, R. (2012). The feeling of being contaminated in adult survivors of childhood sexual abuse and its treatment via a two-session program of cognitive restructuring and imagery modification: A case study. *Behavior Modification*, 36(1), 67–86.

Lee, D. A., Scragg, P., & Turner, S. (2001). The role of shame and guilt in traumatic events: A clinical model of shame-based and guilt-based PTSD. *British Journal of Medical Psychology*, 74(4), 451–466.

CHAPTER FOURTEEN

The head–heart gap

Melody was physically, emotionally, and sexually abused in childhood and developed beliefs that she was 'weak', 'damaged', and 'worthless'. When she reviewed these beliefs in therapy, Melody experienced a head–heart gap; she could identify evidence that she was not worthless, yet she couldn't connect to it emotionally.

Head–heart gap, or rational–emotional dissociation (Stott, 2007), describes the experience of knowing something to be true intellectually, yet not feeling it is true emotionally. Most people can recognise this experience in their everyday lives in the form of 'irrational' emotions. For example, many people feel guilty when they walk past a police officer, even though they are not behaving illegally, or know that drinking and smoking are harmful but still find them enjoyable. In PTSD, the experience is integral to the condition; people know that their trauma is in the past, but feel like it has just happened, or is about to happen. Indeed, important parts of therapy are about reducing the head–heart gap. Updating trauma memories, for example, aims to join together elements of cognition and emotion that aren't yet fully linked.

Head–heart gaps commonly emerge in therapy after what seems like useful cognitive work. For example, after helping our client calculate the probability of experiencing another trauma to discover it is infinitesimally low, we may find little change in their rating of the belief 'the world is unsafe' and the client may feel as anxious as ever. While this can be frustrating, for us as well as our clients, it is not surprising. Human beings do not reason like computers. We are influenced by a myriad of factors besides logic, including emotions, memories, urges, needs, and intuition. When we encounter head–heart gaps clinically, it is generally unhelpful to repeatedly emphasise the rational alternatives to a distressing belief. Instead, we step into our client's shoes and try to understand what else might influence their belief. We then find ways to help them join up what they know in their head, to the feeling in their heart, and their gut. This chapter explains how.

Hot cognitions

- I can see what you're telling me, but I just don't feel it
- I just can't put that feeling into words
- People keep telling me this is true, but I can't accept it
- It makes sense now, but when the memory comes or I'm in a similar situation, I still feel the same as I did then
- I wouldn't think that of someone else, but it feels different when it comes to me
- It's my gut instinct, and I always trust my gut

DOI: 10.4324/9781003288329-17

FIRST STEPS AND CORE TECHNIQUES

ACKNOWLEDGING AND MAPPING THE SPLIT

Clients often feel frustrated, or think that they are failing at treatment, when they cannot 'feel rationally'. They may also struggle to describe the confusing experience of simultaneously holding two positions, one thought and the other felt. We first label and normalise head–heart gap as a common experience, both in PTSD treatment and in everyday life, and give some examples. We then introduce a way to quantify the gap, so encouraging our clients to both accept the divide and work to resolve it. Here Stott (2007) recommends using a two-dimensional belief chart, where the horizontal axis represents their rational judgement and the vertical axis their emotional judgement. There is an example at the end of the chapter. This allows us to disentangle the confusing experience, and monitor the effects of our interventions in a more nuanced way than taking standard belief ratings.

USING THE HIERARCHY

In Chapter 12, we recommend a hierarchical strategy of cognitive techniques, starting with Socratic questioning and moving to seeking new evidence. It is most common for a belief to change logically but not emotionally when we have only used questioning techniques, which is why seeking new, compelling evidence is so important. Often people need to see or experience something to fully believe it, so before you move on to the other techniques described in this chapter, try the techniques at the second level of the hierarchy, particularly behavioural experiments targeting the relevant belief.

> Following a train crash, Carly became terrified of using trains. Together with her therapist, she worked out the probability of being in another train crash. They discovered that around 1.7 billion passenger journeys happen every day in the UK, and crashes are extremely rare, so Carly's chance of being in a similar accident again was tiny. Although Carly recognised how small the risks were, she still felt extremely anxious at the thought of using a train again.
>
> Carly's therapist helped her plan a series of behavioural experiments to target the belief 'trains are dangerous'. They went to a busy train station and observed how many trains arrived and departed the station without an accident. They then took a train journey together and used 'then versus now' discrimination to keep Carly's thoughts and feelings focused on the present, rather than being influenced by her trauma memories. The journey passed without incident, and Carly decided to make the journey back on her own. Carly began to use the trains again more regularly to 'prove the point', albeit still feeling anxious. Over time, however, her belief about being in another accident dropped and she felt less anxious.

UNDERSTANDING AND RESOLVING HEAD–HEART GAPS

There are several potential causes of head–heart gaps, so formulation is key to devising a solution.

THE CLIENT CANNOT ARTICULATE KEY MEMORIES, MEANINGS, AND EMOTIONS

Where trauma memories are very poorly elaborated or lack higher-order cognitive processing, they may be experienced primarily in a highly sensory, almost 'wordless' form. The associated meanings may then be so hard to identify and verbalise that they cannot be restructured. This most often arises when perceptual processing during the trauma is almost entirely 'data-driven' because of dissociation, loss of consciousness, or intoxication during the trauma, or where the client experienced very intense sensations (e.g. extreme pain) or overwhelming emotions (e.g. paralysing fear).

When working with these kinds of memories, we need to find ways to help our client fully articulate their experience, including how they felt then and what their memories mean now. The aim is to develop more concrete and verbally accessible ways to represent their emotional experiences, so providing 'anchors' for discussing and restructuring the associated meanings. We first create a timeline of the event as the client recalls it, and then focus on incrementally adding in details within each level of representation (spatial, sensory, somatic, proprioceptive, emotions, meanings, images etc.), as if we are re-mapping all the lines of a musical score (page 15). In some cases, we must find creative ways to help them articulate their experience. For example, we may ask a client to draw pictures, or create a collage of images from the internet, to represent every element of how something felt or what it meant to them.

Scott, who had a learning disability, was targeted by a group of people who used his flat to deal drugs. They had originally befriended him but later threatened him with violence if he told anyone about the arrangement. Over a year, they repeatedly threatened and bullied Scott. On one occasion, Scott's brother came to check on him and the group believed Scott had reported them and beat him up. When Scott was taken to hospital, social services discovered what had been going on and moved Scott into alternative accommodation. However, Scott remained terrified that the group would find and punish him. He was also having nightmares and flashbacks of the assault.

In therapy, Scott found it difficult to describe how the assault unfolded. His account was disjointed and mainly focused on sensory details, like the expression on the main perpetrator's face. Often he would describe current feelings of pain in his head and body. His therapist wrote the available details into a timeline, then gradually helped Scott fill in additional contextualising information. They started by elaborating the hotspots. His therapist asked Scott to draw their angry faces and they added the pictures to the timeline. They talked about why the group had been angry and wrote this information into the timeline. They drew a plan of Scott's old flat and plotted where each member of the group had been standing during the assault. Scott's therapist asked him more about the pain he had felt. He described it as 'like a train hitting my head'. They found a picture of a train on the internet and stuck it to the timeline, alongside an outline drawing of Scott's head and body, with places he felt pain coloured in red. They realised that the pain was probably due to memories of blows to his head and, as Scott had been lying on the floor, this was most likely from being kicked and stamped on. They added this information to the timeline. As they added more and more ways to represent the different aspects of his experience, Scott began to find more words to talk about his thoughts, feelings, and memories, and the nightmares began to reduce in intensity.

THE CLIENT STRUGGLES TO CONNECT THE OLD WITH THE NEW

One of the most common causes of head–heart gaps in PTSD is when new updating information has not been sufficiently integrated into the trauma memories. In this situation, we need to enhance, or 'amp up', our updates by making sure they address every layer of perception, emotion, and meaning.

Working through the onion

We've talked before about how different emotions and meanings can be like the layers of an onion. Sometimes, with head–heart gaps, our first update hasn't addressed all of the different layers or, as one emotion has reduced, another layer has been exposed.

Irena has been in a violent relationship, and during a particularly horrific assault, her boyfriend raped her at knifepoint. In the first reliving session, Irena reported that her main thought was that she was going to die and the main emotion was terror. Her therapist helped her to update the hotspot with 'I don't die here, I survive to tell the tale. This is old stuff'.

Irena continued to re-experience the memories, and her distress ratings did not reduce. Her therapist spent a session exploring the hotspots in more detail and asking more about what they meant to Irena. She identified more emotions, including helplessness, disgust, and shame, and additional meanings, such as 'I'm not fighting back because I'm weak', 'his sweaty body is all over me' and '(people will think) I'm letting him do this to me and that I'm disgusting'. It took several sessions to generate effective updates for these meanings, including through psychoeducation on the body's threat response, addressing her feelings of contamination, and conducting a survey about others' judgements following rape. These yielded updates including: 'I'm frozen because my body has gone into freeze mode, this is normal survival response when you can't run or fight', 'the safest thing I could do with a knife to my throat was to not move. It was not a sign of my consent or because I am weak', 'I was frozen then but I'm not frozen now', 'there's not an atom of his sweaty body on me anymore', and 'he is the disgusting one for what he's doing, not me, and others agreed in the survey'. When these additional updates were included in the next reliving session, Irena reported a much larger reduction in how distressing the memories felt.

Sewing the past and the present together

It can be difficult for clients to integrate updating information into their trauma memories. Our basic tactic is to bring the memories to mind, say or write the updating information, and try to hold this in mind alongside the trauma memories. If this does not work alone, we ask 'joining' questions to help the client to connect the past and the present, across every modality.

Top tip: Use questions to integrate updates

First, encourage the client to expand on the hotspot to access as much detail as possible, for example asking:

At that moment …

- What am I *thinking*?
- What am I *feeling*?
- What *images or memories* are in my mind?
- What is *happening*?
- What can I *see*, *hear*, *taste*, *smell*?
- What *sensations* are in my body?
- What is my *body position*?
- What am I *doing*?
- What do I *want to do*?
- What do I *need*?

Then, try to expand on the updated information in a similar way, asking:

When I remember it now …

- What do I *think* now about it?
- What do I *know* about what really happened?

- What do I *feel* now when I think of it?
- What can I *hear, see, feel, taste* now?
- What *sensations* are in my body now?
- What *body positions/actions* can I do now?
- How are my *needs* met now?
- What *sense* have I made of it since?
- What does it say about *me as a person*?
- Where does it fit into *my life story*?

Finally, stitch the two layers together by asking questions designed to link the memories and the new information, for example:

- *Knowing* that now, how does it change the way you *feel*?
- *Remembering* that now, how does it change the way you *think about yourself*?
- *Saying* that now, how does it change the way you *understand what happened*?
- *Feeling* that now, how does it change the *sense you make of it*?

Use different modalities

Traumatic events are far less a cognitive–verbal experience, than a sensory and perceptual one. Therefore, verbal updates may in themselves be insufficient; other modalities such as imagery, bodily positions, updating sensory information, and movements can be helpfully incorporated.

Isaac was caught in a firefight while he was based in Afghanistan with the British Army. One of his hotspots involved lying behind a wall with gunfire all around, thinking 'I'm not going to get out of this'. A simple verbal update 'I didn't die, I survive this' was included during his first imaginal reliving session but did not reduce the distress or intensity of the hotspot.

During the second attempt at updating the hotspot, his therapist helped Isaac include updating information across multiple modalities. At the time he had been crouched behind the wall and felt weighed down by his body armour, so they included a physical update by standing, stretching, and moving around to show himself it was now safe to move, while holding the hotspot in mind. At the time, it was unbearably hot and the air had been dusty. During the update, Isaac focused on the cool breeze coming from a fan in his therapist's office and breathed in the clear air. As well as feeling fear at the time of the trauma, Isaac had felt helpless, so they included an update that he was not helpless anymore and coupled this with a recent memory of finding out he had passed an assessment at work, which had made Isaac feel strong and proud. When they updated the memories with the information that Isaac had survived, Isaac also looked at a recent photo on his phone of his son's birthday party to remind himself that he was reunited with his family, something he thought at the time would never happen.

Use imagery rescripting

Imagery techniques can also 'amp up' updates. Visualising an update, represented in a vivid compelling image, can be more emotionally impactful and memorable than holding a verbal update in mind. In Chapter 1, we introduced the idea of 'retrieval competition' (Brewin, 2006), which suggests that better elaborated and more vivid memories will be recalled more readily than other memories. This suggests that if we can help clients create images, via rescripting, that are rich in detail and have powerful emotions attached, they should win the retrieval competition over trauma memories.

Joshua was forcibly recruited as a child soldier in the Lord's Resistance Army in Uganda. He had PTSD re-experiencing symptoms to many different traumas. In treatment for PTSD years later, he identified his most distressing memories related to a mortar attack on their camp, during which many soldiers were killed. Joshua recalled horrific memories of hearing his friends shouting for help, and screaming for their mothers as they died. He was also covered in their blood, and felt terrified, disgusted, and horrified. When he had nightmares of this event, he would awake still feeling and smelling the blood.

Updating the memories verbally did not reduce the nightmares, so Joshua's therapist helped him develop a new ending using imagery rescripting. Joshua's immediate and most important needs in the memories were to feel clean and safe, and for his friends to no longer be in pain and distress. He imagined that, immediately after the massacre, a nearby dam broke and flooded the valley, washing away the bodies and the blood. He imagined hearing the sounds of rushing water, then swimming across the valley and feeling himself washed clean. He imagined building a treehouse nearby where he was safe from attack and looking down to see the massacre was over. The image of the treehouse was particularly vivid for him as it was something he had built as a child. To help the rescripted memory stick, Joshua's therapist asked him to draw it like a comic strip. He kept a copy beside his bed as a reminder and looked at it every night before going to bed.

MEANINGS AND FEELINGS ARE SITUATION-DEPENDENT

Another source of head–heart gaps is when clients can only access key meanings and emotions when they are in situations associated with their trauma memories. We can overcome this in the therapy room by introducing multiple triggers, such as sounds, objects, and images related to the trauma, or by looking at pictures of the trauma site while working on updating. However, sometimes the simplest solution is to deliberately enter similar situations, access the memory, and introduce the updates 'live'. This can be most powerfully accomplished when re-visiting the trauma site.

Stuart was electrocuted by a faulty piece of equipment while working in a factory. After the accident, he became extremely cautious around any sources of electricity. He often had nightmares where he woke shaking, which he confused with the feelings of being shocked. He also panicked and shook when using almost all electrical equipment including light switches. Imaginal reliving and updating failed to decrease his nightmares and physical responses. Although Stuart understood intellectually that he had survived the shock, and that he was highly unlikely to be shocked again, he remained very fearful of electrical devices and his physical response to them.

His therapist realised the updates were not connecting when the memories were activated in imagination and decided to help Stuart activate the memories using triggers instead. They practised first with electrical equipment in the therapy room, touching plug sockets, electrical switches, and cables. Every time Stuart experienced a physical response, they brought in updates that the equipment was safe, that he had survived, and focused on bodily sensations which proved he was not being shocked. They then tried touching the pump in the fish tank in the waiting room (which Stuart perceived as more dangerous due to the electrical device being underwater). Finally, they contacted the factory where Stuart had worked and asked permission to visit. The same machine which had shocked Stuart was still there (now repaired) and Stuart and his therapist spent a session touching the machine and focusing on the updated information that Stuart was no longer in danger of electrocution and that his physical responses were caused by adrenaline.

MEANINGS REFLECTING PRE-EXISTING BELIEFS

The sense someone makes of a trauma is influenced by their previous experiences and beliefs. Sometimes head–heart gaps are due to the influence of earlier memories and/or beliefs, which may need addressing (Chapter 12).

> Karen had PTSD following a medical emergency. After reliving and updating the trauma memories in therapy, her symptoms improved but one hotspot remained highly distressing. When Karen was recovering in hospital, she was briefly left alone in a side room. She tried to call a nurse but no one came and Karen felt desolate and lonely. Updates to this hotspot, that the nurses were busy but still cared about Karen, and that her husband was on his way to the hospital, were helpful on an intellectual level, but Karen still described feeling empty and sad when she remembered this part of the trauma.
>
> Her therapist asked Karen if the feeling reminded her of any previous experiences. Karen revealed that she had often been lonely as a child. She was an only child and her parents worked long hours. Karen had been shy and found it difficult to make friends. She recalled memories of sitting alone in her family home, watching through the window as other children played and feeling sad and excluded. She had felt the same way in the hospital.
>
> Karen agreed to try rescripting the earlier memories by imagining entering the scene as her adult self. She took the younger Karen to the park to play and gave her a puppy, which Karen had desperately wanted as a child, to keep her company and give her love and affection. Older Karen reassured younger Karen that she was loved by her parents, that she would always be there for her if her parents were busy, and told her that she would grow up to have her own family one day. When asked to sum up how this rescript made her feel, Karen used the word 'loved'.
>
> Karen and her therapist then returned to the hotspot of being left alone in the side room. When they brought in the update 'people do care about me', Karen's therapist asked her to remember the rescripted memories and to focus on the feeling of being loved.

UNCONTEXTUALIZED IMAGES DRIVING DISTRESS

Another cause of head–heart gaps is when aspects of the trauma memories, or an associated image of future threat, have been 'constructed'. Examples include peri-traumatic 'worst case' images or imagined 'flash-forward' threat scenarios. In these situations, verbal updates may fail to connect at an emotional level because the powerful image feels more compelling. We discussed in Chapter 10 how to work with constructed memories. Briefly, the therapeutic goal is to create a coherent narrative for the memories, including identifying and labelling when peri-traumatic imagery is experienced. Constructed images can also be addressed through reliving, updating, and imagery rescripting.

> Amina was working in Syria for an aid agency when the building she was in was hit by a shell. As they evacuated, they heard gunfire from outside, and Amina was terrified that she would be killed. Luckily everyone survived, but Amina was plagued by flashbacks and nightmares after the incident.
>
> In treatment, Amina successfully processed and updated her trauma memories. However, her beliefs about vulnerability endured, alongside a recurring nightmare in which Amina was kidnapped by armed men. This had not happened in reality, but had been a constant fear for Amina while she was in Syria. The images in her nightmares represented 'worst-case scenario' constructed images, fuelled by stories she had heard from other aid workers. Amina's therapist helped her relive and update the nightmare with information that she had not been kidnapped and was now safe. She also rescripted the nightmare, giving herself magical powers to repel the armed men and create an invisibility shield that allowed her to feel safe.

SELF-ATTACK TRUMPS RATIONALITY

As discussed in Chapter 13, some people with PTSD experience powerful self-attacking negative thoughts. These may arise as trauma-related appraisals (e.g. 'I'm disgusting for letting the trauma happen') or may be long-standing beliefs that have been amplified by the traumatic experiences. A tendency to self-attack can lead to head–heart gaps because new, less threatening appraisals of traumas are understood intellectually, but fail to neutralise the toxic feelings of shame and self-hatred. Repeated cognitive reappraisal is unlikely to weaken long-standing self-attack and can lead to disengagement so, instead, we explore the origins of toxic self-attack and help the client develop their capacity for self-compassion as an antidote using techniques such as 'perfect nurturer' imagery (page 150) and chair-work techniques (e.g. Pugh, 2018).

Jian's parents had been very strict, demanding, and critical, and he had grown up hating himself and never feeling 'good enough'. As an adult, Jian was bullied by a work colleague, culminating in a violent and humiliating assault. Jian felt he was a disgrace for being assaulted and struggled to generate any alternatives to this appraisal. When his therapist suggested a more compassionate appraisal, he rejected it as 'pathetic'.

Rather than pursue this cognitively, Jian's therapist asked him to describe and imagine the qualities of a perfect nurturer. Jian explained there was a Buddhist goddess of compassion, mercy, and kindness, called Guan Yin, who was thought to watch over children and people in trouble. Jian had grown up hearing stories of Guan Yin in Chinese folklore. Jian and his therapist decided to use an image of Guan Yin to represent a compassionate viewpoint when Jian became self-critical. His therapist asked Jian to imagine what she would say to comfort him, and how it would feel to be unconditionally cared for by this compassionate being. They used Guan Yin's perspective to address Jian's thoughts such as 'I'm a disgrace' and to update moments in the trauma when Jian had felt ashamed. As he felt more able to access compassionate self-beliefs, Jian's therapist encouraged him to practise speaking to himself with Guan Yin's kindness, replacing her voice with his own.

Notes from the therapy room: Melody

Melody sought treatment in her mid-twenties with a history of multiple traumatic experiences starting in childhood. She had been raised alone by her father after her mother died. Her father used drugs and, when intoxicated, he was frequently physically and emotionally abusive towards Melody. He also allowed some of his friends to sexually abuse Melody when they came to 'parties' at the house. Melody left home at 15 years old and was homeless for several years. During this time, she was physically and sexually assaulted several times.

When she started treatment, Melody was living in temporary hostel accommodation. She was terrified of ending up back on the streets and having to resort to sex work to survive. She described a powerful sense of disconnection from her body, saying it had been 'used and abused' for so long that it was no longer her own. She self-harmed by cutting and burning herself, usually after flashbacks. Her formulation is in Figure 14.1.

Early therapy sessions focused on developing the therapeutic relationship, teaching grounding skills, and reducing Melody's self-harm behaviour. Melody dissociated frequently into immersive flashbacks in response to trauma triggers. She also described periods of disconnecting from her environment when she felt unsafe, as well as episodes of feeling and acting as if she was a child again. Melody's therapist helped her to label and track how these various forms of dissociation arose, and they practised applying different grounding strategies for each kind. Melody also learnt stimulus discrimination to help cope with her triggers.

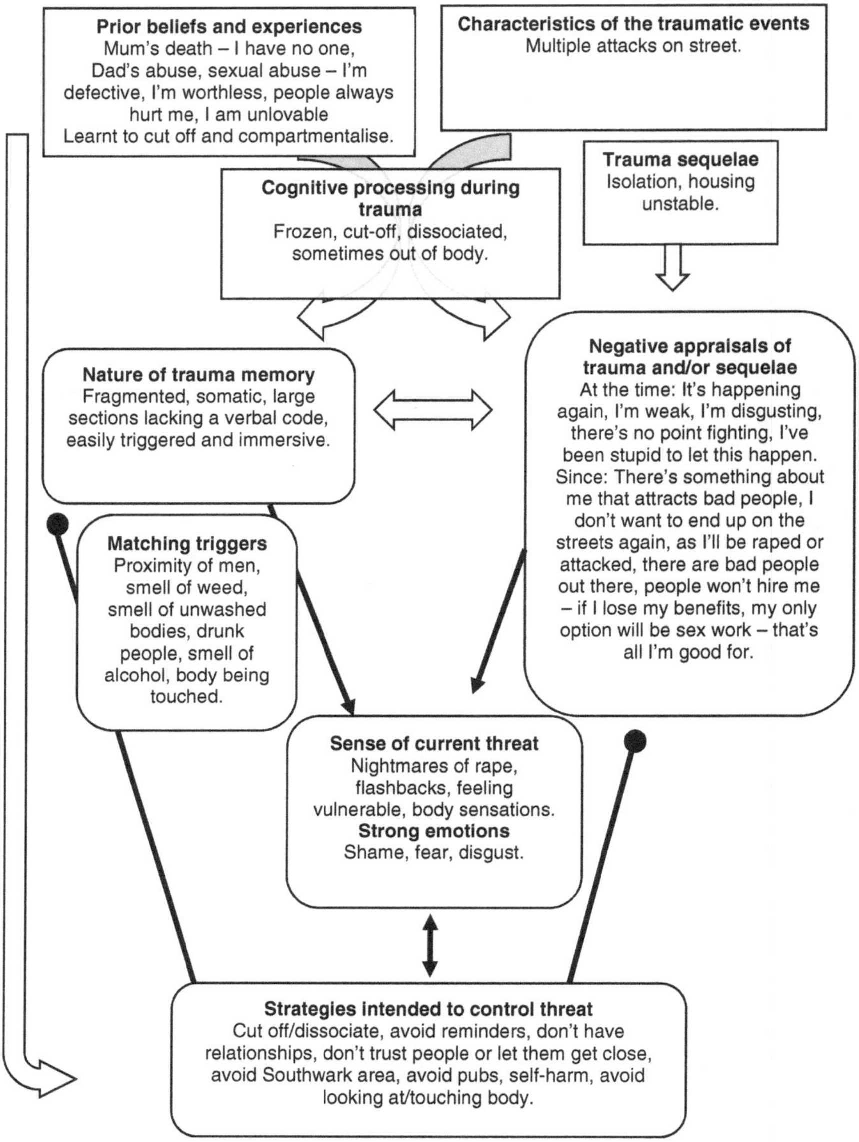

Figure 14.1 Melody's formulation

Melody and her therapist created a timeline of her life to identify her key trauma memories. Melody had most PTSD intrusions of a violent rape she had experienced while she was homeless. The memories were very disjointed and confused, dominated by sensory recollections, and extremely difficult for Melody to talk about without dissociating. She described an out-of-body experience during the rape, where she felt like she was watching it from the sky above the alleyway.

The next task was to construct a more elaborated and coherent trauma narrative. Melody had previously done art therapy and had enjoyed making collages. Her therapist encouraged her to make a collage that represented all of her feelings associated with the rape. They then discussed each picture she had chosen and what they represented to her. Melody gradually became able to put more words to her physical sensations and emotions, without dissociating. They also used a 'bird's eye view' version of reliving to map out the events before, during, and after the trauma.

The main beliefs Melody associated with the trauma were that she was entirely 'weak', 'disgusting', and 'worthless'. Melody also believed that she was 'damaged' by her early experiences and could never be 'normal'. Melody's therapist approached these beliefs using guided discovery techniques to help her gather relevant evidence and then place herself on a belief continuum. They also anonymously surveyed other people's opinions on how much they considered Melody to be 'disgusting' and 'weak' because of her experiences. However, Melody struggled to connect emotionally to these new perspectives.

Melody's therapist explained this 'head–heart gap' was a common experience and gave some examples in everyday life. They developed an alternative belief that Melody was a 'survivor' and 'deserving of love' and made a graph of how much she thought versus felt this to be true. They identified some factors contributing to her head–heart gap, including Melody's long-standing self-attacking thoughts and the influence of her childhood experiences, in particular her father's total disregard for her safety and wellbeing.

Melody and her therapist decided to address her self-attack using the image of a perfect nurturer to provide a compassionate viewpoint. Melody believed in guardian angels, so they imagined what her guardian angel would look like, how she would sound and behave, and what she would say to Melody. Melody made a collage to represent her guardian angel and saved a photo of it on the lock screen of her phone, so she was frequently reminded of this compassionate perspective. She began to consult her imagined guardian angel whenever she doubted herself, felt an urge to self-harm, had an intrusive memory, or a self-attacking thought. With her therapist's help, Melody also brought her guardian angel into her trauma memories. She imagined the angel holding and comforting Melody after the rape, and intervening to protect Melody when she was a child.

Melody and her therapist tracked her head–heart gap on the graph (Figure 14.2). Over time, her belief in the new perspective that she was a survivor and deserving of love began to increase, both in her head and her heart.

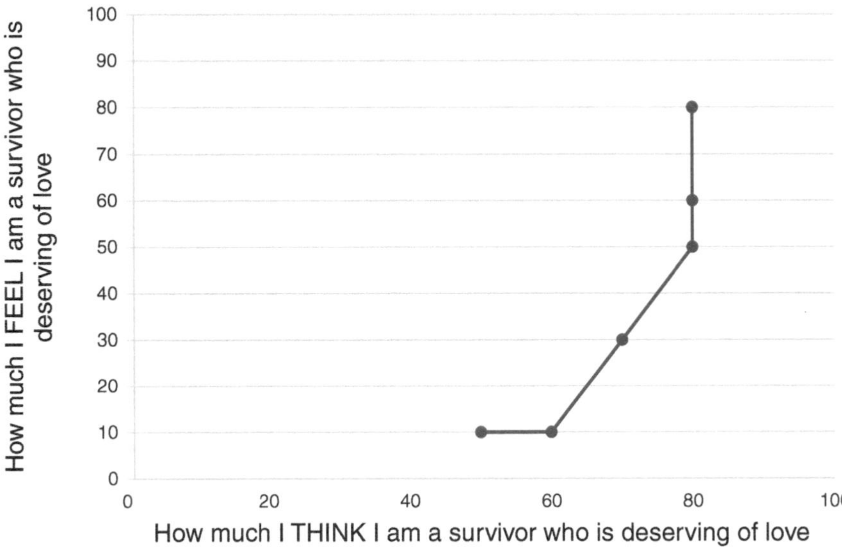

Figure 14.2 Melody's head–heart gap

Recommended reading

Lee, D. A. (2005). The perfect nurturer: A model to develop a compassionate mind within the context of cognitive therapy. In P. Gilbert (Ed.). *Compassion* (pp. 338–363). Routledge.

Stott, R. (2007). When head and heart do not agree: A theoretical and clinical analysis of rational–emotional dissociation (RED) in cognitive therapy. *Journal of Cognitive Psychotherapy*, 21(1), 37–50.

CHAPTER FIFTEEN

Loss

Callum saw his sister Lily die in a sudden accident when they were children. Callum was pulled away from his sister's body by his parents and never saw her again. As an adult, he continued to experience intrusive images of her body and felt guilty that he had survived when Lily had died. In therapy, Callum explored how he wanted to remember Lily, and his therapist helped him relive and then rescript the images of her death.

Traumatic events can lead to loss in different ways. Some traumas include the death of another person, and grief can be an important part of the clinical picture. Other losses include changes to an individual's life, such as fleeing a country and the resulting losses in home, community, social networks, employment, and often status. PTSD symptoms can lead to losses, such as a job or relationship. Lastly, some traumas result in physical changes, such as chronic pain, disability, and disfigurement. Treatment must then include helping clients acknowledge and mourn what has been lost, and find meaningful ways of moving forward and rebuilding their lives.

Traumatic bereavement

PTSD can arise from witnessing the death of another person or people, or learning about the violent or accidental death of a close friend or family member (APA, 2013). Survivors of these types of traumas may therefore not only be battling the usual PTSD symptoms but also grieving for a loved one.

GRIEF DISORDERS

We often use the term 'traumatic grief' to describe the psychological symptoms that arise after a traumatic bereavement, but it is not an official diagnosis. However, grief disorders have recently been included in diagnostic manuals: 'prolonged grief disorder' in ICD-11 and prolonged grief disorder in DSM-5-TR (Prigerson et al., 2021). Critics argue that grief disorders risk pathologising normal distress, but these new disorders reflect evidence that around 10% of people struggle to recover from bereavements, and experience long-lasting and disabling psychological symptoms (Lundorff et al., 2017).

When working with people who have experienced traumatic bereavements, the clinical picture often includes a mixture of prolonged grief and PTSD symptoms. PTSD symptoms may block 'normal' grieving; for example, where thinking about the deceased person triggers upsetting intrusions of the way they died, people may entirely avoid all memories and reminders of them. The 'nowness' of these death memories may also contribute to a persisting sense of disbelief, as if the person 'only died yesterday'. When beliefs about the manner of death lead to guilt or anger, people may become preoccupied with those aspects and struggle to come to terms with their loss.

DOI: 10.4324/9781003288329-18

Recent CBT models of prolonged grief disorders have been heavily influenced by the cognitive model of PTSD, and conceptualise similar core maintaining processes, namely insufficient integration of the loss into the autobiographical knowledge base, negative beliefs about the loss and its consequences, and unhelpful avoidant, safety-seeking, and ruminative coping strategies (Boelen et al., 2006; Duffy, & Wild, 2017; Smith, & Ehlers, 2021). It follows that treatments include many similar elements to CT-PTSD, such as imaginal reliving of memories of the death, identifying and modifying excessively negative or anxious appraisals, and discriminating and reducing avoidance of reminders of the deceased (Boelen et al., 2007; Duffy, & Wild, 2017; Shear et al., 2005). Other models have highlighted the role of attachment processes (Shear, & Shair, 2005), and meaning reconstruction (Neimeyer, 2001), and have generated some useful strategies which we integrate into treatment.

TREATING TRAUMATIC GRIEF

Early sessions

As usual, we spend early sessions of therapy developing a shared understanding of presenting difficulties through formulation and psychoeducation. With traumatic grief, we give time and space in early sessions to the expression of loss and yearning, gently encouraging the client to tell us about their loved one, if they feel comfortable, without moving too quickly into more structured parts of treatment.

As well as the usual psychoeducation and normalisation of PTSD symptoms, we highlight early on that a loss can provoke a huge mixture of emotions, from sadness to anger to guilt to emptiness to relief, and everything in between. We want our clients to know that all emotions are acceptable and can be expressed. Metacognitive beliefs such as 'I shouldn't feel angry with the person who died', or 'feeling happy is betraying what we had', may need addressing early in therapy.

Rebuilding your life

'Reclaiming your life' is important following a traumatic bereavement but needs to be approached sensitively. Duffy and Wild (2017) suggest that terms like 'rebuilding your life' or 'reconnecting' can feel more appropriate for people who shared many previously valued activities with the deceased and do not feel they can be reclaimed.

As well as re-engaging with previously valued activities where possible, we also encourage new activities in line with an individual's values. New interests can create memories of positive experiences without the person who has died, challenge beliefs such as 'I'm nobody without them', and help the establishment of a self-identity separate from the deceased (Maccallum, & Bryant, 2013).

As usual, we should be alert to blocking beliefs. In traumatic grief, these may include that it is unfair or disloyal to experience pleasure (usually Socratic questioning reveals that the deceased would want them to be happy), concerns that people will ask about the deceased (it can be helpful to prepare and practise how to manage this), and/or fear of being overwhelmed by emotions. Behavioural experiments can be useful in testing out these predictions.

Reconnecting with others is often an important part of rebuilding. Many people avoid social contact after a bereavement as they are worried about others' reactions to them, believe they have changed, and feel more comfortable alone (Smith et al., 2020). These concerns may need to be addressed. We also recommend discussing with clients how to set boundaries with loved ones about how and when they would like to talk about the deceased, and practising asking for how they wish to be supported. It can be useful to consider with the client how, and with whom, they want to talk about their grief. It might be with certain friends or family members, or with understanding strangers. Some people like support groups, or prefer anonymous internet forums, blogging, or journaling. Expressions of grief differ between families, communities, and cultural groups, and clients will need to decide how to negotiate their needs within these contexts.

> Jeremy and his wife Claire lost their son Josh to cancer. Jeremy developed PTSD and struggled to talk about or remember Josh as he found it upsetting and believed it would worsen his symptoms. This led to conflict with Claire, who wanted to remember and talk about Josh to 'keep his memory alive'. Jeremy's therapist asked if he was comfortable inviting Claire to a therapy session. They discussed their different preferences for dealing with the loss and agreed some compromises. Jeremy agreed to experiment with allowing himself to think and talk about Josh more, and found that the increase in distress he experienced was only temporary and did not seem to worsen his PTSD.

Meaningful remembrance

Another early task in therapy is to establish how and when the client would like to remember the deceased, and agree dedicated time and space to do so. This helps to allay fears that reducing PTSD symptoms means that the person is forgotten, and aims to replace the constant rumination which can be a feature of traumatic grief with purposeful, meaningful remembrance. In general, clients agree that the best way of honouring the deceased person is by remembering positive memories of them 'at their best', that highlight their strengths and qualities, rather than focusing on the moment of their death. Certain activities can be used as part of deliberate remembrance, such as visiting the grave, looking at photos, speaking to the person in imagination, or journaling. Neimeyer (2017) and others have written about 'legacy' work in grief, such as creating an online memorial for an individual (others can also be invited to add photos and messages), contributing to a relevant charity or organisation, or doing an activity that was valued by the deceased 'in their memory'.

The therapist and client can discuss how much time to dedicate to meaningful remembrance, and try to reduce rumination at other times, akin to a 'worry time' intervention. The need for planned remembrance may reduce over time. For example, in the early stages of treatment, clients may want to spend a certain amount of every day or every other day remembering the person who has died and eventually reduce this to one hour a week. They can also plan how to mark special occasions like birthdays and the anniversary of the death.

Memory work

Intrusive memories following a traumatic bereavement may be of witnessing the death, constructed images of the death (Chapter 10), the moment of learning about the death, when they last saw the person alive, or moments where they feel they could have intervened to prevent the death (often associated with feelings of guilt and regret).

Where the sense of loss is considerable, and grief is a large part of the clinical picture, we do not rush into memory work. In early sessions, we ask for a few details about the nature of the trauma, but delay imaginal reliving until we have worked on some of the main cognitive themes and generated some relevant updates. Before reliving, we agree a point of safety at which to end the narrative. Where a significant emotional loss has occurred, this endpoint should ideally include an image that encapsulates an antidote to this sense of loss or that strengthens the connection to the deceased (page 172–3).

Melanie lost her partner Neil to suicide. She arrived at the scene of his death shortly after an ambulance arrived and witnessed paramedics trying to revive Neil. Melanie had frequent intrusions and nightmares about the scene, accompanied by strong feelings of helplessness, guilt, and loss. Melanie's therapist did not initially relive the trauma with her, but first worked on the main beliefs that Melanie had about Neil's death: that she should have got to him sooner and prevented his death, and that she was now completely alone. Once they had worked on Melanie's guilt cognitions and created an image of Neil watching over her, peaceful and full of love, they returned to the trauma memories.

Not all traumas involving a death lead to a strong sense of loss. For example, in cases where the deceased was a stranger, the main emotions associated with the trauma may be fear related to threat to their own life, or horror or disgust related to witnessing the death or finding a body. In these examples, delaying reliving is usually unnecessary.

Hot cognitions

- It isn't fair
- I didn't do enough to save them
- The medical staff let them down/made mistakes
- If I let go, they are forgotten
- My life is over now
- They are still suffering
- If I let my grief in I will lose control
- Life is meaningless without them

Cognitive work

The 'hot cognitions' illustrate some common cognitive themes associated with traumatic grief:

Unfairness: Beliefs about injustice are common, and often linked to frustration and anger. First, we help clients vent these feelings, and empathise with unfairness before gently exploring the facts. Sometimes there has been genuine wrongdoing, such as medical errors. Here we offer to support our clients in raising formal complaints if they so wish, or channelling their anger into positive action or improving things for others (e.g. campaigning for improved safety or volunteering for a charity). Sometimes a sense of unfairness is more existential, and exploring beliefs around fairness often leads to the conclusion that life is sometimes not fair, and the messages we often receive as children like 'good things happen to good people, and bad things happen to bad people' are not always true. Where rumination is maintaining distress, we help our clients consider the advantages and disadvantages of dwelling and brooding, ask what the deceased would want them to do, and experiment with reducing rumination.

Self-blame: Clients sometimes blame themselves for not preventing the death of another. Others regret some aspect of their behaviour, such as arguing the last time they saw the deceased. Often these beliefs are influenced by hindsight bias (although see Chapter 16 for working with genuine responsibility). Our usual strategies for working with guilt apply, such as responsibility pie charts, and examining what information was available to the client at the time (Chapter 13). It can also be useful to ask the client to list what they *did* do to help the person who died; very often they did as much as possible. Surveys can help consolidate this. We also encourage clients to tell the story of their relationship with the person who died; this often reveals how much care and love has been shared.

Loss: For many, the most painful aspect of losing a loved one is simply missing them and their shared life. People can fear that coming to terms with the death, and recovering from PTSD, will mean forgetting them. We often emphasise that overcoming grief doesn't mean 'getting over' the death or 'letting go' of the person, but accepting the reality of their death and the permanent change to that relationship, while nurturing a new connection with them as part of moving forward. This may include planned remembrances, consulting them in imagination about big decisions, symbolic gestures which represent what they meant to them (such as wearing a personal piece of jewellery, doing activities in their memory), and thinking about what qualities they brought out in our client, and how they can stay connected with them. Memory-focused techniques can be used as behavioural experiments to test whether the deceased is forgotten if the client's PTSD symptoms reduce. In general, clients find that they remember the deceased differently (but not less) after PTSD treatment, with a greater ability to access positive memories.

Ongoing suffering: When the last memories or images of the deceased are of their death, re-experiencing these memories often makes it feel as if the deceased is still suffering. Socratic questioning generally reveals that this is not in keeping with the client's beliefs about death, so we use imagery exercises (next section) to encapsulate this, by running the memories past the point of suffering to a more peaceful place. Many clients believe their loved one is in heaven, which can be a useful imagery update. Others believe there is no life after death, but rather an absence of being where the deceased is at least no longer in pain or suffering. Some of our clients have other fears, for example, that their loved one is in limbo, alone and aware in the grave, or has gone to hell. Sometimes it can be helpful to consult a religious authority (such as a local faith leader) if the client has concerns about the afterlife, although we recommend speaking to them first if possible to ascertain their views.

Top tips: How to treat survivor guilt

Guilt about surviving when others did not is common. In some cases, guilt relates to foreseeability or preventability of a death, which can be addressed with our usual tools for trauma-related guilt (Chapter 13). However, survivor guilt can be more existential; clients know logically that nothing they did affected the fact that someone else died, but continue to feel guilty, simply for surviving.

Existential survivor guilt often relates to beliefs that the survivor has somehow unfairly benefitted to the detriment of others. They may report thoughts like 'the other person was more worthy of surviving than me' or 'I took their place'. People often have a sense that the world should be fair, and that things happen for a reason, so their survival feels like it broke the rules. In treatment, we can help people consider other explanations for why they survived. Often survival is just a matter of chance, and the world is not always fair. Some clients develop the alternative belief that 'maybe I survived for a reason'.

If you want to read more about survivor guilt, along with treatment recommendations, try Murray et al. (2021).

Imagery work

Although we have separated them in this chapter for convenience, imagery work is intertwined with work on cognitions throughout treatment for traumatic grief, and both can be used to update trauma memories.

Conversations with the deceased: A useful technique is to ask what the deceased person would want for the client and, conversely, if the client had died in similar circumstances, what they would want for a loved one who had survived. In general, this is for them to be happy, not to blame themselves, and to move forward in their lives. Having a conversation with the deceased in imagery can be a helpful way to access this perspective and to connect with updates at an emotional level. The basic procedure is to choose a place where they often spent time with the deceased, or 'somewhere between here and the hereafter', and to imagine meeting them there. In the conversation, they say 'hello', give them their news, explain their difficulties with moving on after their death, for example telling them that they feel responsible for not doing enough or feel lost without them, and ask the person for advice. They can also ask any questions they are struggling with. They then end the image by saying 'goodbye for now' and making an arrangement to visit again.

FAQ: What if the deceased person says something unhelpful?

When we started doing these imagery conversations, we worried that this might happen, but it is very rare! To guard against the possibility, we ask clients 'what do you think [the deceased] would say about that?' before suggesting the imagery conversation. In general, we know a bit about the person who died and the nature of their relationship already and we wouldn't suggest an imagery conversation if, for example, they have always been highly critical of our client.

In the rare event that the deceased person says something unhelpful in imagery or the conversation becomes hostile, we first check whether this response was what the deceased would say, or reflective of the client's appraisals, and use other techniques to generate a fair and accurate appraisal of events. If the hostility is realistic, this may lead the conversation towards confronting them about attitudes they held which were unhelpful or abusive. When a client has been responsible for the death, they can use the imagery conversation to apologise and ask forgiveness (Chapter 16).

Running the memory on: Where peri-traumatic hotspots relate to the moments of death or images of the body after death, it can feel as if the person is somehow frozen in suffering. We can use imagery rescripting to run past the moment of death and to imagine the person now at peace in whichever way feels most fitting for the client, for example, in heaven with others they love, or in a peaceful sleep.

Resolution imagery: Sometimes, clients were unable to do things they wanted or needed at the time of the trauma, such as saying goodbye, so we can use imagery rescripting to do so. If the scene of the death was very disturbing, clients may choose to repair it in some way, such as by cleaning and tending to the body. For clients who were unable to hold or attend a funeral, this can be done in imagery or through a symbolic act to commemorate the death.

Images to strengthen updates: For every alternative belief that we create, we can generate an image to strengthen it. For example, if we have an update that 'they are at peace now', we can help the client generate an image to represent this, such as the person peacefully sleeping in a beautiful place.

Images to represent the deceased: Similarly, we can ask clients how they would like to remember the deceased and generate a representative image. We ask the client to imagine the deceased 'at their best', their valued qualities and what they meant to them, then ask what images come to mind (Duffy, & Wild, 2017).

> Max created an image to represent their partner Justin after he died. Max had always felt protected and comfortable around Justin and this brought to mind an image of being wrapped up in a warm blanket. They imagined keeping the blanket in a cupboard at home and when Max wanted to feel close to Justin, they imagined taking it out and wrapping it around them. Max felt comforted knowing that the blanket was always there if they wanted to remember Justin and the love they had shared.

A NOTE ON SELF-CARE

Working with traumatic grief can be tough on therapists, not least because most of us will experience bereavements ourselves. If you have had a recent bereavement, consider taking a break from this work for a while. Even if a loss isn't recent, working with grief can bring back feelings of sadness, so it is important to prioritise self-care and to use supervision and our support networks to acknowledge and express our feelings (Chapter 26).

LIFE CHANGES AFTER TRAUMA

Traumas may result in, or occur at a similar time to, significant life changes. People may need to flee their country of origin, change or lose their job, become separated from friends or family, lose relationships, or their homes. As with other types of loss, we need to spend time in therapy acknowledging and grieving these changes, before working with our clients to move forward, while retaining what was meaningful about what was lost.

REBUILDING YOUR LIFE

When significant life changes have occurred, we refer to 'rebuilding' rather than 'reclaiming' your life. Re-engaging with some activities may be physically or practically impossible. Instead, we ask our clients what they previously valued or enjoyed, then explore ways to replicate or replace this where possible, as well as encouraging the development of new goals, interests, and activities aligned with their values.

> Abdul fled Afghanistan after an attack on his family and travelled to the UK. In Afghanistan, he had worked as an engineer, but he was unable to work in the UK while claiming asylum so had little money. In Afghanistan, Abdul lived with his large family and had many friends, but in the UK he lived alone and felt isolated.
>
> Abdul's therapist asked what activities he had previously valued and whether there were ways of replicating them in the UK. Abdul missed his family, so arranged to video call them once a week during family dinner, and ate a meal alongside them. His therapist helped him find a local Afghan community group and Abdul started attending their social events. In Afghanistan, Abdul had enjoyed watching cricket and football on the television and liked walking in the local park, things he could still do in the UK. His therapist helped him apply for a Freedom Pass so that he could use public transport for free and Abdul also tried out new activities, including visiting a local technology museum.

DECIDING WHAT TO KEEP AND WHAT TO LEAVE BEHIND

Clients may not wish to keep all aspects of their previous way of life. It can be helpful to list what they would like to keep, and what they would like to leave behind. This helps reduce the idealisation of the past and helps establish continuity of connection to previous values.

> Patrick retired from the military after 22 years and struggled to adapt to civilian life. In therapy, he made a list of the aspects of military life that he wanted to retain (discipline, physical activity, connection with others, and pride in the job), and those he wanted to leave behind (causing worry to his family, being away from home, and discouragement of individuality). They planned how Patrick could retain aspects of what he had valued about military life. He joined a cycling club to keep up his physical fitness and make new friends. He joined a Facebook group for his old regiment to stay in touch with his friends. Lastly, he started volunteering for a military charity, which was something he felt proud of. He took pleasure from activities that he had missed in the past, such as being at his children's birthday parties and school plays, and growing his hair long.

PHYSICAL CHANGES AFTER TRAUMA

Some traumas result in physical changes such as pain, disability, or disfigurement (see also Chapter 21). Again, these need to be recognised and mourned, before moving too quickly into change strategies.

REBUILDING YOUR LIFE

Physical changes can limit participation in some activities. These may need to be adapted or replaced with alternatives that give equivalent meaning and pleasure. We are also alert to potential blocking beliefs and address these with cognitive techniques, including behavioural experiments.

> Tracey lost the use of her legs following a car accident. She had previously been very active and had enjoyed netball, and playing with her daughter. When Tracey's therapist asked what had been important to her about those activities, she listed spending time with her friends from the netball team, feeling fit and healthy, and having fun with her daughter. They made a list of alternative activities which could achieve these same outcomes including going for meals with her netball team and supporting them at matches, participating in wheelchair sports, going to the park with her daughter, and reading her stories. Tracey initially expressed thoughts like 'there's no point, I won't enjoy it', but tried a behavioural experiment of rating her mood before and after taking her daughter to the park, and found that she still got pleasure and satisfaction from watching her play.

PHYSICAL TRIGGERS

Where traumas have involved physical illness or injury, physical sensations often become triggers to trauma memories. Similarly, associated re-experiencing symptoms are often highly sensory and somatic. We use stimulus discrimination techniques, helping people to notice the differences between now, and at the time of the trauma, including how their body felt.

> Costas avoided taking showers as he found the sensation of warm water running down his body triggered trauma memories of bleeding heavily from his chest after he was stabbed, accompanied by intense pain. His therapist taught him to tune his attention to all the differences between the shower and when he had been stabbed, including by gently massaging the site of the entry wound. In the session, they put warm water on their arms, while practising the technique, and Costas tried it in the shower between sessions.

Many clients will avoid reminders of the trauma, including looking at parts of their own body, or their scars. This can mean that memories of the body as it was at the time of the trauma are not updated, so we encourage people to interact with their bodies, including the marks left by the trauma. For example, homework tasks could include applying moisturiser to their scars for ten minutes every day, paying attention to how the wound sites look and feel different.

Another common safety-seeking behaviour is to mentally scan the body for signs of illness or pain, which can fuel a sense of current threat. Exercises in switching attention to different parts of the body (similar to those used in cognitive therapy for health anxiety, e.g. Salkovskis et al., 2003) and to external stimuli can be useful in demonstrating how the role of self-focused attention can amplify bodily sensations, and help test beliefs about a physical sensation being a sign of impending danger (Chapter 21).

PHYSICAL UPDATING

Hotspots can include strong physical sensations which can be difficult to update verbally. For example, clients often report re-experiencing the sensation of an impact or pain, and may not recall a conscious thought. In these cases, we can update the hotspot using physical sensations, such as gently touching or stroking the place where the impact or pain occurred, to provide a different sensation, linked to the meaning 'it isn't happening now', 'there's nothing there' or 'the wound has healed'. We can also use imagery updates to introduce these meanings, for example imagining wounds healing and the body repairing itself, or a recent memory where the client felt strong or healed.

COGNITIVE WORK

It is important to use the downward arrow technique to understand the underlying meaning of a physical change to a client. For example, a belief such as 'I look different now' may be accurate, but often has a distorted meaning attached, such as 'I am completely unattractive and will never meet someone'. The following themes are common following physical changes.

Socially anxious beliefs and negative self-image

For some clients, physical changes lead to concerns about how other people will perceive them, for example as unattractive, damaged, or embarrassing. Here we can draw on interventions from social anxiety disorder treatments including behavioural experiments, surveys, and video feedback (Wild, 2009).

> Farida was badly burned in a house fire, and was extremely self-conscious about her appearance, believing that others would stare at her scars if she revealed them, and would think she was disgusting. She wore thick make-up on her face and hands to disguise the scars, and clothes which covered her whole body.

Farida's therapist helped her design a survey including photos of her scars, asking people whether they would stare at someone with such scars or find them disgusting. Most people responded that they might briefly look at someone with a visible difference out of surprise or curiosity, but not out of disgust. Farida and her therapist also read stories on the website for the charity 'Changing Faces' to investigate how other people with visible differences perceived themselves.

This helped Farida feel confident enough to try some behavioural experiments in revealing her scars. With her therapist, she went to the supermarket without make-up on her hands and they observed peoples' reactions. Farida also experimented with wearing less make-up on her face and shorter sleeves to test how others responded. She found that people did sometimes look at her scars but, if she smiled at them, they usually smiled back, which showed Farida they did not find her disgusting.

Beliefs about unfairness

Understandably, many clients hold beliefs about unfairness and feel angry about physical losses. As with grief, we need to listen, empathise, and validate these experiences. In some circumstances, it may be possible to raise complaints or seek compensation, but not always. Anger is often maintained by rumination and, when the costs and benefits of holding on to anger are reviewed, clients generally find that it causes them difficulties and has little benefit. Working towards an alternative perspective, such as 'it is unfair and I can't change that, but I can make the best of my life moving forward', opens up the possibility of rebuilding your life activities and reducing rumination.

Beliefs about permanent change and loss

Clients will often express understandable sadness about what they have lost, and describe feelings of hopelessness attached to appraisals such as 'I'm not myself anymore'. As well as acknowledging what has been lost, we help our clients recognise what has not been lost (Wild, 2009). For example, changes to physical appearance and abilities do not alter the core values and personality traits that make us who we are. We also identify any excessively negative beliefs and help the client to challenge them.

Zara was forced to retire from the navy when she was injured in a training accident. As well as leaving a career she loved and had worked hard for, the accident left her with chronic pain and unable to engage in many of the activities she enjoyed. Zara reported thoughts such as 'my life is over' and 'I've nothing to live for'. Her therapist helped her to express her deep sadness and anger about what had happened. She then asked Zara if there was anything she hadn't lost. To start with, Zara couldn't think of anything, but with encouragement was able to talk about her friends and family, who had been very supportive, her new dog, and the fact that her mind was still sharp. As therapy progressed, Zara began to express more hope for the future and to make some plans for a career outside the navy.

Beliefs about vulnerability

People with PTSD have a heightened sense of threat and this can be further intensified by physical changes. For example, clients may report beliefs such as 'I wouldn't be able to run away now', or 'people will see me as an easy target'. These beliefs can be addressed in a similar way to other beliefs about risk, by trying to estimate a realistic likelihood of the feared outcome, alongside identifying factors that would support them in coping with threats. Evidence can be gathered by internet searches, speaking to experts or others affected by a similar physical change, or conducting a survey. Behavioural experiments can then be used to test fears about further threat.

Notes from the therapy room: Callum

Callum's younger sister, Lily, died when he was 12. Lily was hit by a car while playing on a bike outside the family home. Callum was nearby and witnessed the accident. He tried to help Lily, but family members quickly arrived and pulled him away. He never saw Lily again, as his family did not believe he should see her at the hospital or attend the funeral.

Callum sought treatment in his thirties. He reported longstanding intrusive images of the accident and frequent dwelling about what Lily's life might have been. He also described significant survivor guilt, saying 'it should have been me'. His formulation is in Figure 15.1.

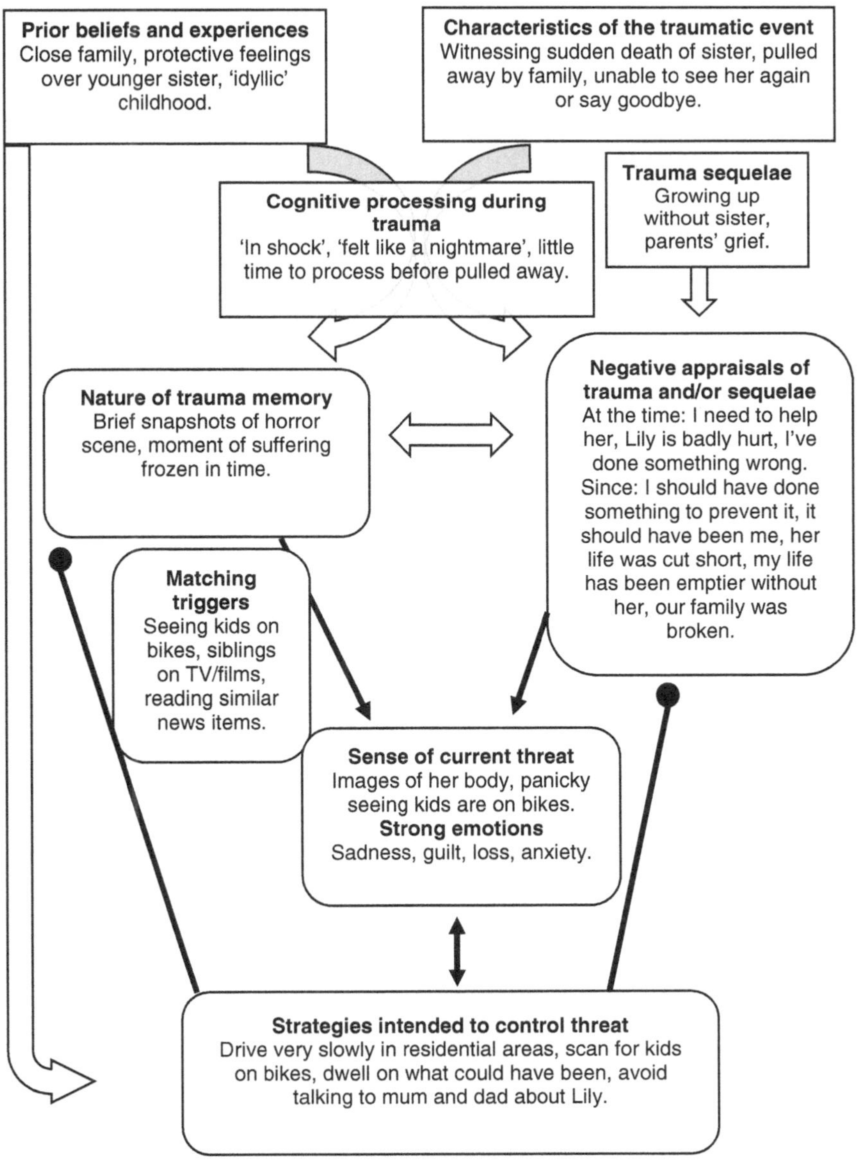

Figure 15.1 Callum's formulation

In therapy, Callum's therapist encouraged him to speak about Lily and express his sadness. They discussed how Callum wanted to remember Lily. He talked about happy memories of family holidays and said that he wanted to remember her that way, rather than the unpleasant images of her body. They agreed a plan to dedicate an hour a week to happy memories of Lily, such as looking at photos and sharing stories within the family. Callum also generated a positive image of Lily playing on a beach in Cornwall, where she had been happiest, to represent the meaning 'she's in a happy place now'.

To address the memories of Lily's death, they used imaginal reliving of the accident and worked on the meanings attached to the hotspots, updating them with new information such as 'she was knocked out immediately and wouldn't have felt any pain', 'she's at peace now', and 'it was an accident, that no one could have prevented'.

One source of distress for Callum was that he never had the chance to say goodbye to Lily. They rescripted the memories to allow Callum to spend time comforting and saying goodbye to her. Callum also changed the scene of the accident to make it less distressing by 'cleaning' his sister so that there was no blood or glass on her body. He wrapped her in her favourite blanket with her teddy bear and imagined his mother comforting his younger self and leading him gently away. He then transported his sister's soul to the beach in Cornwall and imagined her playing there happily.

Callum described a decrease in his intrusions of Lily's death after working on the memories. However, he continued to feel guilty for surviving, and still had a sense of 'it should have been me'. On exploration of this belief, Callum realised that he had felt protective over Lily as an older brother, and remembered his parents telling him to look after her. He felt that he had let them down and that his parents might have preferred him to die over Lily. As an adult, Callum could see rationally that this wasn't true. They used an imagery exercise for Callum to comfort his younger self, telling him that it wasn't his fault, it was a tragic accident, and that his parents loved them both equally.

Recommended reading

Duffy, M., & Wild, J. (2017). A cognitive approach to persistent complex bereavement disorder (PCBD). *The Cognitive Behaviour Therapist, 10*, 1–19.

Ehlers, A. (2006). Understanding and treating complicated grief: What can we learn from posttraumatic stress disorder? *Clinical Psychology: Science and Practice, 13*(2), 135–140.

Wild, J. (2009). Cognitive therapy for post-traumatic stress disorder and permanent physical injury. In N. Grey (Ed.). *A casebook of cognitive therapy for traumatic stress reactions* (pp. 147–162). Routledge.

CHAPTER SIXTEEN

Moral injury

Liam developed PTSD after an incident in Bosnia, where he was serving with the British Army. He believed he was responsible for the deaths of multiple civilians, as well as for killing in anger. After leaving the army, Liam experienced moral injury, ruminating, and punishing himself for what had happened. His therapist helped him to contextualise the incident and find ways to move forward.

Moral injury describes the profound psychological distress that can arise after perpetrating, witnessing, or failing to prevent events that transgress an individual's morals (Litz et al., 2009), or by a sense of betrayal by others, particularly leaders (Shay, 1994). The majority of research into moral injury has been carried out with military populations. Exposure to potentially morally injurious events is extremely common in combat, such as close-quarters killing, witnessing extreme human suffering, failing to help injured civilians, or feeling 'sent to die' by leaders. However, moral injury can also affect other occupational groups such as healthcare workers, journalists, aid workers, prison officers, and social workers, particularly where they have made mistakes or been unable to help people for whom they feel responsible. Moral injury from betrayal also arises within occupational settings, such as when emergency service personnel feel let down by leaders during or after serious incidents (e.g. the shortage of protective equipment during the COVID-19 pandemic). Moral injury is also common for our refugee clients, in the context of conflicts and wars, experiences during torture such as naming other people, witnessing others being tortured, or being forced to kill (Ehlers et al., 2000). Other potentially morally injurious events include accidents where another person was killed or seriously hurt, disasters or terrorist attacks where someone failed to help others, perpetration of crimes which are later regretted, when people have unwittingly passed on a serious illness to loved ones, or following personal betrayals such as discovering that a partner or family member has abused one's child.

Studies have shown that morally injurious experiences such as killing and witnessing atrocities are associated with more severe PTSD, increased use of alcohol, and suicidality (Bryan et al., 2014; Maguen et al., 2010). Moral injury can be an important part of what makes a traumatic event distressing so is a potential target in psychological treatments for PTSD. Despite this, treatment research has been relatively sparse, particularly outside the military, and some have argued that trauma-focused CBT interventions are unsuitable (e.g. Williamson et al., 2021) particularly because not all appraisals linked to moral injury are distorted (for example, genuine wrongdoing may have occurred). Our experience has been that CT-PTSD can be successfully used with people who have moral injury-related PTSD, with some adaptations, as discussed in this chapter.

Understanding moral injury

Moral injury arises when someone is unable to accommodate their traumatic experiences within the moral standards they hold for themselves, others, or the world. Indeed, many people who

DOI: 10.4324/9781003288329-19

develop moral injury hold very high standards of conduct for themselves or others, and a strong sense of personal responsibility (this fits in the top box of the cognitive model). Therefore, although many appraisals linked to moral injury are accurate, e.g. 'I've taken a life' or 'this person has betrayed me', it is the added meaning and generalisation of these beliefs which creates distress, e.g. 'and therefore I have lost my soul' or 'I can never trust anyone again'.

Sometimes events are reappraised later on and the meaning shifts. For example, the experience of killing during warfare may feel acceptable, or even thrilling, at the time, given that it is an expected, encouraged, and sometimes rewarded aspect of the job. Much later, for example, after leaving the armed forces, the meaning may be reappraised negatively. Similarly, meanings can build up over time. For example, a medical professional may feel intensely distressed the first time they witness a patient's death, but become numb to death over time, leading them to question 'have I lost my humanity?'.

Peri-traumatic detachment is common during moral injury-related traumas, particularly those which are occupationally related, as people learn to shut down their emotions to operate effectively, cope afterwards, and continue to do their jobs. As well as leading to post-traumatic negative self-evaluation (e.g. 'I'm a monster because I felt nothing'), this may also mean that trauma memories are particularly poorly processed. In situations of extreme and sustained mental pressure or maltreatment, such as torture, mental defeat is a common emotional experience. Defeat may also be re-experienced when the memories are triggered, leading to negative evaluations (e.g. 'I am destroyed as a person'), and affecting memory processing (Wilker et al., 2017).

Typically, behavioural and cognitive strategies associated with moral injury perpetuate the problem. Rumination on negative cognitive themes is particularly common, strengthening appraisals. Many people withdraw from others, fearing judgement or further betrayal, and so never experience opportunities for corrective or restorative experiences. Attempts at 'atonement' through self-punishment, in the form of self-harm and self-sabotaging behaviour, are often linked to meanings such as 'I deserve to be punished'. These fail to resolve the negative feelings as no punishment feels sufficient, and instead fuel further shame (Chapter 18). Toxic negative emotions also lead to avoidance, such as emotional numbing, distraction, and substance use, which in turn prevent the trauma memories and associated emotions from being processed.

How to help

NORMALISATION

Labelling and providing psychoeducation about the experience of moral injury helps to normalise it. It can also reduce the sense of isolation and defectiveness that people often feel. Areas to mention include how common morally injurious events are in various environments (depending on the client's experience), and how psychologically damaging they can be to anyone exposed to them. Knowing that moral injury is an area studied and treated by psychologists can reinforce the message that it is both common and understood, and that the therapist will not be shocked by the client's experiences.

Top tips: Find accounts from others

Reading the accounts of others who have had similar experiences helps normalise moral injury, is a useful starting point for a conversation about the nature of their moral injury, and as a precursor for Socratic questioning about their self-evaluations, e.g. 'do you judge the person in this account as harshly as you judge yourself?'. Here are some examples of books that recount moral injury:

- *Complications: A surgeon's notes on an imperfect science* (Gawande, 2010) gives a first-hand account of the challenges doctors face in their work, and the human errors they make.
- *A soldier's song* (Lukowiak, 1993) includes stories of ethical challenges facing the author when he fought in the Falkland Islands.
- *Journalists under fire* (Feinstein, & Phil, 2006) records the emotional impact of the work journalists do, based on their accounts.
- Not a book, but the website 'Accidental impacts' (https://accidentalimpacts.org/) provides support for people who have caused accidents that have harmed others.

FACILITATING DISCLOSURE

Moral injury is characterised by high levels of shame and withdrawal (Litz et al., 2009).Therefore, people with moral injury may struggle to disclose their experiences to anyone, including their therapist. Common anxieties include:

- *Fear of judgment from the therapist*: Clients with moral injury may fear others' negative judgements and often closely observe their therapist for signs of disgust or rejection. We try to address this pre-emptively by saying that this is a common concern and remind clients that our role is to help them, not to judge.
- *Fear of harming the therapist*: Some of our clients worry that their therapist will be distressed or damaged by hearing about their experiences, and may want to protect us from upsetting details. Using the metaphor of scientists working with toxic substances in a laboratory (page 55), we offer reassurance about our training and experience in hearing about highly unpleasant events, and explain that the structure of therapy provides us both with the necessary 'psychological protective equipment' to support us in managing our emotional reactions.
- *Concerns about breaking the Official Secrets Act*: Some military clients are concerned about disclosing events that are covered by the Official Secrets Act. If so, we ask them to omit details such as dates, names, or locations, which would make the events identifiable. We explain that we are concerned with their experience of the events and how they affected them, rather than with specific facts of time, place, and person.
- *Concerns about being prosecuted*: Morally injurious events sometimes include perpetration of serious crimes. For example, some of our military clients report participating in or witnessing acts that fall outside the rules of engagement or international laws of armed conflict. Although rare, there have been prosecutions for crimes committed during wars, sometimes many years later, so some of our clients are understandably concerned about disclosing such information.

It is important to make clear to the client the limits of confidentiality before they make any disclosures, not least to maximise trust in the therapist by ensuring decisions to break confidentiality never come as a surprise. In the UK, this includes the responsibility for clinicians to report serious historical crimes (NHS code of practice; Department of Health, 2003) although these decisions are made on a case-by-case basis, balancing the public good achieved by the disclosure with the obligation of respecting confidentiality. Guidance varies in different countries, so therapists should be aware of relevant guidelines and discuss decisions with colleagues. If clients know the responsibilities of the therapist, they can decide what they wish to disclose. It can still be possible to work with issues associated with the incident and implement some of the intervention techniques we discuss in this chapter, without requiring full disclosures of the event. See Williamson et al. (2020) for a detailed discussion of the clinical, ethical, and legal issues.

MEMORY WORK

As usual, we develop a detailed account of trauma memories to access important peri-traumatic meanings and emotions. However, as with other types of memories where the dominant emotions are shame, guilt, or anger, once the details of the narrative are clear we move quickly into working on the meanings associated with key hotspots, rather than reliving the memories repeatedly without including updating information.

There may be discrepancies between how the client thought and felt at the time of the incident compared to later. For example, some people report feeling numb, angry, or excited at the time of an incident, and only later begin to question the rights and wrongs of what happened and how they reacted, and come to feel ashamed or bitter. Where there is considerable distress caused by the peri-traumatic experience (this is usually apparent when re-experiencing symptoms are very distressing), the usual reliving and updating procedures should be prioritised. However, for other clients, the most distressing symptom is the guilty or angry rumination that emerges after an event (sometimes years later). Although it is still useful to hear the trauma narrative to help us understand the context and to update any peri-traumatic hotspots, the bulk of the intervention will focus on the post-traumatic appraisals that contribute to moral injury.

> Jock fought in the Falklands War. It was his first overseas deployment and he was initially very excited. However, the reality of warfare was frequently scary and unpleasant. Towards the end of the war, Jock became numb to the pain and suffering around him. When he came for treatment many years later, it wasn't the moments of fear that troubled him. Instead, it was the times when he had transgressed his morals. Firstly, he had seen people from his unit beating up and humiliating prisoners and blamed himself for not intervening. Secondly, Jock had killed an injured Argentinian soldier and felt good about it at the time. Jock believed he had lost his sense of humanity by the end of the war, and it troubled him deeply that he had enjoyed killing and seen others inflicting pain.

COGNITIVE WORK

One criticism of cognitive approaches to moral injury has been that they presume that trauma-related appraisals are distorted, when they may be accurate (Gray et al., 2017). CT-PTSD does not aim to promote an unrealistic perspective on traumas or to assume that all trauma-related appraisals are excessively negative. Instead, we work with the client to assess the validity of their appraisals, and to develop alternatives if the appraisal is distorted. Where there is genuine responsibility for moral transgressions, or appraisals are accurate, we don't challenge them, but work instead on coming to terms with and accepting the implications, then finding ways to move forward despite them.

However, we do often find that clients overestimate their (or others') responsibility for what has happened and/or have generalised the meaning of an isolated, or extreme, event into a global appraisal. Therefore, our usual cognitive techniques remain useful to developing an accurate perspective. Here are some areas to focus on.

Contextualisation

One common pattern is that clients do not contextualise their/others' actions within the situation they faced. For example, behaviour which would not be appropriate or acceptable in civilian life is necessary and encouraged in a combat situation. A desire to intervene to help others may be denied, such as journalists who are instructed to observe and not intervene when reporting on a story; or overwhelmed by basic survival needs, such as accident survivors who push others out of their way to escape. Commonly, people face a 'no-win' situation; all the available options lead to awful outcomes. Socratic methods can be used, as well as 'zooming out' or 'bird's eye view' reliving to help people view the event from a detached observer standpoint, hopefully therefore appreciating the impossibility of the situation. It can also be helpful to ask clients to describe the various options available to them, and the pros and cons of each, based on their knowledge at the time. This usually reveals that people took the best, if not the only, of several bad options (Young et al., 2021).

Clara worked for an overseas aid agency in a temporary refugee camp and was tasked with triaging the medical needs of arriving refugees. Resources were limited, and only a small proportion of those needing medical treatment could be seen immediately by doctors. Clara had to make a quick assessment of who would die if they weren't seen quickly, and who could wait. Occasionally, somebody she had triaged as lower priority died, and Clara always blamed herself. Working on this in therapy, Clara began to appreciate the impossible situation she had been in. Many of those arriving had complex medical needs, and she had little access to equipment or sufficient time to properly assess them. Ideally, Clara would have requested immediate medical help for many more of the people she triaged, but resources simply could not match the need.

Psychoeducation on why people do bad things

Many people describe a sense of incomprehension about what people are capable of, whether because of atrocities they have witnessed or their own actions. Psychoeducation is often useful here, for example drawing on social psychology experiments like those of Milgram (1963) and Zimbardo (Haney et al., 1973) to explain the capacity for humans to harm each other, given the right conditions (i.e. when instructed to by people in authority or when in positions of power). These provide a useful alternative for the appraisal 'because I have done this, it means I must be a psychopath/evil/a monster'. It is also sometimes worth noting that someone truly 'evil' or psychopathic would be unlikely to experience remorse or emotional pain after an event. Psychoeducation on learned helplessness, dissociation, compliance, and torture-induced defeat can also be helpful where people have judged their peri-traumatic reactions negatively.

Another useful resource is a BBC documentary called 'Five steps to tyranny' (McDonald, 2000), which describes the processes through which ordinary people end up committing acts of extreme brutality. We have sometimes watched this with clients in session or suggested it as a homework task (with the warning that it shows images of war and genocide which may be triggering), when we are addressing appraisals like 'how could they/I have done this?'.

Developing a realistic estimate of responsibility

Responsibility appraisals are common in moral injury, and responsibility pie charts are a good way of highlighting the shared responsibility that underlies most situations. The goal is for a balanced perspective to be reached where the client is afforded an appropriate slice of the pie; neither overstating nor understating their responsibility (page 137).

Watching out for thinking errors

Common thinking errors in moral injury include superhuman standards (e.g. 'I should have been able to save them' when it was impossible), hindsight bias (e.g. 'if only I hadn't changed my route to work, then the accident would never have happened'), and overgeneralisation (e.g. 'because I lost control in that moment, it means I can no longer trust myself').

Socratic questioning and other guided discovery techniques can be used to elucidate and gently challenge these thinking patterns. For example, where an individual is defining themselves by an event (e.g. 'because I killed someone, it means I am rotten to the core'), it is helpful to bring awareness to the broad range of characteristics, experiences, actions, and values which define a person. Continua methods can be useful here (Chapter 12). Litz et al. (2009) summarise the goal of cognitive work is to generate

> a new way to view the world and the self in it that takes into account the reality of the event and its significance, without giving up too much of what was known to be good and just about the world and the self prior to the event.
>
> (p. 703)

In CT-PTSD, this involves helping people develop more flexible personal standards that can accommodate the morally injurious event.

Hot cognitions

- I've lost my soul
- If people know what I did, they will reject me
- I've let myself and others down
- Now that I know what people are capable of, I can't trust anyone

Seeking out others' opinions

Surveys can be used to gather a range of opinions on morally injurious events. However, as some events are outside the common realm of experience for many people, and may include distressing details, surveys will not always be appropriate.

An alternative is to ask the opinion of others in imagery. In 'adaptive disclosure', a treatment developed for moral injury in military personnel (Litz et al., 2017), clients are encouraged to select a person whose opinion they respect, and who has 'always had their back', imagine explaining the moral injury event to them and how they feel about it, then ask their opinion. Where a betrayal has occurred, the client explains this experience and asks for advice about how to move forward.

Dom was a teacher supervising a school trip during which a child drowned. Although the inquest ruled the death was accidental, Dom felt he was personally to blame. In therapy, Dom had a conversation in imagery with Michael, a senior teacher he had always respected.

THERAPIST: Where was a place you and Michael would often talk?
DOM: The staffroom at my old school.
T: Ok, so I want you to imagine you are talking to Michael in the staffroom. Can you picture it?

D: Yes, clearly.
T: Where are you sitting?
D: In the corner on the soft chairs, sitting opposite each other.
T: Ok, good. Can you tell Michael what happened in Wales?
D: He knows, he already knows about it.
T: Ok, so tell him about your role in what happened.
D: Ok. Mike, it was my idea to take the shortcut because everyone was soaking and miserable. I shouldn't have changed the plan. We hadn't done a risk assessment on the lower route, only the higher one. I should have warned the kids to stay back from the river. They were messing around, pushing each other, running. I shouted at them to stop but they are kids, they were never going to listen. I should've gone back there and stopped them. Then, well you know what happened.
T: Well done. How does Mike look when you tell him that?
D: Sad.
T: Does he look angry, upset at you?
D: No, he's just sad about Jayden.
T: Tell him how this has affected you.
D: I think about it all the time. I am so angry with myself. I let him down. The parents … they have been so kind considering it all. But I can't forgive myself. I carry him with me all the time. I just think about that day over and over. I left the job, I couldn't face the responsibility anymore.
T: What does Mike say when you say that?
D: He says 'I'm sorry'.
T: What's he sorry about?
D: About the whole mess. That I'm not teaching anymore. That so many people are hurt by what happened.
T: Including you?
D: Yes.
T: What would he want to say to you?
D: You loved those kids.
T: Is that true?
D: Yes, I always loved the job and it was because of the kids.
T: What else would Mike say?
D: You didn't do it deliberately. You never have wanted anyone to get hurt.
T: How does he look when he says that?
D: There are tears in his eyes. He looks sad.
T: What is his voice like?
D: Kind, caring. He wants me to feel better.
T: What do you want to say to him?
D: I didn't want anyone to get hurt, but that isn't enough. I had responsibility for those kids and I made a mistake, and one of them died, and that's on me.
T: What does he say to that?
D: He says 'you've got to forgive yourself.'
T: Does he forgive you?
D: Yes.
T: How does that feel, that he forgives you?
D: It feels good. It does feel good. I know he would feel that way. I just don't know how to forgive myself.
T: Why don't you ask him?

Where clients have struggled to access a compassionate response from an imagined other, an alternative is to imagine a friend coming to them to confess a similar incident and imagining how they would respond.

Moving forward

Once excessively negative beliefs have been identified and addressed, and new information has been reintegrated into the trauma memories via updating, the next challenge is often to help clients move forward from the event. In many cases, this will include accepting responsibility for areas in which they were genuinely at fault.

Blocks to moving forward include beliefs about the self or others deserving ongoing punishment (e.g. 'if I move on from this, I am forgetting about/letting down the people who were hurt' or 'I am letting myself/others off the hook'). Reviewing the costs and benefits of ongoing self-punishment or angry rumination often reveals that it benefits no one. Instead, focusing energies on moving forward by making meaningful change can be encouraged.

Making amends

Where genuine responsibility has been identified, it can be helpful to discuss ways to make amends or, in the case of betrayal, seek reparation. Possible strategies include:

- *Writing letters*: It may be possible to apologise to a wronged party, or complain to a perpetrator in reality by letter (if appropriate) but, even if this is not practicable, writing an unsent letter allows the client to express their remorse or anger.
- *Imagery*: Similarly, imagery exercises can be used to express regret to the wronged party, or anger to a betrayer, through imagined conversations or empty chair exercises. Although plans for genuine revenge should be risk assessed and discouraged, taking revenge through imagery rescripting can be a valuable exercise.

FAQ: Is it safe to do violent rescripts?

Revenge fantasies are common where people have been wronged and can increase a sense of injustice (Lillie, & Strelan, 2016). There is a risk that encouraging our clients to rescript memories to exact justice may fuel rumination about revenge. Another, more grave, concern is that it may lead them to take real revenge. A study by Seebauer et al. (2014) provides some reassurance – they found that rescripting with violence did not lead to an increase in aggressive emotions. However, this was a study of non-clinical participants using an analogue design, so we need to be cautious in generalising to a clinical sample.

To err on the side of caution, we tend not to encourage violent rescripting with our clients who have a history of perpetration of violence, and especially where they have access to the perpetrator. We also monitor the impact of the rescript on their angry emotions and rumination. If, following a revenge rescript, anger increases or stays the same, we try another approach. Interestingly, there is evidence that incorporating forgiveness into a rescript is more effective than revenge rescripting (Watson et al., 2016), although clients may not choose this approach, especially early on. We find that many clients ultimately decide not to choose violent rescripts as they do not wish to stoop to the level of the perpetrator, or initially choose violent rescripts but then prefer alternative approaches in subsequent rescripting sessions.

- *Reparation*: Sometimes, it is possible to take actions that make amends for wrongdoing. Depending on the individual situation, this may directly benefit those who were negatively affected or reparation may be symbolic (such as volunteering for a charity), or in imagination via imagery rescripting. Following betrayal, practical steps may be possible like reporting a perpetrator to the police, raising a formal complaint, or seeking compensation.

> Colin was convicted of causing death by dangerous driving and sentenced to three years in prison. He had PTSD following the accident and felt huge remorse for his actions. In prison, Colin attended courses on restorative justice. As part of the programme, he wrote a letter to the family of the woman who had died, apologising and expressing his regret. His psychologist also helped him to do an imagery exercise in which he apologised to the woman who had died and imagined her in heaven. Colin decided to volunteer for the restorative justice charity which had helped him after his release, giving talks about his experiences, to help other victims and perpetrators.

Rituals for closure

Whether or not there is genuine responsibility, some clients benefit from conducting a ritual to commemorate the incident. Rituals can help counteract fears that moving on means dishonouring, forgetting, or minimising the suffering of those affected. The type of ritual chosen depends on the client's experiences and their spiritual or religious beliefs but may include funerals held in imagery, a symbolic act such as planting a tree or laying flowers, commemorating the anniversary, imagining a person in afterlife, or a site visit to see how a place has moved on since the trauma.

> Saskia was caught up in a terrorist incident in which multiple people died. As Saskia ran away, she stepped on bodies of people who had fallen in the rush. She never knew if those people survived or not, or whether being trampled had injured or killed them. Saskia had been too distressed to attend any funerals of those who had died or the inquest. She felt guilty about surviving, stepping on people, and not helping injured people.
>
> In therapy, Saskia decided to commemorate those who had died. She made a scrapbook of news reports about the incident and found pictures and information about those who had died. She lit a candle and said a prayer for each of them, wishing them eternal peace and to be reunited with their loved ones. She planned to do the same every year on the anniversary of the attack. She also visited the scene to place a bunch of rosemary she had cut from her garden.

Reclaiming your life

'Reclaiming your life' can complement work on appraisals by asking clients to choose activities that fit with their values and morals. This is particularly important when the client has come to define themselves by an event that does not represent their qualities or values. We emphasise that while the client cannot change their past, they can live in a way that represents their values in the present and future.

Who and how to tell

People with moral injury are often wary of sharing their experiences with others and may have faced negative reactions in the past. Depending on the trauma, there may be mixed reactions to disclosure, so it can be helpful in therapy to discuss who to tell, and how to broach the subject. Surveys to get insight into likely responses, and behavioural experiments in disclosure, can also lay the groundwork before telling loved ones.

> Charlotte was raped when she was a teenager. She didn't report it to the police and later found out that the man had gone on to rape several more women. She believed that the other attacks could have been avoided if she had reported the rape. This idea had been strengthened when Charlotte reported the rape months later, as the police officer who took her statement told her it was 'a bit late now'. Charlotte was worried that others would blame her for the later attacks if they found out.
>
> With the help of her therapist, Charlotte designed a survey to ask what people would think of someone in her situation. Although some of the respondents were critical of Charlotte for not reporting, most took a sympathetic view that she had been young, vulnerable, traumatised, and afraid of reprisal which made going to the police very difficult. Charlotte felt confident enough to tell one of her close friends what happened and received an understanding response. She decided not to tell all of her friends or extended family but planned to tell a few of her close circle.

Dealing with awkward questions

Many clients with moral injury withdraw socially to avoid people asking them about their experiences. A helpful task when planning social reintegration is to consider how to deal with awkward questions and conversations. For example, military veterans are often asked 'have you killed anyone?' which can trigger strong emotions. It can be helpful for clients to remember that such questions are generally a sign of curiosity, rather than intentionally antagonistic or judgemental, and to role-play with their therapist ways of answering such questions or moving the conversation on.

> Eric was born in Rwanda and lost many of his family in the genocide. In the UK, he found that, when people found out he was Rwandan, they often asked about the genocide which triggered upsetting memories. With his therapist, Eric prepared some different answers to awkward questions. If people asked Eric where he was from, he said 'I live in London'. If they asked where he was from originally, he would answer 'Africa' and then ask, 'have you ever been?' to move the conversation on. If they asked which country in Africa he was from and asked about the genocide, Eric would answer 'it was a difficult time in my country and I don't like to talk about it' and then ask a question to change the subject. After practising this a few times with his therapist, Eric felt more confident to interact socially.

Issues for the therapist

Working with moral injury can present various challenges for the therapist. The therapeutic relationship needs to be strong to enable disclosure of painful and shameful memories, so as therapists we need to demonstrate we are compassionate, trustworthy, and capable of tolerating distressing information. Yet, some incidents will naturally trigger an emotional response in us, such as disgust or horror. Good supervision and team cohesion, as well as actively monitoring our reactions and addressing our wellbeing, are therefore even more important than usual (Chapter 26).

Our own moral and ethical outlook may be challenged when we hear certain stories, and maintaining the 'unconditional positive regard' often considered a basic requirement of a therapeutic relationship may feel challenging. But unconditional positive regard doesn't mean we have to always like our clients or approve of everything they have done. It means accepting them as an imperfect human being rather than globally judging them, and supporting them in their efforts to move forward in their life.

Notes from the therapy room: Liam

Liam came for treatment six years after leaving the army. He had encountered several traumatic experiences during his career. The most distressing occurred when he and some others had spoken to some civilians in Bosnia to gather intelligence. When they later revisited the area, many had been killed as punishment for speaking to the army, and the bodies mutilated as a warning. Liam and his colleagues found those responsible and killed them. Liam felt deeply responsible for the death of the civilians and also guilty for feeling satisfaction when he killed the perpetrators because he felt he had acted out of anger and revenge and was not in control of his emotions at the time.

Liam presented with nightmares and intrusions of the incident, and pervasive feelings of anger and shame. Since leaving the army, he had struggled to keep a job and his marriage had broken down. He had been drinking heavily and was arrested twice for fighting. His formulation is in Figure 16.1.

Early stages of treatment included addressing Liam's alcohol intake and replacing it with alternative ways of coping with PTSD symptoms, as well as anger management techniques to reduce his risk of getting into fights. Alcohol intake and aggression were monitored throughout treatment. Liam's therapist gave information about PTSD and moral injury to normalise his experiences and reactions.

Initially, Liam felt able to give only brief details of the incident, and instead of prioritising a more complete narrative, they worked on some of the key appraisals, including Liam's belief that he was fully responsible for the deaths of the civilians. Using a responsibility pie chart helped Liam to see that the perpetrators held most of the responsibility for the murders. He was also able to acknowledge that he had not intended the civilians to be harmed and could not have predicted it. They addressed Liam's belief that because he had killed the perpetrators when he was angry and felt satisfaction, it meant he was out of control, unprofessional, and was becoming like his father, who had himself been violent. He spoke to a friend who had also served in the army, who said that he would have also gained pleasure in killing the people responsible for such a terrible massacre.

Liam had a conversation in imagery with a major he had served under and had always respected. He explained the incident and sought his advice. The major told him that the massacre reflected the brutality of the war in Bosnia and showed why the army needed to be there. The major reminded Liam that he had been there to do a job, and it was not his decision where the army went.

After this exercise, Liam felt able to talk in more detail about the trauma. He was distressed by mental images of the massacre and agreed to try an imagery rescript where he and colleagues

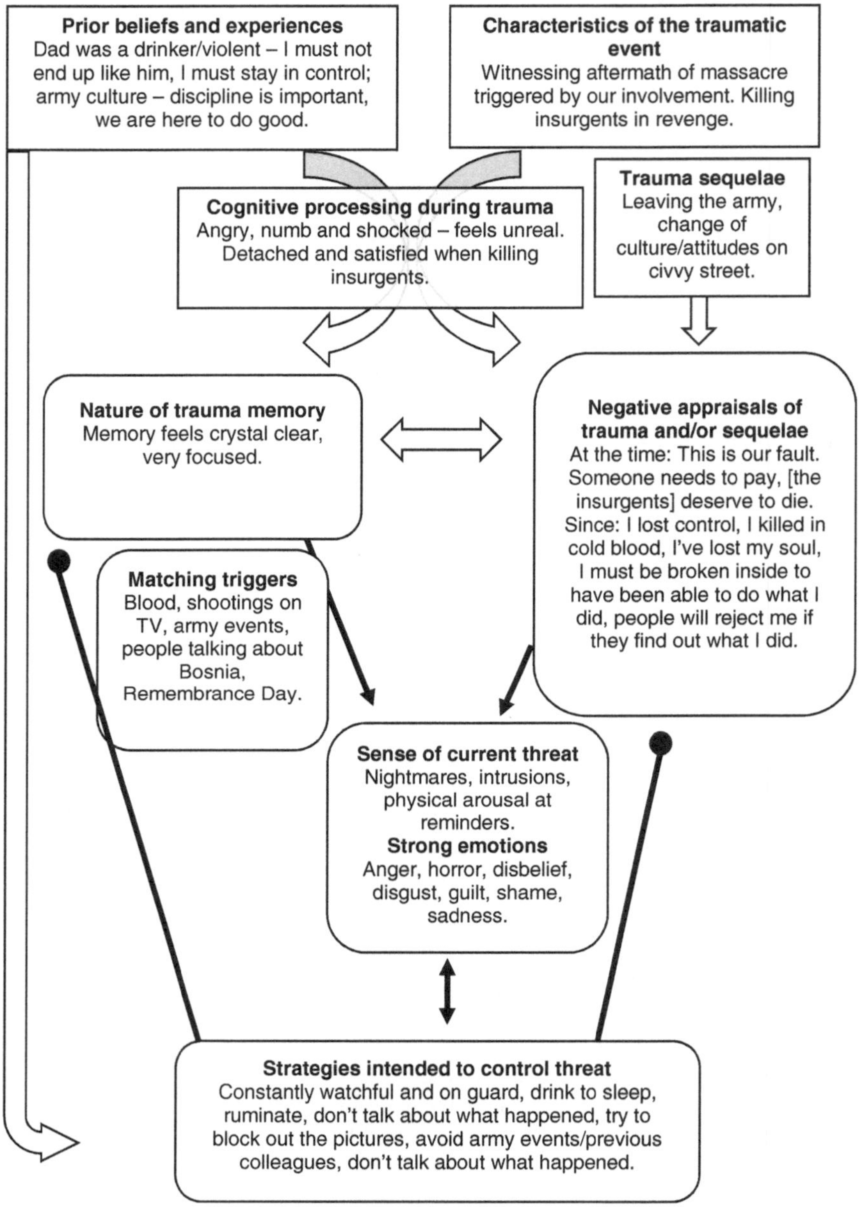

Figure 16.1 Liam's formulation

'cleaned' the scene. He imagined repairing the bodies, covering them carefully and respectfully, and arranging for them to be buried in line with local customs. He wrote a letter to the civilians apologising to them, and commending their bravery, and buried it underneath a tree he planted in his garden, along with one of his medals.

Recommended reading

Griffin, B. J., Purcell, N., Burkman, K., Litz, B. T., Bryan, C. J., Schmitz, M., Villierme, C., Walsh, J., & Maguen, S. (2019). Moral injury: An integrative review. *Journal of Traumatic Stress*, 32(3), 350–362.

Litz, B. T., Stein, N., Delaney, E., Lebowitz, L., Nash, W. P., Silva, C., & Maguen, S. (2009). Moral injury and moral repair in war veterans: A preliminary model and intervention strategy. *Clinical Psychology Review*, 29(8), 695–706.

Murray, H., & Ehlers, A. (2021). Cognitive therapy for moral injury in post-traumatic stress disorder. *the Cognitive Behaviour Therapist*, 14, e8.

PART FOUR

Complexity in coping strategies

CHAPTER SEVENTEEN

Drugs and alcohol

Brendan had a long history of excessive alcohol use, which worsened after he developed PTSD and depression following the sudden death of his wife. He was taking opiate-based pain medication for back pain, and also using it when he felt stressed. Brendan's therapist helped him understand how PTSD and substance use could keep each other going, and they developed a plan to create a 'window' of three alcohol and pain medication-free days a week around their PTSD treatment sessions.

Many people with PTSD misuse drugs or medication, or drink alcohol to excess. This can complicate treatment and, in some clinical services, may exclude people from trauma-focused treatment. However, where PTSD and substance use have become mutually maintaining, clients may struggle to reduce their substance use while their PTSD remains untreated. Hence, our treatment interventions ideally need to address both problems simultaneously rather than sequentially. This chapter will explain how.

Why are substance use and PTSD often co-morbid?

People with PTSD are more likely than the general population to also have a substance use disorder or SUD (Jacobsen et al., 2001) and the two problems can interact in various ways. Firstly, many people use substances (whether it be alcohol, nicotine, caffeine, illicit drugs, or medication) to manage their PTSD symptoms. For example, to numb distress caused by memories, get to sleep, manage tiredness, cope with anxiety, or increase readiness for perceived threats. This may be a new coping behaviour or an exacerbation of pre-existing substance use, problematic or otherwise. This 'self-medication hypothesis' is supported fairly consistently by research (Chilcoat, & Breslau, 1998). There is also some evidence that people with SUDs are at increased risk of trauma (the 'high risk' hypothesis, Chilcoat, & Breslau, 1998). For example, people may be more likely to get into conflicts leading to assaults, take risks, or have accidents when they are intoxicated.

Finally, substance misuse may interfere with recovery from PTSD (Kaysen et al., 2011). Alcohol and drugs affect the emotional and cognitive processing of trauma memories; so where substances are used to block out PTSD re-experiencing symptoms or numb associated painful emotions, the memories are never processed and continue to intrude. Substance misuse may also inadvertently exacerbate PTSD symptoms, and/or maintain trauma-related beliefs such as 'I'm a lousy coper'. For example, a client who uses alcohol to get to sleep may have less refreshing sleep leading to lower mood and energy the following day. A client who smokes cannabis to feel less anxious may instead feel more paranoid and suspicious, driving increased hypervigilance behaviours. A client who drinks 'energy' drinks to overcome tiredness may instead feel agitated and irritable, and then struggle to get to sleep. A client who binges on cocaine may become more

DOI: 10.4324/9781003288329-21

aggressive and reckless while 'high', and more depressed and suicidal afterwards. Clients who misuse prescribed medication to alleviate emotional or physical pain may experience unwanted side effects, withdrawal symptoms, or accidental overdoses. Substance misuse may also contribute to secondary psychological problems such as depression, as well as financial, occupational, health, and relationship problems.

Treatment approaches

From a treatment perspective, not all substance use is problematic. Moderate levels of alcohol, nicotine, caffeine, or occasional recreational drug use are unlikely to interfere with recovery from PTSD. Equally, we support appropriate and targeted use of medication such as adherent use of a prescribed antidepressant or taking a single benzodiazepine dose to cope with a dental or gynaecological procedure.

However, where substance use is habitual, dependent, and/or is being used to self-medicate PTSD symptoms, trauma-focused treatment risks worsening it. Distress and temporary PTSD symptom exacerbation, caused by working on trauma memories, may lead to a harmful increase in substance use with associated risks. In turn, substance misuse may exacerbate PTSD symptoms directly, or interfere with the effective components of trauma-focused therapies, limiting benefit or prolonging exacerbation. While it is preferable, requiring our clients to stop using alcohol or drugs entirely before starting treatment is also often ineffective if this is their primary means of coping with their PTSD symptoms. Instead, it may result in them 'bouncing' between services, as untreated PTSD leads to relapsing substance misuse, which in turn prevents them accessing PTSD treatment.

An alternative approach is to integrate treatment for both problems, and several programmes have been developed with this aim (e.g. Back et al., 2014; Coffey et al., 2016; Najavits et al., 2005). Systemic factors, including the type of service offering treatment, will be relevant in shaping how treatment can be delivered. For example, multidisciplinary teams, specialist drug and alcohol services, and residential units may see clients with more significant substance use, and have greater capacity to provide PTSD therapy safely alongside interventions for substance misuse, compared to psychology-only primary care teams. Treatment decisions are therefore made on a case-by-case basis, depending on the client's needs and the clinical setting.

How to adjust treatment

The nature and extent of substance use determine how we adapt treatment. For example:

- *Minimal interference with treatment:* The client is motivated to attend and engage with therapy tasks, substance use is low, or the client is prepared to stop or minimise use except for clearly circumscribed contexts, e.g. a glass or two of wine at social events. Medication is taken as prescribed, with no evidence of withdrawal cycles, 'topping up', or impairment in cognitive functioning. Here, treatment proceeds as usual.
- *Historical misuse:* The client has previously misused substances, but is currently abstinent. Here, we make a concrete safety plan around how to recognise and respond to a relapse.
- *Problematic misuse:* The client is using at a problematic level and/or substance use is exacerbating PTSD symptoms, interfering with treatment, or leading to additional problems. We explore the functions and costs of substance use, bringing the client's attention to interactions with

PTSD and treatment. To support the delivery of trauma-focused treatment, we negotiate to create a 'window' in their day or week where they can minimise or abstain from substance misuse.

- *Moderate to severe substance use disorders*: The client uses high quantities of substances, in a frequent, prolonged or dependent manner, with significant impairment in health and functioning. In these cases, multidisciplinary team input is needed (psychology-only services should liaise with specialist services), including medical professionals to support withdrawal and address physical dependence. More sessions are likely to be needed, with components drawn from existing evidence-based treatments that address comorbid PTSD-SUD presentations, e.g. 'Seeking Safety' (Najavits, 2002).

ASSESSMENT

Asking about drugs and alcohol is a standard aspect of a clinical assessment. Where alcohol is being used to excess, any non-prescribed drugs are being used, or there is an overuse of prescribed drugs such as benzodiazepines or opiate-based painkillers, we use standardised tools such as the SCID-5 module for substance use disorders (First et al., 2016), and the AUDIT (Alcohol Use Disorders Identification Test; Babor et al., 2001) to learn more about the extent and impact of the use.

To plan treatment and gather information for our formulation, we need to assess:

- *How much is being used?* It can be difficult to get an accurate measure of substance use retrospectively, so diaries are useful. Clients may feel embarrassed or ashamed and minimise their use, so we need to foster a supportive and collaborative therapeutic relationship, and emphasise the importance of transparency in working together effectively.
- *How is it being used?* Diaries can also help us to understand how and when substances are being used, particularly in relation to PTSD symptoms, other emotional and mental states such as low mood, dissociation or stress, and situations such as social interactions. This information helps us formulate the functions of substance use. More detailed chain analyses can also be used to understand the factors leading up to an episode of substance use and its consequences (Rizvi, & Ritschel, 2014).
- *How did use develop over time?* Knowing how substance use has developed over time, particularly in relation to life events and the emergence of psychological problems, allows us to understand how these various elements interrelate.
- *What is being used, how does it affect them?* Different drugs will have different cognitive effects and can stay in an individual's system for varying amounts of time (depending on the drug, how much is used, the client's age, weight etc.). Cognitive functioning may be impaired by chronic drug use. These variables will help understand the potential impact on treatment.
- *How does it contribute to maintaining PTSD?* The effects of substances on PTSD (and other symptoms) should also be assessed. Diaries and behavioural experiments in reducing substance use and monitoring the impact on symptoms can be useful.
- *What risks does it pose?* Substance use can place people at significant risk of harm to themselves or others, and from others. Where present, these risks take immediate priority before treatment proceeds.
- *What other coping strategies/resources do they have?* The capacity of an individual to engage with treatment will depend in part on their personal resources, including support networks, overall level of functioning, and alternative coping strategies.

Top tips: Watch out for opiate-based pain medication

The excessive use and misuse of opiate-based pain medications such as Tramadol, Co-Codamol, and Fentanyl have been well-documented in the United States and, increasingly, in the UK. Many of our PTSD clients experience chronic pain, sometimes caused by trauma-related injuries, and may have been prescribed strong pain medication. Not everyone takes it as prescribed. Some clients find it has an appealing psychological effect, helping them sleep or taking the edge off strong negative emotions, so use the medication to manage their PTSD symptoms as well as their pain.

One problem with opiate painkillers is that they interfere with cognitive processing (Elrassas et al., 2020), which may reduce the effectiveness of trauma-focused treatments both by reducing learning capacity and, potentially, by blunting the necessary activation of trauma memories, appraisals, and emotions. Ideally, we prefer our clients not to take opiates during treatment but significant pain is clearly also a potential obstacle to treatment. We approach this by negotiating with the client and whoever manages their pain medication (preferably a specialist pain service) to trial an alternative (non-opiate) pain medication, at least for the day of the session and the following day, to create a window for unimpaired learning and cognitive and emotional processing.

If other pain medications are ineffective and pain is an obstacle to treatment, or switching medications causes unwanted effects, then we ask clients to take opiate medication at regular intervals and stable dosages, only as prescribed, and not in response to emotional distress or PTSD symptoms. It can be helpful to ask their doctor to dispense medications in pre-loaded 'dosette' boxes to help the client stick to a stable dose regime.

FORMULATION

The information from our assessment informs a shared formulation. As well as guiding treatment, this opens a conversation about how PTSD and substance use may maintain one another, and hopefully normalises and de-stigmatises both problems.

Formulations may be as simple as a single maintenance cycle. Using a recent example of an episode of problematic use is a good place to start. Other formulations are more complex. Multiple maintenance cycles may be relevant. Longitudinal formulations may also be helpful, particularly for clients with a long history of drug and/or alcohol use which has interacted with traumatic experiences throughout their life.

Ian explained that he had 'always been a drinker', dating his alcohol use back to his time in the police. Ian remembered senior members of his unit encouraging younger officers to have a drink after a difficult day, and had found it an effective way of coping. He had also enjoyed drinking socially with friends.

After he retired, Ian's alcohol use increased and he reported drinking up to a bottle of whiskey most days. He was no longer drinking socially, but alone. Since leaving the police, Ian had been plagued by nightmares and distressing intrusions of traumatic experiences and he found the whiskey was a useful way of getting to sleep and 'keeping the demons away'.

Ian's therapist shared some information about PTSD, including how avoidance could maintain trauma memories and sketched a simple diagram to illustrate this (Figure 17.1).

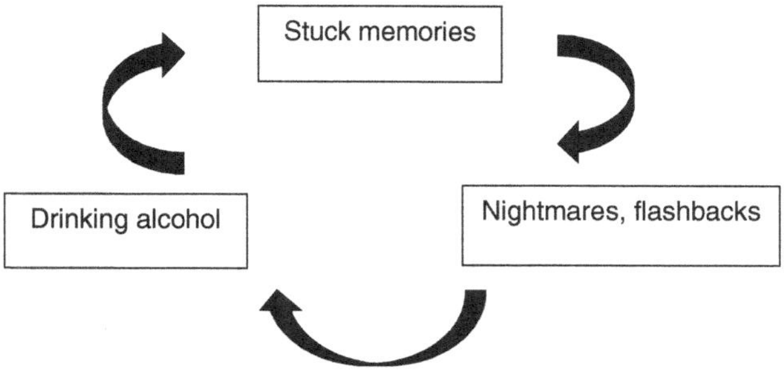

Figure 17.1 Ian's formulation

> Ian quickly understood that alcohol was only a temporary solution to managing his trauma memories and did not solve the underlying problems. He expressed concerns about what would happen if he didn't use alcohol, but was willing to consider a treatment plan that included learning other ways of dealing with his problems.

INCREASING MOTIVATION TO REDUCE SUBSTANCE USE

In early sessions, we address the client's motivation to reduce their use of drugs and alcohol. Considering the costs and benefits (short- and longer-term) of substance use is often helpful. We validate the reasons for use and help clients recognise the consequences, including maintaining PTSD as well as other problems in their life. We include relevant psychoeducation on the effects of alcohol and drugs, including on mood, sleep, and PTSD symptoms.

> Tara had smoked cannabis with friends since her early teens. She found it made her feel more relaxed in social situations. After she was raped by an ex-boyfriend whilst at university, Tara began smoking cannabis every day, starting from the morning.
>
> Tara and her therapist drew up a list of pros and cons of using cannabis. Tara found it made her feel more relaxed and less anxious, particularly in social situations. However, she knew that smoking was bad for her health, reduced her motivation to study, was expensive, made her hungry and had led to weight gain, and she didn't like having to hide it from her parents.
>
> Together, Tara and her therapist researched the effects of cannabis on mood. They found that it can make people paranoid and Tara had noticed experiencing this. Tara's therapist explained that PTSD could often make people feel under threat and the cannabis might be exacerbating this feeling. They also learned that cannabis can impact people's ability to learn new things. Tara's therapist explained that treatment would probably be more effective if Tara had a clear head. Tara agreed to not smoke on the evening before, the day of, and the day after an appointment. They agreed to monitor the effect this had on Tara's PTSD symptoms, her mood, and concentration.

We draw on techniques from motivational interviewing (Miller, & Rollnick, 2012) in this work, i.e. use of empathy and a non-judgemental understanding of the client's perspective, helping the client to explore discrepancies between their current behaviour and the lives they would like to lead, avoiding arguments, rolling with resistance, and supporting self-efficacy as the client moves towards making changes.

Top tips: Involve family, friends and partners

Involving supportive family members, friends, and partners in PTSD treatment is often valuable, and especially so when we are working with substance misuse. We sometimes talk about identifying a 'cheerleader' who can provide encouragement, maintain momentum between sessions, and prompt the use of healthy coping strategies and techniques such as stimulus discrimination. This person can be invited to some therapy sessions (with agreement from the client) and recruited to help with homework assignments.

Be alert to the wellbeing of others in the client's network; they may be vulnerable to mental health problems themselves. Relapses may also occur when people within the client's network misuse substances themselves, so identifying and problem-solving this risk early is important.

BEHAVIOURAL EXPERIMENTS

Behavioural experiments are used to test the effects of substances on particular symptoms. For example, people may use substances to help them sleep and prevent nightmares. Experiments in dropping the strategy and measuring the impact often reveal that some substances help people get to sleep initially, but sleep quality is poorer and they feel more fatigued the next day. Broken sleep caused by substances can actually increase the number of nightmares experienced. Some symptoms may temporarily increase when substances are reduced, so it is worth repeating an experiment on several occasions to get clear data.

Krishnan felt anxious leaving the house after he was assaulted. He would often have several drinks before he went out to 'take the edge off' his nerves. He planned a behavioural experiment where he recorded his anxiety levels while out every day for a week and whether or not he had a drink. Krishnan found that, initially, he felt slightly more anxious without alcohol, but the feeling quickly reduced, and he felt less shaky and jittery.

LEARNING ALTERNATIVE WAYS TO MANAGE SYMPTOMS

Using substances to manage PTSD symptoms may be a deliberate strategy, but some clients do not realise what triggers the urge to use, so diaries and functional analyses can be useful to understand the link. Recognising triggers allows a more conscious decision to cope in an alternative way. For example, stimulus discrimination can be an alternative way of coping with memory triggers, sleep hygiene to fall asleep, and self-care and emotion regulation strategies to cope with painful emotions. As usual, we only spend as much time as is needed on teaching effective coping for the client to safely proceed to trauma-focused treatment, which will hopefully resolve symptoms more effectively. We try to avoid replacing substance use with other safety-seeking behaviours. For example, if someone is using amphetamines to increase their awareness of danger, we wouldn't replace that with an alternative vigilance behaviour, as this maintains the belief that excessive vigilance is necessary to prevent future harm. However, we would encourage adaptive coping strategies that reduce the impact of symptoms.

For many clients, a few sessions on this type of work is sufficient. However, for others, a more thorough approach is needed, particularly when clients meet criteria for a SUD. If so, we recommend the 'Seeking Safety' approach (Najavits et al., 2005). Clients and therapists choose problem-specific modules to work on from 25 topics relating to SUD and PTSD, such as 'When

Substances Control You', 'Healthy Relationships', and 'Healing from Anger'. 'Seeking Safety' doesn't include work on trauma memories, but can be used as a precursor to trauma-focused work.

ADDRESSING BARRIERS TO CHANGE

Identifying, formulating, and problem-solving barriers to change is an important aspect of this work. Clients may have previous experiences of unsuccessful treatment and limited hopes of success, or lack self-belief in their capacity to make changes, or stick to them. Others feel very ashamed about their problems. We must show consistency, patience, compassion, and optimism in our approach, and identify and address these internal barriers.

Other barriers may be external, such as factors in the client's life and interpersonal network which support substance misuse. Where possible, we engage others in the client's system and support them to problem-solve difficulties.

> Michaela's children were taken into care due to domestic abuse. After Michaela's ex-partner was sent to prison, the local authority decided that the children should stay in foster care due to Michaela's history of substance misuse.
>
> In therapy, Michaela reported a strong motivation to get her children back. She met criteria for PTSD and SUD. Initially, she made good progress in treatment. However, Michaela had a series of negative interactions with social services, making her feel judged and stigmatised despite her efforts to recover, and she relapsed into substance use to cope with these difficult feelings. The relapse made her feel even worse about herself. Michaela's therapist helped her to map out this vicious cycle and they discussed ways to break it.
>
> Michaela's therapist arranged a joint meeting with her caseworker from social services and a representative from a family rights charity who had agreed to advocate for Michaela. They discussed the processes involved in the care system clearly and calmly, which allowed Michaela to understand her rights, what social services needed her to achieve, and the support available. They also agreed a plan for Michaela to update her caseworker regularly, and how and when she was allowed to contact the children. Although no promises were made to Michaela about getting her children back, she felt more in control and better supported as a result of the meeting, and better able to engage in her recovery.

Hot cognitions

- I need alcohol/drugs to get to sleep/cope with my feelings and memories
- I need to stay sharp to avoid being hurt again
- If I admit how much I am drinking/using, my therapist will say I can't have therapy
- I've tried to stop so many times, it doesn't work for me
- If I stop drinking/using drugs, my anxiety will be out of control

FLEXIBILITY IN TREATMENT

The flexible, formulation-based approach of CT-PTSD means that we can target whichever processes are most problematic for a client, including those which trigger substance misuse. For example, if shame is a trigger, we can address the related beliefs and memory hotspots as a priority. If substances are used to reduce anxiety in certain situations, the associated appraisals can be addressed and tested using behavioural experiments.

Flexibility may also be needed in treatment delivery. Clients with SUDs have higher dropout rates from PTSD treatment (Bedard-Gilligan et al., 2018), so extra efforts to engage them may be needed. This includes listening carefully to the client's goals, priorities and concerns, remaining transparent and collaborative about all aspects of treatment, and being prepared to adjust the treatment plan to deal with problems as they emerge and change.

RESPONDING TO RELAPSES

Clients may relapse into heavy alcohol or drug use during treatment. If so, we pause work on trauma memories and work on understanding what triggered the relapse and how to manage these triggers differently if they arise again. We avoid 'telling off' or shaming our client, or overstating the significance of a setback. Equally, we avoid minimising the relapse, its consequences, or the client's feelings about it. We positively reinforce their disclosure and hence their commitment to 'working together' to address it, and frame the relapse as a 'bump in the road' rather than being 'back to square one'. We use it as an opportunity to better understand the functions of relapses through a chain analysis of the events leading up to it, and support our client to re-establish their coping plan and 'get back on track'. As soon as possible, and with the agreement of the client that they feel ready, we return to trauma-focused work.

FAQ: What do I do if someone shows up to an appointment intoxicated?

If a client has used drugs or alcohol before a session, we usually stop the session and rearrange the appointment. At the next session, we discuss what triggered the use, taking a non-judgemental stance. Often clients feel anxious before a session and have used a substance to manage this. We address the appraisals underlying the anxiety and plan behavioural experiments to test alternative ways to cope.

If a client is repeatedly coming to sessions intoxicated, it may be an indication that they require an intervention focused on substance misuse before revisiting trauma work. We never want to give someone the impression that they have failed, or that they will never be able to get through a course of treatment. Instead, we discuss the current goals and priorities, and how to address these, with a plan to return to trauma-focused treatment when possible.

NOTES FROM THE THERAPY ROOM: BRENDAN

Brendan was referred to mental health services by his GP. He had a long history of alcohol use disorder and had attempted several courses of outpatient treatment with a drug and alcohol service, as well as two residential 'detoxes', but had relapsed each time. In his twenties, Brendan had used drugs recreationally, including cocaine and ecstasy. Now in his fifties, Brendan no longer used non-prescribed drugs. However, he took Tramadol for chronic back pain, which he described as a 'crutch' that helped with his psychological problems.

Brendan had grown up in Northern Ireland. His father had been violent towards Brendan's mother and their five children. Brendan left home as soon as possible and moved to England, where he worked in the building trade throughout his adult life. He described a culture of heavy drinking amongst his peers, and would routinely go to the pub after work and drink up to ten pints of beer. When Brendan was in his thirties, his wife died suddenly while they were on holiday. Brendan described a 'dark year' that followed where he became very depressed, his drinking escalated, and he came close to suicide.

At assessment, Brendan reported PTSD symptoms related to his wife's death, including intrusions of her face as she was dying, nightmares where she begged him for help, and strong feelings of guilt for not saving her. He had been signed off work due to his back pain and was spending a lot of time at home 'stewing'. Brendan described other stresses in his life including conflict with his second wife, from whom he was separated, money worries, and concerns about his health. Brendan was overweight, with type II diabetes. His GP had told him that, unless he changed his lifestyle, he was likely to die early. Brendan had an 11-year old daughter from his second marriage and described a strong motivation to 'sort himself out' so he could live to see her grow up.

Brendan's therapist asked him to keep a diary of his alcohol and Tramadol use. Several patterns emerged. He tended to drink when his mood was low and when he was dwelling on 'where it all went wrong'. Brendan was doing very little with his time and it appeared that boredom and inactivity were also triggers for alcohol use. He used Tramadol to cope with back pain, but also in response to intrusive memories and the associated feelings of guilt and sadness. His formulation is in Figure 17.2.

Brendan and his therapist discussed a simplified version of this formulation and agreed some initial treatment targets, including cutting down his alcohol use. They wrote down the pros and cons of his drinking, and Brendan kept a copy of this on his fridge and his phone for when he was tempted to drink. They also worked on triggers for drinking, decreasing rumination, and introduced 'reclaiming your life' to increase Brendan's meaningful activities. This included problem-solving ways for Brendan to spend time with his friends outside of the pub. With help from his GP, Brendan agreed to begin switching from Tramadol to a non-opiate painkiller. They worked on stimulus discrimination to deal with his intrusions differently.

As guilt was another common trigger for Brendan's drinking, they addressed his appraisals about his wife's death. She had suffered from an undiagnosed heart problem and had been complaining of tiredness and swelling in her ankles. Brendan believed he should have recognised there was something seriously wrong, got her medical help, and delayed their holiday. In addressing his hindsight bias, Brendan and his therapist distributed a survey that revealed that most other people did not recognise these were symptoms of heart disease in a young woman. Brendan also remembered that his wife had suggested the holiday and had not thought her symptoms were serious.

After five sessions, Brendan had reduced his alcohol use and had stopped using Tramadol. However, he suffered a relapse following an argument with his brother and missed several sessions. When he re-engaged, Brendan admitted he had been drinking heavily for a few weeks, and they agreed to pause trauma-focused work and spend a few sessions on interpersonal conflict, as this was a common trigger for Brendan's drinking. Brendan decided to put a pull-up bar in his garage and agreed to a behavioural experiment where he did pull-ups for five minutes instead of drinking when he felt angry. He found this a useful strategy, and his alcohol use stabilised.

Once Brendan was having three alcohol-free days a week again, they returned to work on the trauma, including having a conversation with his wife in imagery. This unexpectedly led to an improvement in Brendan's alcohol use, as he realised that his wife would have hated him drinking so much. It also helped to generate meaningful updates about his wife's death, as Brendan realised that she would not have blamed him, and would not want him to feel guilty, which they inserted into a written narrative of the trauma. Brendan's PTSD symptoms began to decrease and his mood improved. This facilitated further work on 'reclaiming your life'. Brendan realised that his job prospects in the building trade were now limited due to his back condition and took steps to look for alternative work. His therapist helped him access a charity to support him finding work, and Brendan also decided to start attending Alcoholics Anonymous, to continue his recovery.

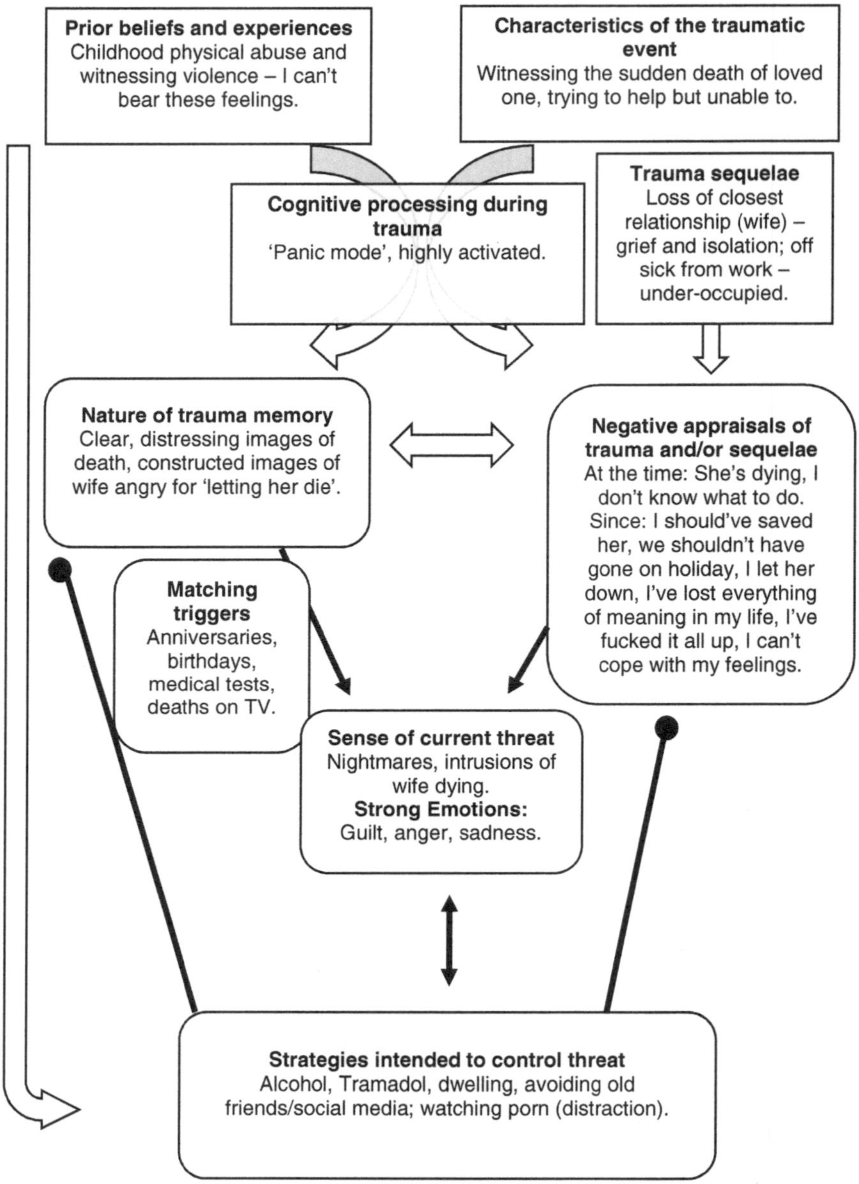

Figure 17.2 Brendan's formulation

Recommended reading

Baschnagel, J. S., Coffey, S. F., & Rash, C. J. (2006). The treatment of co-occurring PTSD and substance use disorders using trauma-focused exposure therapy. *International Journal of Behavioral Consultation and Therapy*, 2(4), 498–508.

Improving Access to Psychological Therapy. (2012). *IAPT positive practice guide for working with people who use drugs and alcohol*. Available at: www.uea.ac.uk/documents/746480/2855738/iapt-drug-and-alcohol-positive-practice-guide.pdf

Najavits, L. (2002). *Seeking safety: A treatment manual for PTSD and substance abuse*. Guilford Press.

CHAPTER EIGHTEEN

Reckless behaviour

Julia had experienced abuse within relationships in childhood and as an adult. She now engaged in several risky behaviours, including self-harm by cutting, 'rough' sex, and having contact with her abusive ex-partner. Her therapist helped her explore and understand the functions of these behaviours. They worked together to address Julia's guilt which drove an urge to punish herself, finding alternative ways to manage her intense feelings and make sense of her traumatic experiences.

Some people with PTSD engage in unintentionally risky and/or intentionally self-destructive behaviours, and this may reflect a personality-related 'externalising' (Miller, & Resick, 2007) or behaviourally 'reckless' PTSD subtype (Contractor, & Weiss, 2019). Examples include non-suicidal self-injury (NSSI), high-risk sexual behaviour, dangerous driving, disordered eating, drink/drug bingeing, criminality, gambling, 'cyber addiction', and aggression. 'Reckless and self-destructive behaviour' was added as a symptom of PTSD in DSM-5 (APA, 2013). In this chapter, we have used the word 'reckless' to encompass the full range of behaviours, in keeping with the DSM phrasing, but recognise that it represents a subjective label which some may find stigmatising, and use our clients' words in therapy to describe specific behaviours.

Only a minority of people with PTSD present with reckless behaviour (Carmassi et al., 2013). It appears to be associated with more severe presentations of PTSD (Contractor et al., 2017), and particularly those who have experienced multiple and interpersonal traumas including military veterans (Killgore et al., 2008), refugees (Spiller et al., 2017), survivors of sexual assault (Deliramich, & Gray, 2008), and people abused in childhood (Briere, 2019). Reckless behaviours are also associated with other disorders, including personality disorders. We discuss how to work with comorbid personality disorders in Chapter 20, so we focus in this chapter on reckless behaviours associated with PTSD.

Reckless behaviours require attention in treatment. They can place people at risk of experiencing further traumas (Lusk et al., 2017) and may partly account for the increased mortality rates in people with PTSD through accidents, substance misuse, cardiovascular disease (Drescher et al., 2003; Flood et al., 2010), and suicidality (Armour et al., 2017).

Behaving recklessly may seem counter-intuitive, given that people with PTSD generally take excessive precautions to feel safe. Similarly, although most people with PTSD avoid trauma reminders, some deliberately seek out and expose themselves to memory triggers (Bellet et al., 2020). Reckless behaviours can often be understood as a form of 'reactive avoidance'; a means to reduce emotional pain which is effective in the short term but, as with other forms of avoidance, creates vicious cycles which maintain the problem longer term (Briere, 2019). For example, people may feel ashamed of their behaviour, which compounds their distress and self-attack; or be exposed to further adverse events and their consequences.

DOI: 10.4324/9781003288329-22

In this chapter, we will cover reckless behaviours that are not overtly motivated by a wish to die. Although there are areas of overlap, we discuss working with suicidality, risk from others, and occupational risk in Chapter 23.

Why do some people with PTSD take excessive risks?

Several theories have been proposed for why some traumatised people take risks (Ben-Zur, & Zeidner, 2009), and people with PTSD give wide-ranging explanations for their reckless behaviour. Different kinds of reckless behaviours often co-occur, and equally may serve different functions and be associated with different PTSD symptom clusters (Armour et al., 2020). For example, re-experiencing symptoms may be associated with substance misuse and NSSI; numbing symptoms with thrill-seeking; negative emotions and anhedonia with gambling, spending, and smartphone use; and arousal symptoms with aggression or risky sexual behaviour. We need to conceptualise the idiosyncratic functions of our client's reckless behaviours and their relationship to PTSD symptoms. Here are some common mechanisms.

SYMPTOM MANAGEMENT AND EMOTION REGULATION

Many people with prolonged traumatic experiences in childhood, especially abuse or neglect from a primary caregiver, lack adaptive skills in regulating their emotions. Outside the PTSD literature, there is significant evidence that difficulties regulating emotions underlie a range of reckless behaviours (Weiss et al., 2015). Symptoms of PTSD are intrinsically aversive and often feel overwhelming, so clients may use reckless behaviours to manage intense emotional states. These may represent an individual's best available means to self-soothe, by releasing emotional tension or distracting from emotional pain. There are neurobiological correlates to this mechanism; NSSI, for example, temporarily increases levels of endogenous opioids, which induce calm feelings and reduce pain, and are often depleted in survivors of chronic trauma (Groschwitz, & Plener, 2012).

Clients with emotional numbing symptoms may use behaviours such as gambling, dangerous driving, or criminality to experience an adrenaline rush; a preferable alternative to feeling flat or empty. NSSI is sometimes also used to control dissociation; either to feel 'real' when experiencing depersonalisation/derealisation or to 'ground' and terminate dissociative flashbacks.

> Irina struggled with feelings of contamination after a sexual assault. One way she coped was by restricting her eating, which made her feel 'cleaner' inside. She had felt powerless and defeated during the trauma, and counting calories, 'clean eating', and exercising hard made her feel more in control. She also liked the sense of being detached from her body which arose when she was hungry. Unfortunately, restricting was having severe negative effects on Irina's health. She began to have fainting episodes, and blood tests showed that her potassium and sodium levels were dangerously low. She was physically exhausted, and often felt 'foggy' and confused, which in turn made her feel more vulnerable.

SELF-TRIGGERING AND AFFECT MATCHING

A similar process occurs with 'affect matching', where clients choose external experiences or manage feelings in ways that match or enhance their negative internal experience. For example, depressed people often choose emotion-regulation strategies that increase their feelings of sadness (like listening to sad music), rather than those that lift their mood (Millgram et al., 2015), because negative feelings are also reassuringly familiar, and match their sense of themselves as depressed. In PTSD, this process can motivate reckless affect-matching; for example, risky sexual behaviours that make an individual feel used and degraded to match a debased sense of self; or seeking out road rage encounters to match an internal aroused rage state.

For others, intentional 'self-triggering' may provide a sense of mastery over PTSD symptoms, by making external triggers come under their control and therefore become predictable or by maintaining a constant and tolerable level of symptoms rather than experiencing unexpected 'spikes' (Bellet et al., 2020).

Some clients deliberately re-enact traumas or self-trigger trauma memories to 'make sense' of an event, perhaps to fill in gaps in their memory, work out why it happened, or if they could have coped better and achieved a different outcome (Bellet et al., 2020).

THRILL-SEEKING AND DISINHIBITION

For some people, the feeling of being flooded with adrenaline, whether through danger or excitement, can become addictive. Clients who have been repeatedly exposed to danger may find themselves deliberately seeking it out to achieve the same 'buzz', counter negative feelings, or simply feel 'normal'.

There are also inherent rewards to some reckless behaviours, such as positive feelings generated by drugs, alcohol, sex, or food, and excitement related to dicing with danger or gambling. PTSD symptoms can make it more difficult to inhibit risky behaviours in such rewarding situations (Ben-Zur, & Zeidner, 2009). PTSD also affects information processing through narrowing attention and reducing concentration, making it more difficult to properly evaluate risks and potential negative consequences. Some clients, especially those with early trauma histories, or prolonged periods of living in risky situations, may also lack the skills to recognise and respond to risk. Their recklessness may be inadvertent; some situations simply do not feel subjectively risky when they are. These patterns can interact with personality variables, such as impulsivity, which pre-date the traumas (James et al., 2014).

> When Lee left the army, he missed the excitement of living and working in a high-risk environment, as well as the bonds he had formed with others. Lee described himself as an 'adrenaline junkie' even before the army and had always enjoyed extreme sports. After he left, he felt out of place and bored in civilian life and tried to find ways of getting his 'fix' of excitement. He started going out a lot with friends, taking and dealing drugs, getting into fights, and visiting sex workers. He began working as a bouncer in a rough pub but ideally wanted to go back to Iraq to work as a private security contractor.

SELF-PUNISHMENT OR REPAIRING SELF-ESTEEM

Reckless behaviours may operate as a form of self-punishment, usually relating to feelings of guilt, shame, and/or self-hatred. This may lead to NSSI, deliberate self-triggering, or seeking out abusive relationships. Some clients tell us this is what they feel they 'deserve'.

Others with low self-esteem may use reckless behaviours as a means of repairing their self-image. They may also place themselves at risk by doing things for others, to keep a relationship rather than be alone. This pattern has been suggested as a reaction against awareness of mortality which often follows a life-threatening trauma (Ben-Zur, & Zeidner, 2009). For example, 'picking up' a stranger for sex may initially make someone feel powerful and desirable, and provide a brief, intense interpersonal connection. However, after the initial self-esteem enhancement, reckless behaviours can lead to further self-criticism, perpetuating the cycle.

PASSIVE SUICIDALITY

Some clients tell us that, while they have no concrete plans to kill themselves, they don't care if they live or die and are passively reckless; for example, crossing roads without looking, driving dangerously, or not taking medications that keep them healthy. These behaviours may be a way of 'letting it happen', or even making their death seem like an accident rather than suicide, to avoid upsetting loved ones.

Hot cognitions

- This is the only thing that makes me feel something
- I deserve to be hurt/treated this way
- It doesn't matter if I die/this will make it look like an accident
- I don't know why I do it, but it feels right
- It's the best way of releasing the bad feelings/emotional pain
- I'm pathetic/disgusting because I can't control my cutting/eating/sexual behaviours/ gambling etc.

RECKLESS SAFETY-SEEKING AND RECLAIMING

Finally, some of our clients inadvertently put themselves at risk when responding to trauma triggers. For example, veterans may drive dangerously to escape perceived threats such as getting 'boxed in' by other vehicles, or someone who experienced a car accident may switch lanes suddenly to avoid a vehicle similar to one which hit them (Possis et al., 2014). Safety behaviours intended to reduce threat may inadvertently increase danger, for example, repeatedly checking mirrors may take attention away from traffic ahead.

Cameron was assaulted and robbed by two men. He became hypervigilant when out in public, wanting to ensure that he was not targeted again. If Cameron saw anyone looking at him, he would stare them down and, on several occasions, he had aggressively confronted people who he believed were planning to rob him. He also got into a fight with a man who he believed was following him. Cameron's behaviour, while intended to prevent a further assault, inadvertently increased his risk, and also his perception of current threat.

People may also prefer to 'self-determine' their exposure to further harm, reasoning that if it is going to happen anyway, it is better by their own choosing. Others may engineer risky situations as a way of 'reclaiming their life' or 'getting over' their PTSD symptoms. For example, a client who was sexually assaulted by an acquaintance deliberately arranged internet dates at strangers' houses to 'not let it beat me'.

In summary, reckless behaviours may operate as a form of self-medicating, self-regulating, making sense, self-punishing, or gaining mastery after trauma. Through reinforcement, they may become increasingly compulsive and even addictive (Blasco-Fontecilla et al., 2016). Strategies intended to increase a feeling of control may instead contribute to feeling out of control. Reckless behaviours may directly exacerbate PTSD symptoms as well as the sense of the trauma being central to the client's life and identity. The client's appraisals of their behaviour, for example, that they are damaged, defective, or stupid for acting recklessly, and other people's responses, including blame, stigmatisation, and rejection, may create further vicious maintaining cycles.

How to help

ASSESSING AND FORMULATING

Standard clinical assessment will detect a subset of reckless behaviours, particularly substance use, aggression, and NSSI. Assessment tools based on the DSM-5 PTSD criteria will include an item on recklessness and, if this is endorsed, we comprehensively assess the full range of reckless behaviours as different types will frequently co-occur. Clients may feel ashamed, defensive, or secretive about these behaviours, or may not recognise them as reckless and so not report them spontaneously. They may have experienced negative reactions from others in the past, including blaming, accusations of 'attention seeking', criticism, or rejection. We discuss reckless behaviours in a non-judgemental, compassionate, and matter-of-fact manner, providing examples to check whether they might apply. We also use additional measures, such as the Posttrauma Risky Behaviours Questionnaire (Contractor et al., 2020), as a basis for further exploration.

As reckless behaviours have a range of well-intentioned functions, normalising, validating, and collaboratively formulating them with our clients is crucial before we attempt to modify them. Exploring the intended functions, and unintended consequences, of reckless behaviour helps to validate them as attempts to cope or recover, in the face of feeling powerless to control emotional pain or make sense of their experiences. This helps tackle stigma, promote self-compassion and understanding, and enhance motivation for change, as well as guiding us to possible interventions.

We use guided discovery techniques alongside functional analysis of recent examples to understand the 'chains' of situations, emotions, cognitions, and physical states that precede and follow the behaviours. Helping clients to recognise the triggers (which may be situational or more subtle internal triggers such as certain bodily sensations), alongside potentially reinforcing consequences, is a first step towards implementing changes.

If, as well as PTSD, a person's difficulties meet criteria for a personality disorder, with lifelong interpersonal difficulties alongside dangerous impulsivity, then consider whether evidence-based treatments such as dialectical behaviour therapy are more appropriate, or a better first step, before trauma-focused treatment for PTSD (see Chapter 20).

ADDRESSING MOTIVATION

The factors that determine whether trauma-focused psychological therapy is possible when a client is engaging in reckless behaviours include the type of behaviour, the level of risk, the service/treatment context, and the level of appropriate support in the client's network. If PTSD is effectively treated, the drive to engage in reckless behaviours should reduce. However, if they are functionally related to PTSD symptoms, then working on trauma memories may increase the behaviour temporarily, increasing risks. We share this dilemma with our clients and, if the behaviour presents an immediate risk, focus preliminary sessions on reducing it to a 'good enough' level, minimising harm, or stopping it completely. Behaviours that may prove fatal, such as driving very dangerously, extreme fasting, or potentially lethal NSSI are addressed in a safety plan (Chapter 23). This may involve negotiating a voluntary 'ban' on some activities to give treatment a chance, with the acknowledgement that, after treatment, it will be their choice whether to resume the behaviour.

Some behaviours can become compulsive and difficult to stop. Clients may be highly motivated already to change their behaviour; others may see no benefits. Many are ambivalent, torn between wanting and not wanting to change. Motivational interviewing techniques can be helpful here (Miller, & Rollnick, 2012). Drawing out a 2x2 table and listing the short-term and long-term costs and benefits of the behaviour is a valuable exercise, especially given that traumatised individuals are more likely to perceive greater benefit and fewer risks of reckless behaviours

(Smith et al., 2004). For some, this includes acknowledging and accepting that behaviours that feel good and 'right' may nevertheless lead to unwanted outcomes and prevent recovery, while more healthy alternatives may be less enjoyable, powerful, or rewarding.

> Sylvie was meeting men through dating apps for sex. She enjoyed the lead-up to the encounters, including messaging and flirting, which made her feel attractive and excited. She would stay up very late using her smartphone, which she preferred to sleeping and having nightmares. She also liked the 'edgy' feeling before dates and being in 'date-mode'. However she often felt 'used' afterwards, as some men would stop contacting her, or it would emerge that they were in relationships. Sylvie sometimes wanted men to be rough with her during sex, which she enjoyed, but also acknowledged that it could be risky if proper boundaries hadn't been established and Sylvie didn't know the person well. When she reviewed the costs and benefits of these behaviours with her therapist, Sylvie realised that, although she found the encounters exciting and distracting, they were not good for her self-esteem and could place her at risk. She agreed to try going on dates with people who she met through friends and to focus on shared interests and having fun, rather than on sexual chemistry.

ADDRESSING THE FUNCTION

Since many clients use external situations and stimulation to regulate their emotions, whether to improve mood, distract from unbearable affect, or 'affect match' internal states, we explore alternative ways of meeting the same need. For example, for people who use reckless behaviours to 'feel something', we experiment with 'reclaiming your life' activities that reduce numbing or produce positive feelings with fewer risks. For people who dissociate, we experiment instead with grounding strategies, attention shifting, applied tension, and movement.

Where clients have a limited repertoire of emotion regulation strategies, we support them to build both emotion-focused and problem-focused coping skills. We integrate modules targeting specific skills deficits from packages such as DBT-PE (Harned et al., 2012) or 'Seeking Safety' (Najavits et al., 2005), including 'opposite action', self-soothing strategies, distraction, boundary-setting, interpersonal skills, problem-solving, cost-benefit evaluation, and positive self-statements (page 45). We encourage clients to make written, pictorial, or audio-visual flashcards with a specific skill for each trigger or behavioural urge. Where relevant, we focus on mechanisms common to other PTSD symptoms, such as rumination, withdrawal, and self-attack. As before, our goal with skills-based work is to increase an individual's 'window of tolerance' just enough to permit trauma-focused treatment. Treating core PTSD symptoms as rapidly as possible will also reduce urges to behave recklessly. Hence, we may either work sequentially or concurrently, depending on the relative risks.

> Simon developed a gambling problem after the death of his wife. He found himself feeling flat and blank most of the time, or troubled by distressing intrusions of her death. He used online gambling as a way of feeling some positive emotions, like excitement, and to distract himself from the memories. In therapy, he experimented with alternative ways of managing his feelings. His therapist helped him increase reclaiming your life activities that he had previously enjoyed, like playing World of Warcraft with friends, and taught him stimulus discrimination as an alternative way of managing intrusive memories. He installed software on his computer and phone to block gambling sites and bought a games console so he could play video games when he had an urge to gamble.

Other mechanisms of reckless behaviours are addressed as part of CT-PTSD and these treatment elements can be prioritised. For example, where self-triggering forms part of understanding a trauma, filling in gaps, or mastering triggers, we can focus on the relevant cognitive themes, update hotspots, practise stimulus discrimination, seek new information through surveys and so on.

Where reckless behaviours function as self-punishment, preserving identity or repairing self-esteem, the beliefs underlying these can be addressed using cognitive strategies (e.g. cognitive-behavioural chairwork; Chapter 13). Clients whose safety behaviours inadvertently place them at risk of harm can benefit from addressing related risk appraisals (e.g. 'I'm safer when I carry a weapon'), and undertaking behavioural experiments in dropping the behaviours or replacing them with less risky precautions.

It is not always possible for clients to completely stop their reckless behaviours early in treatment, so we may need to accept some level of risk while we push the treatment forward. Depending on the service context, we can attempt to minimise the harm that the behaviour poses, rather than stopping it entirely, at least to the extent that treatment can be safely completed. Examples of harm minimisation include: replacing high-risk self-harm, such as blood-letting, with superficial cutting, keeping wounds clean, and seeking medical help if needed; replacing alcoholic spirits with beer, or strong 'skunk' cannabis with lower grade alternatives; or agreeing limits to high-risk thrill-seeking or sexual behaviour.

Lee missed the adrenaline and bonding experiences in the army and was seeking them in reckless ways in civilian life. He had limited motivation to change. Although he saw the potential risks of getting into fights and visiting sex workers, he also enjoyed the thrill of it and wasn't prepared to stop going on nights out with his friends. He planned several harm minimisation strategies with his therapist. He agreed to always use condoms when he had sex. He gave his friends permission to tell him to walk away from a potential fight on nights out. Lee also agreed to test out other activities to see if he could get an adrenaline rush more safely. He had a friend who ran a go-karting track and started helping out there at weekends in exchange for driving the karts for free. Lee also enjoyed weight training and decided to start training for a bodybuilding competition to help motivate him to prioritise his health, and to bond with others in the bodybuilding community.

Occasionally, our interventions take a more didactic approach. Some clients struggle to accurately assess risks, especially if they have spent much of their life in traumatic environments. For example, people who have grown up without models of healthy relationships may struggle to recognise warning signs of potentially abusive partners or respond effectively to abusive or controlling behaviour (Chapter 23).

Jyoti was born in India and was orphaned at a young age. After a period of being street homeless, she began working as a servant for a family, who treated her very badly. She was later trafficked to the UK to work as a servant for another family. In therapy, it became apparent that Jyoti had little experience of living in a safe environment and sometimes misjudged the risk in situations. For example, she tended to do whatever she was told because she was used to being punished for disobedience. However, this led to risky situations, and people took advantage of her vulnerability. Jyoti's therapist helped her learn how to evaluate which situations or requests from others were dangerous and which were safe. They role-played assertive statements and taking a 'zero tolerance' approach to mistreatment, then used behavioural experiments to test Jyoti's fear that she would be punished if she said 'no' to people in different settings, both public and private.

Notes from the therapy room: Julia

Julia had a history of multiple traumas in childhood and adulthood and now reported a range of reckless behaviours. She had grown up in a chaotic household. Her main caregiver was her mother, who had untreated bipolar disorder and struggled to care for Julia or her twin sister Chloe. Both girls were sexually abused by one of their mother's partners over several years. Chloe died by suicide when Julia was in her early twenties, and her mother died from cancer a few years later.

After the deaths of her sister and mother, Julia married an Italian man and moved to Italy for 'a new start'. However, she found it difficult to settle in a new culture, and her husband became increasingly jealous and possessive, so Julia left him and returned to the UK. She formed a new relationship but her boyfriend began to control Julia emotionally and financially. On one occasion, Julia tried to leave but he found her and persuaded her to come back. After this, he locked Julia in the house and became increasingly physically and sexually violent. Most of Julia's PTSD re-experiencing symptoms related to this time.

When Julia came for treatment, she had ended the relationship and moved to a different area of the country. However, she remained in touch with her ex-partner and had also formed a new relationship with a man who showed signs of becoming controlling and emotionally abusive. Julia described other behaviours which placed her at risk. She asked her partner to slap and choke her during sex. She also self-harmed by cutting her legs and breasts and described feeling that she had little control over this.

Julia's therapist helped her to explore these behaviours and together they began to understand their functions. Julia described being attracted to men who were controlling. This, and her desire to be hurt during sex, seemed to be self-triggering behaviours, as a way of making sense of her childhood traumas and as punishment for not protecting her sister Chloe. She reported low self-esteem and saw herself as 'broken' and 'worthless'. Self-punishment was also a motivation for self-harm, but Julia also felt it worked to release her 'bad' emotions and to feel physical pain which matched her emotional pain. Her formulation is in Figure 18.1.

Julia was motivated to change her behaviour but had struggled to in the past. She could identify no advantages to her risky behaviours, except that they 'felt right'. Her therapist explored with her the idea that 'things that feel right may not always be good for us', suggesting it might help to work on what makes them feel right, and try alternatives. Julia was open to this idea. She agreed to some harm minimisation strategies, including not seeing her ex-boyfriend or telling him her new address, not asking for higher-risk sexual behaviours such as choking while she was in therapy, and managing her self-harm safely (using clean blades and seeking medical help if she accidentally cut deeply).

Rather than work on the trauma memories immediately, they agreed to address Julia's beliefs about herself, as they seemed to underpin her urge for self-punishment. They worked on her belief that she should have protected her sister using a responsibility pie chart and a survey, and used continuum methods to address her beliefs about herself as 'broken' and 'worthless'. Julia had difficulty accepting an alternative, more compassionate view of herself as a 'survivor' with intrinsic worth and many positive qualities. Her therapist asked what she would have said to her sister, who had been through the same childhood experiences, and Julia was able to write a compassionate letter to them both, which she read out loud while holding a photo of herself and her sister as children.

Alongside this work, Julia's therapist helped her learn and practise emotion regulation strategies to help her manage distress. She enjoyed yoga and started using yoga postures and breathing when she felt upset, as well as listening to a meditation tape that her yoga instructor had recorded for her. They also experimented with ways to release the bad feelings other than self-harm, and

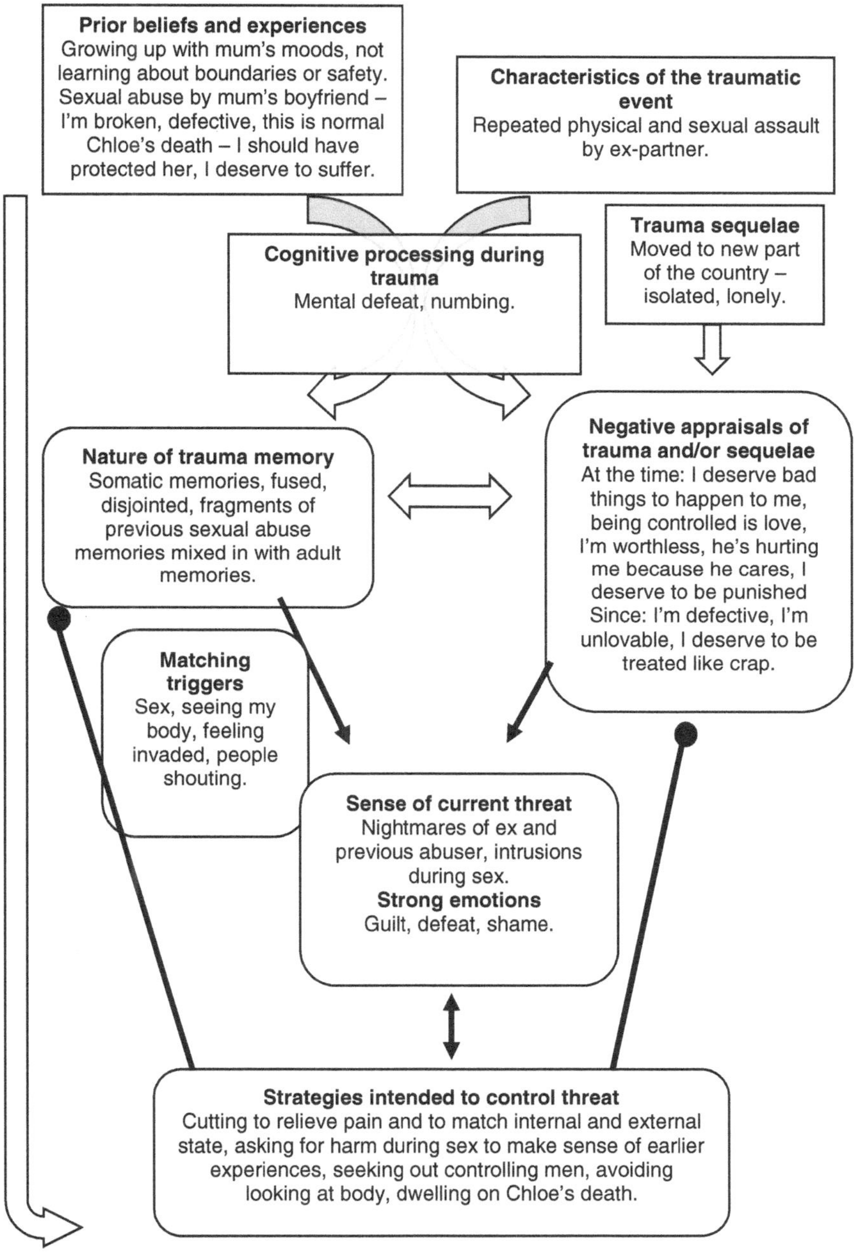

Figure 18.1 Julia's formulation

Julia found that running fast on the spot, doing squats, and lifting weights helped release the build-up of tension. Using these strategies, and with an improved sense of self-worth, Julia was able to reduce her self-harm episodes.

Julia felt ready to confront her trauma memories. She prepared a written narrative of her childhood trauma experiences. Julia's therapist normalised her experiences of confusion as a child about her mother's changing moods and the sexual abuse, and they focused on making sense of what had happened. They also used a written narrative with hotspot updates to address Julia's adult trauma memories. This work helped Julia to understand why she felt attracted to men who controlled her, and why she liked to be hurt during sex, as these dynamics felt familiar to her, and allowed her to re-enact and master past abuse memories. Processing the trauma memories in therapy presented an alternative way for Julia to deal with her past experiences. She also began to recognise other ways that she had been cared for in the past, and how she could seek these out in the future.

In the final stage of therapy, they explored Julia's relationship patterns, and how to identify the type of man who might end up hurting her. Julia had by now ended her relationship and resolved to stay single and to break off contact with her ex-boyfriend until she had worked out what she wanted from a partner. She planned instead a series of activities to reclaim her identity and build friendships.

Recommended reading

Bellet, B. W., Jones, P. J., & McNally, R. J. (2020). Self-triggering? An exploration of individuals who seek reminders of trauma. *Clinical Psychological Science*, 8(4), 739–755.

Briere, J. (2019). *Treating risky and compulsive behavior in trauma survivors*. Guilford Press.

CHAPTER NINETEEN
Avoidance

Cora developed PTSD after regaining consciousness during an operation. She strenuously avoided any reminder or conversation about her experience, as she rapidly felt overwhelmed with distress. In treatment, she did not want to work on trauma memories or undertake behavioural experiments. Her therapist formulated the beliefs which underlay Cora's avoidance and addressed these in treatment.

Everyone with PTSD avoids trauma memories, thoughts, feelings, or reminders, as reflected in the avoidance cluster of the PTSD diagnosis. People will cognitively and emotionally avoid the most upsetting details of their trauma memories. Most avoid specific situations or activities, such as being alone with a strange man in an office. For some, avoidance becomes much more generalised, such as avoiding strangers entirely or feeling pervasively numb and detached. Avoidance may come to dominate their life to the extent that they withdraw entirely from activities and relationships.

As avoidance is a crucial factor in how PTSD is maintained, much of our therapeutic work involves supporting our clients to reduce avoidance in all its forms. However, as therapy itself is a trauma reminder, clients understandably, and almost invariably, feel the urge to avoid therapy sessions or important tasks, reducing potential benefits from treatment. As therapists, we may also wish to avoid hearing details of horrendous traumas, or fear upsetting our clients by encouraging them to approach trauma memories, leading us to collude with their avoidance. These dynamics can set up an unhelpful feedback loop whereby ineffective treatment reinforces a client's beliefs that they are permanently damaged or beyond help and that traumatic material is unbearable for both parties.

In this chapter, we consider the reasons why clients avoid reminders of the trauma, including certain aspects of treatment. Understanding these reasons helps us to address them in therapy.

Understanding avoidance in PTSD

Avoidance includes any behavioural or cognitive strategy used to inhibit distressing thoughts or feelings. Behaviourally, this involves avoiding and escaping from people, places, and activities that elicit distress. In PTSD, these stimuli are associated with highly aversive memories, so intentionally talking or thinking about memories seems counterintuitive to our clients who, above all else, want to feel less distressed. People, therefore, use a range of cognitive strategies to control memories, including effortful distraction, thought suppression, emotional detachment, self-isolation, and intentional dissociation. For some people, both 'inward' rumination (e.g. repetitively dwelling on 'why me?' and 'if only …' thoughts) and 'outward' verbal rumination, may also function as ways of avoiding thinking or talking about the distressing details of their trauma memories (Moulds et al., 2020).

DOI: 10.4324/9781003288329-23

As part of a broader repertoire of coping, avoidance can be an adaptive way to manage negative feelings following trauma, so it is not intrinsically problematic. However avoidant coping becomes problematic when it is to the exclusion of other adaptive coping strategies, has unforeseen negative consequences, or prevents distressing experiences resolving. In particular, avoiding trauma memories prevents them from being properly processed, and means people never access new information that could update them.

Avoidance and escape are also entirely healthy survival responses to threatening situations, so appraisals of threat naturally lead to avoidance. If we believe that a certain situation, place, or person is dangerous because it has been so before, it makes sense to avoid it to stay safe. But avoiding objectively 'safe' situations or activities means that people with PTSD lose the opportunity to naturally test out their trauma-related fears; of the situation, of their and others' reactions. This understandably strengthens their efforts at avoidance over time because, when expected fears don't materialise, it seems as if their efforts to avoid or manage the perceived threats kept them safe.

Although conceptually different, safety-seeking behaviours are related to avoidance. In PTSD, these tend to be behaviours intended to prevent further trauma, including hypervigilance and taking excessive precautions. People may also have specific concerns about the consequences of remembering the trauma or encountering trauma-related reminders, such as becoming overwhelmingly upset or violent, being sick, or making a fool of themselves in front of others, and so deploy safety-seeking behaviours to prevent these threats.

These appraisals may have their roots in earlier experiences, such as how emotions were dealt with in the family, or experiences of seeing others overwhelmed, and they are often shaped by cultural influences. Peri-traumatic appraisals are also relevant. People who felt helpless and defeated during a trauma may re-experience these emotions when memories are triggered, and so feel powerless in the face of them. This can make avoidance harder to overcome and contribute to beliefs about permanent change, e.g. 'I will never recover', further eroding confidence and increasing defeat. These factors can be added to the relevant boxes of the CT-PTSD formulation.

Usually, people avoid in deliberate and explicit ways, making strenuous efforts to anticipate and rapidly escape reminders. However, over time, avoidance can become so habitual that it feels automatic, with triggers more implicit and outside of awareness, making avoidance harder to notice and control. Emotional detachment and numbing may also develop as overlearned ways of coping with adverse developmental experiences, and so be automatically triggered to manage distress following a later trauma. In therapy, numbing can make work on the trauma memories more challenging as the 'therapeutic window' is harder to access (Chapter 5).

Lastly, there may be systemic and cultural factors that support avoidance. Where PTSD is longstanding, the client's lifestyle and relationships may have changed to accommodate the problem. Reducing avoidance may introduce unwanted changes to the status quo, such as an expectation to return to work for someone who has been on long-term sick leave, receiving less care or attention from a partner, or unwanted changes in how they are viewed by others.

Shpresa escaped to the UK from Kosovo when her father and husband were both killed in the Kosovo War. In therapy, Shpresa was highly avoidant of her emotions and of talking about her problems. Her therapist was curious about how Shpresa's background influenced her beliefs about emotions, so asked how difficult experiences were talked about when she was growing up. Shpresa explained that her family, and others she knew, were very private about difficulties and that she had been taught that talking about your problems made them worse. Her therapist mentioned an English expression 'a problem shared is a problem halved', and Shpresa responded that in her culture, the expression was the exact opposite, that sharing problems 'doubled them' by burdening two people. This context helped Shpresa's therapist to better understand her avoidance of discussing difficult feelings and opened up a conversation about how this approach might help cope with everyday stresses, but be unhelpful for PTSD symptoms.

Helping clients overcome avoidance

Assessing and formulating these various factors helps us understand how to address avoidance with our clients. Here are some important interventions.

THERAPEUTIC ALLIANCE AND DEVELOPING A COMPELLING RATIONALE

In treatment, we are asking a lot of our clients to override their strong instincts to avoid and, instead, deliberately approach horrific memories and feelings, as well as putting themselves in situations that feel dangerous while dropping their precautions. This is more achievable if they trust us and the treatment, and understand the rationale for how it will help.

It is important when we work with avoidance to adopt a stance that is neither cajoling nor pressuring the client; instead, we need to maximise their control of the therapy. Nor do we want to collude with avoidance, avoid naming it, or shy away from memories that are difficult for us as well as the client. Together, we formulate the role of avoidance in maintaining PTSD, using metaphors (see 'top tips') to aid understanding. Inherent to these discussions is validation of avoidance as an understandable way to cope with frightening and overwhelming symptoms of PTSD. We then explore with our clients the costs and benefits of avoidance, acknowledging that in the short term it is often effective, but can have significant longer-term costs, not only in preventing recovery from PTSD but also in causing their lives to shrink, limiting their ability to live a full and rewarding life.

Given the central role avoidance plays, we keep it on the agenda from the start of treatment and throughout. We begin with assessing and exploring all the avoidance strategies our client uses. We discuss in advance that they will likely have an urge to avoid therapy at times and normalise this experience. We also foster our client's (and our) 'avoidance radar', actively looking for subtle signs of avoidance, like changes in awareness or demeanour, where they stand or look. Asking yourself 'what might I do if I felt threatened in this situation?' can help you both to identify more subtle avoidances and safety-seeking.

For behavioural avoidance, we put together a list of avoided situations, setting 'reclaiming your life' tasks that also involve approaching avoided stimuli or dropping specific safety-seeking. Starting with small tasks, like stepping onto the doorstep for one minute (we sometimes call these 'dares'), and celebrating these successes, helps build momentum and confidence. Helping our client identify their long-term 'blue-sky' goals, like going shopping on Oxford Street at Christmas, is also important, not because they are necessarily achievable during treatment, but because they 'set the bar' as to what is achievable and so generate hope.

Top tips: Metaphors to explain avoidance

As overcoming avoidance may seem counterintuitive to our clients, metaphors can help explain its role in PTSD treatment. Here are our favourites:

- *The messy linen cupboard (to explain avoidance of trauma memories)*: The memory system is like a cupboard where we store experiences away. The trauma memories are like an enormous blanket that has been hurriedly stuffed into the cupboard but keeps falling out. Instead of trying to jam the door closed (avoidance), we need to sort out the contents of the cupboard, fold and tidy the blanket, and find a proper space for it in the memory system, so that the doors can close and stay closed.

- *The builder's apprentice (to explain safety-seeking)*: A young apprentice starts work at a building site and the other builders, as a joke, tell him to hold up a wall they have just built while they go to lunch, which he does. We ask our clients: 'what would you say to him?' and 'what can he do to discover if the wall will fall down?', and draw the metaphor back to ways in which they may be unnecessarily 'holding up the wall', such as through safety-seeking behaviours.
- *Being bitten by a dog (to explain behavioural avoidance)*: If a child has been bitten by a dog, it makes sense that they would be frightened of dogs and avoid them. We ask the client 'how would you help the child get over their fear?' (Stott et al., 2010), and use their answers to draw parallels with how they may overcome their trauma-related avoidance.

ADDRESSING APPRAISALS AND WIDENING THE WINDOW OF PROCESSING

Identifying and addressing any appraisals which motivate avoidance is crucial, especially when it blocks progress in therapy. The usual cognitive strategies can be employed, including guided discovery, psychoeducation, and surveys, tailored to idiosyncratic beliefs. These will often relate to overestimation of risk (and/or underestimating capacity to manage it), so strategies such as risk calculations, that foster a balanced appraisal of risk, are useful. Behavioural experiments are a central part of this work, helping clients to test out what happens when they reduce or drop both cognitive and behavioural avoidance. Many clients will struggle with these experiments alone so, rather than set only them for homework, we first do experiments during therapy sessions whenever possible. This also helps us spot other safety-seeking behaviours which the client may not report or be aware of.

Philippa expressed concerns about therapy at her first session, explaining that she was only attending due to the insistence of her GP. She had 'tried CBT' in the past and found it unhelpful, dropping out after the first few sessions. Alert to the risk of disengagement, Philippa's therapist explored her concerns. Philippa explained she was struggling to cope emotionally following the loss of her husband from suicide the previous year and felt that she was only managing to cope by avoiding the difficult emotions associated with her grief. She felt that talking about his death would 'push her over the edge'.

Philippa agreed to an experiment. They would spend the session discussing PTSD, but without discussing the death in detail. Philippa would arrange a pleasant activity for after the session. Later that day, she would rate whether she felt any closer to 'the edge'. At the next session, Philippa reported that, although she had been tired after the session, she had not felt overwhelmed emotionally and had enjoyed her chosen pleasant activity. Her therapist commended Philippa on the experiment. They agreed an agenda for the session that Philippa was comfortable with, including discussing a little more about her husband's death, before working on 'reclaiming your life'. Philippa would again rate her distress after the session and would feed back to the therapist if she felt overwhelmed.

Appraisals linked to helplessness are particularly important to address, as they may interfere with engagement if clients feel they have no control over their PTSD. Peri-traumatic appraisals linked to mental defeat can be updated, for example 'I was helpless then, but I'm not helpless now', and post-traumatic appraisals, such as those linked to permanent change ('I'll never get over this'; 'my life is ruined') can also be identified and addressed. Where these beliefs also relate to earlier distressing memories which have been reactivated, it can be helpful to bring the client's awareness to this link and address them using updating and/or imagery rescripting (page 140, 162).

Even when avoidance is habitual or pervasive, such as numbing, it can help to explore its origins and associated beliefs, and identify when and why the strategy occurs now. As discussed in Chapter 5, we may need to 'turn up the volume' on trauma memories when we use memory-focused techniques such as imaginal reliving. In vivo work will also be particularly important, such as introducing triggers during reliving or when working on stimulus discrimination, and activating and updating the trauma memories 'live' in avoided situations and when returning to the scene of the trauma.

Hot cognitions

- I won't be able to cope if I don't avoid my memories/feelings
- I need to control myself otherwise I will go mad/fall to pieces
- It is too risky to go to that place/do that activity/see that person
- My life has changed too much – there is no way I can go back
- Treatment is too hard/too much for me
- If I no longer have PTSD, I may lose something important

MAXIMISING LEARNING AND GENERALISATION

Behavioural experiments focused on avoidance work best when the therapist takes steps to maximise the learning gained from them in various ways (see also page 138 and Murray, & El-Leithy, 2021). Clients may need explicit support to generalise the learning gained from experiments. We ask questions to promote reflection, consolidate learning, and encourage generalisation, e.g. 'what do you make of that?', 'how does that compare to what you expected to happen?', 'how does that relate to your belief about x?', and 'in what other situations could that also be relevant?'. We listen carefully for 'yes, but ...' statements, where clients discount results, and repeat experiments in different situations as needed. Operationalising and testing individual predictions via behavioural experiments is a cornerstone of CT-PTSD, but research into the mechanisms underlying exposure therapies has led to similar conclusions: that the more a threat expectancy (or feared outcome) is violated by actual experience and the more surprising the outcome, the greater and more long-lasting the extinction of fear via inhibitory learning. Inhibitory learning can also be maximised by dropping safety behaviours, adding additional triggers, varying the timings, intensity, and context of exposure (Craske et al., 2014), just as we try to do in our behavioural experiments.

PRE-EXISTING DETACHED/AVOIDANT COPING STYLE

Post-traumatic avoidance may be particularly rigid or intransigent in clients with pre-existing or lifelong tendencies towards avoidant and detached coping. Here trauma-related meanings have often 'confirmed' long-standing negative beliefs (Chapter 12) or schemas about themselves as defective, vulnerable, or unlovable, and others as untrustworthy or abusive. Organised clusters of these negative schema, emotions, and their corresponding coping behaviours, termed 'schema modes', evolve where basic emotional needs, such as feeling safe and connected, are unmet or threatened in childhood (Young et al., 2006). For example, children who experience bullying or emotional neglect may develop powerful mistrust and defectiveness schemas associated with shame and helplessness, and so learn to cope by detaching from the emotional pain of their unmet needs, and avoiding 'opening up' emotionally to others. As adults, these modes then arise moment-to-moment in response to emotional events. Most relevant to avoidance are the 'detached protector' mode, characterised by disconnection, emotional, and psychological withdrawal; and the 'detached self-soothing' mode, characterised by excessive and repetitive distraction.

Schema modes, and their historical origins, can be readily integrated into CT-PTSD formulations. Schema therapy involves working with these modes, combining cognitive therapy techniques with experiential methods, including exploring, emotionally processing, and reinterpreting memories of relevant early childhood experiences through imagery rescripting and chairwork (Arntz & Weertman, 1999; Pugh, 2018). Aspects of schema therapy can be incorporated into CT-PTSD, including identifying the unmet needs within childhood that seem linked to adult schemas and are motivating avoidance, then addressing those needs through imagery rescripting. The goal is to weaken unhealthy detached coping modes and enhance 'healthy adult' modes that can experience, express, tolerate, and soothe negative emotions.

Constance grew up in a strictly religious family and was badly bullied at school. As an adult, Constance was extremely fearful of negative evaluation from others and avoided friendships and relationships. When Constance sought therapy after an assault, her therapist noticed that she avoided eye contact, and would not discuss her thoughts and feelings. Constance feared being assaulted again and struggled to leave her home, but also described a longstanding sense of social inadequacy, and beliefs that others disliked her and would target and humiliate her. These pre-existing beliefs were added to her formulation, and treatment was broadened to include work on earlier beliefs using surveys and continua methods, as well as imagery rescripting of Constance's bullying memories. As Constance's beliefs about being disliked changed, she felt more able to engage in behavioural experiments with leaving her house and being around other people.

COMORBID PROBLEMS

Difficulties associated with comorbid problems can feed into, and reinforce, PTSD avoidance. For example, clients with social anxiety disorder may avoid situations for fear of embarrassing themselves. Clients with depression may lack energy or motivation to undertake behavioural experiments between sessions. As we discuss further in Chapter 20, we can incorporate elements of other disorder-specific treatments, especially when the symptoms of that disorder are interfering with effective PTSD treatment. For example, a client who avoids busy situations for fear of having a panic attack, rather than a trauma-related fear, may benefit from some of the strategies from cognitive therapy for panic disorder (Clark, 1986).

FEARS ABOUT CHANGE

Over time, a stable network of relationships, identities, and roles can develop around a person with PTSD. Changing a central element of the network, by overcoming avoidance or recovering from PTSD, can have negative consequences. Improvement in one area (like feeling less frightened to go out) may lead to unwanted effects in another (such as increased pressure from family and friends to attend stressful social events).

It helps for these changes and losses to be discussed in therapy, with an explicit acknowledgement that not all changes will be positive. We ask clients to think through what their life would be like if they were no longer avoiding situations and make it acceptable to express concerns about aspects of those changes. This helps put the issue 'on the table' and enables clients to weigh up the pros and cons of change.

We also help clients consider what might be lost, and how they can recover or compensate for losses. For example, for those who fear that they will lose closeness or care from those around them, we discuss how to nurture those aspects of their relationships in other ways. Concerns may relate to earlier losses, for example, childhood experiences of neglect. Often relationship dynamics do change as the client does, often for the better, but sometimes for the worse. We try to articulate these issues with our clients and involve relevant others in therapy as needed.

> Conrad started a new relationship soon after a sexual assault but avoided sex with his new partner, Ali. By the time he started therapy, Conrad and Ali had been together for two years and had never had a sexual relationship. Conrad reported they were both 'fine' with the situation and was reluctant to attempt behavioural experiments in decreasing his avoidance of sex. His therapist explored with Conrad how his PTSD symptoms had affected their relationship and how things might be different if he recovered. Conrad revealed fears that, as Ali had been so accepting of the situation, he may not want a sexual relationship with Conrad, and may feel platonic love for him rather than sexual attraction. He had never discussed these fears with Ali, so agreed to invite him to a therapy session where Conrad's therapist could support him to explain his concerns. Ali was surprised that Conrad felt that way, and explained that he had wanted to be supportive and not pressure Conrad into sex, but he was attracted to him and would be delighted for them to have a sexual relationship. They agreed a plan to gradually increase intimacy through touching and massage and to keep communicating about how they felt as their relationship progressed.

For some of our clients, PTSD has become a central aspect of their identity. Centrality of meaning (Berntsen, & Rubin, 2006) refers to the extent to which a traumatic experience becomes key to an individual's identity, and their life organised around it. Event centrality has been found to predict PTSD development (Boals, & Ruggero, 2016). Losing this sense of meaning and identity presents an often difficult to articulate threat to some clients. If so, we help them consider aspects of their identity which are separate from the traumatic experience. We use 'reclaiming your life' tasks to nurture these areas, and to develop new interests which represent the client's values beyond those related to the trauma. In many cases, clients can keep some aspects of what they valued about their trauma identity, without keeping PTSD itself.

> Ben served in the British Army for five years before being discharged due to PTSD. Ben's therapist noticed his identity was very closely linked to the army. He always wore army surplus clothing to appointments, referred to his army experiences regularly, and much of his social life was spent with other ex-soldiers. Ben expressed motivation to reduce his PTSD symptoms but was difficult to engage in therapeutic tasks. His therapist wondered if change represented a threat to Ben's identity as a military veteran with PTSD and, furthermore, if not having PTSD would force him to confront other uncomfortable issues in his life. Ben's therapist spent a session focusing on 'reclaiming your life' and used it as an opportunity to discuss Ben's identity and values. They discussed what would change and what would remain the same if Ben no longer had PTSD. Ben's social life with other veterans would remain, and Ben could envisage using his experiences to help others recover. They also discussed the impact of Ben's PTSD symptoms on his marriage and his work. Ben could see that the impact was largely negative but that some of his difficulties would not fully resolve if he recovered from PTSD. They problem-solved ways to address these, such as seeking relationship counselling.

FAQ: How can I resist colluding with avoidance?

Therapists may naturally prefer to avoid some aspects of PTSD therapy, including hearing about horrific traumas, causing their clients distress, or having 'awkward' conversations. It can be hard to strike the balance between being appropriately validating, empathic, and supportive without colluding with avoidance. Here are some ideas:

- *Be self-aware*: Use reflective practice, especially through supervision, to examine your own beliefs and behaviours around avoidance, and how these may interact with your client's. Recognise what you bring to the therapeutic relationship (Chapter 24).
- *Remain collaborative*: Try to tackle avoidance as a shared therapy task, with you and your client against the PTSD, and not against each other; and doing things *with* your client, not *to* or *for* them.
- *Agree your involvement*: Ask your client's preferences for how you can support them to reduce avoidance. For example, ask for 'permission to pester' if you notice avoidance, including sending messages between sessions to remind them of homework tasks.
- *Use treatment contracts*: Agree session limits and regular reviews. Foster some sense of urgency and momentum in the treatment and, if progress stalls, initiate conversations about why (in a spirit of shared discovery, not criticism).
- *Use avoidance as data*: Avoidance is not failure, it is an opportunity to learn something important about your client and their PTSD. Raise it for discussion in sessions and use this to improve your shared formulation.
- *Use your responses as data*: Clients' avoidance can leave us feeling frustrated, and this can affect our alliance. The same thing may be happening in their other relationships, so your reactions can give you clues about systemic maintenance factors.
- *Try paradoxical interventions*: Your client may be used to one form of encouragement, which isn't working, so try another, for example, suggesting 'we *could* try this, but then again it may be too much for you'. Agree temporary bans of avoided activities, such as penetrative sex, to reduce your client's anticipatory anxiety and enable them to safely focus on alternative ways of being intimate.

Notes from the therapy room: Cora

Cora was referred for PTSD treatment several years after she woke up during an operation. Cora reported nightmares and flashbacks of the experience and was easily triggered by reminders of the trauma, especially medical appointments, lying flat on her back, and certain physical sensations. She also described ongoing abdominal pain and nausea. Cora was highly avoidant of medical settings and would only attend appointments accompanied by her husband or adult children. She slept propped up by pillows. Due to anxiety about someone knocking her stomach, Cora avoided busy places, including the supermarket and public transport.

In the early stages of therapy, Cora responded well to psychoeducation about PTSD, including the role of avoidance. However, she rarely completed homework tasks and missed several appointments, giving a range of reasons. In sessions, she was reluctant to participate in behavioural experiments or memory work and often focused on her physical health or worries about her children.

Cora's therapist decided to gather further information about what factors might contribute to her avoidant style. Her parents had moved to the UK from Greece before Cora was born. Cora was the fifth of six children and always believed she was different from her siblings, as she was quieter. Cora felt that she was ignored by her family in childhood and often felt uncared for. They added this to her formulation (Figure 19.1).

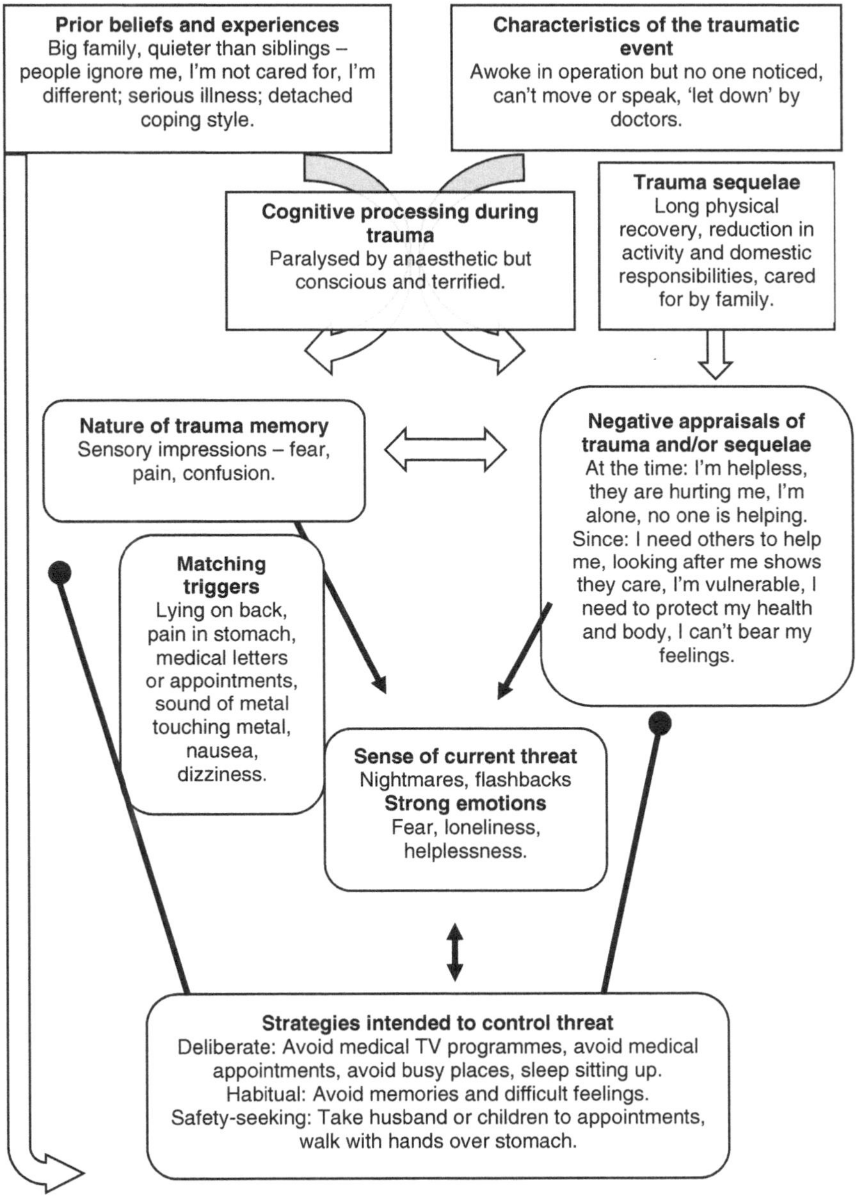

Figure 19.1 Cora's formulation

Cora married in her twenties and worked briefly as a seamstress before giving up work to raise her family. Two of her children had now left home but the younger two lived with Cora and her husband. Cora had developed womb cancer in her early fifties and, following a course of chemotherapy, had a hysterectomy. It was during this operation that Cora regained consciousness due to a medical error. She could not move or speak but was aware of her surroundings and in physical pain. She was horrified that no one was noticing or helping. Family life changed considerably to accommodate Cora's illness and recovery. Her husband and children now managed the household jobs which had been Cora's responsibility, her youngest daughter had delayed going to university, and her other children called and visited regularly.

Cora's therapist hypothesised that she was fearful that her emotional needs would no longer be met if she was seen by her family to have recovered. They returned to Cora's therapy goals and normalised the possibility that both positive and negative changes would occur in Cora's life if she recovered from PTSD. Cora acknowledged that having her family around made her feel cared for and had brought them closer, but she was also worried about 'holding them back'. They discussed the ways that the family could stay connected without this happening. Cora began to engage in 'reclaiming your life' activities that didn't involve her family, such as sewing and reading.

Themes of being helpless and uncared for were present in Cora's experiences in hospital, as well as her childhood memories. In addition to adding updates to a written narrative of Cora's trauma, they also used imagery rescripting to address her childhood memories. Cora imagined visiting her younger self, hugging her and explaining that her parents and siblings loved her, and it didn't matter that they were different in some ways. Cora developed a new belief, that 'I'm loved and I'm getting stronger every day'. She became more willing to engage in behavioural experiments that involved dropping avoidance. With her therapist's help, Cora began to notice times that her family felt proud of her, rather than worried about her which made her feel good. Cora's therapist also helped her use 'then versus now' in relation to her abdominal pain, as this seemed to be 'fed' by her trauma memories. They were able to experiment with Cora lightly tapping her stomach and learning that it did not damage her and with going into busier places. Cora learnt that she was rarely knocked in the stomach and, if she was, no serious harm was caused.

Recommended reading

Boterhoven de Haan, K. L., Fassbinder, E., Hayes, C., & Lee, C. W. (2019). A schema therapy approach to the treatment of posttraumatic stress disorder. *Journal of Psychotherapy Integration*, 29(1), 54–64.

Zoellner, L. A., Marks, E. H., Jun, J. J., & Smith, H. L. (2014). Avoidance. In L. A. Zoellner & N. C. Feeny (Eds.). *Facilitating resilience and recovery following trauma* (pp. 237–264). Guilford Press.

PART FIVE
Comorbidity

CHAPTER TWENTY
Psychological comorbidity

Jason had struggled with social anxiety disorder (SAD) before experiencing a serious accident and developing PTSD. Jason's SAD affected how he perceived the accident and its consequences, and so was incorporated into his formulation. Treatment initially targeted his PTSD symptoms, drawing on techniques used to treat SAD when shared beliefs and maintaining behaviours were identified.

Of any psychological disorder, PTSD presents with perhaps the most severe and diverse pattern of psychological comorbidity (Brown et al., 2001). Around 75% of people with PTSD meet criteria for at least one other psychological disorder (Kessler et al., 2005), most commonly depression, anxiety, and substance misuse disorders. Personality disorders are also commonly comorbid, particularly avoidant and borderline personality disorders (BPD; Zimmerman et al., 2005). In this chapter, we outline the principles we use to make treatment decisions when PTSD presents alongside other psychological disorders.

Why is comorbidity so common?

Traumatic events, PTSD, and other psychological problems may interrelate in several ways:

- Some pre-existing mental health problems, particularly anxiety, somatoform, and mood disorders, place people at increased risk both of experiencing trauma and developing PTSD afterwards (Perkonigg et al., 2000).
- Distinct disorders may share biological, social, or psychological vulnerability factors. For example, established risk factors for anxiety and depression, such as low self-esteem, a 'neurotic' personality type, or childhood trauma, also increase the risk of developing PTSD (Elwood et al., 2009).
- Other problems can develop as a consequence of PTSD (Breslau et al., 1997). For example, avoidance of trauma reminders may reduce engagement in valued activities or loss of occupational functioning, leading to isolation and depression. Substance misuse may develop as a way to 'self-medicate' PTSD symptoms such as hyperarousal or sleep difficulties.
- Traumatic events, and their physical and social consequences, can be direct or indirect risk factors for almost all psychological disorders, including personality disorders and psychosis. Hence they may potentially trigger psychological symptoms that fall within several diagnostic categories.

One or more of these relationships between traumatic events, PTSD, and comorbidities may apply to any particular client. Assessing and formulating these patterns ultimately informs our treatment approach, be it a disorder-specific CBT model or an idiosyncratic transdiagnostic approach.

DOI: 10.4324/9781003288329-25

FAQ: Is the PTSD diagnosis valid?

One argument for why comorbidity is so high is that it reflects a problem with the PTSD diagnosis. Perhaps it tells us that reactions to traumatic events are much broader than the PTSD symptoms listed in DSM-5. DSM-5 PTSD criteria overlap with those of other disorders, a problem that ICD-11 has attempted to address by narrowing the definition to just six symptom criteria. Or it may be that assigning symptoms to categorical diagnostic 'silos' is itself a fundamentally flawed approach. Indeed, there has been a long and lively debate on exactly this topic (e.g. Casey et al., 2013). Nevertheless, diagnostic categories can have benefits, such as helping us to research and deliver effective treatments by more reliably establishing what interventions work for which problems and people.

Our approach to diagnosis is therefore a pragmatic one. We find it helpful to categorise symptoms into disorders as short-hand 'problem descriptors'. This assists our treatment planning by directing us towards problem-specific CBT models with demonstrated effectiveness, as starting points for developing our formulation and intervention. However, given that many clients experience symptoms that relate to several different diagnoses, we also draw on models and techniques from different disorder-specific CBT approaches and use an individualised formulation-derived approach rather than a single protocolised treatment.

This approach will be familiar to therapists; protocolised treatments need to be followed carefully in research trials but, in routine practice, most therapists are adept at working flexibly when needed. The key is remaining watchful for 'drift' away from evidence-based CBT models, relying too much on therapist intuition rather than formulation, or simply implementing CBT techniques without a formulation to guide them. We should always know why we are using a given intervention and which process we are targeting in our formulation.

We are also mindful that we need to discuss diagnoses sensitively with our clients. For many clients, explaining how their apparently disparate set of problems fits with a recognisable and treatable diagnostic disorder can destigmatise it and instil hope. For others, it can contribute to their sense of being mad, damaged, or stigmatised, and these interpretations are both highly individual and culturally bound. If clients don't like the PTSD label, we don't need to use it and focus instead on using our client's own words to describe their problems, and on achieving their treatment goals rather than a diagnostic 'cure'.

Approaches to comorbidity

Disorder-specific CBT approaches have the most robust evidence base and, reassuringly, CT-PTSD delivered as a stand-alone treatment appears effective despite psychological comorbidity. Comorbidity (including personality disorders) appears not to moderate PTSD treatment effects, typically alongside large improvements in comorbid symptoms of anxiety and depression (Ehlers et al., 2013). One explanation for these findings is that the CT-PTSD model already incorporates flexibility to adapt for comorbidity. That said, comorbidity may produce poorer outcomes if it means the treatment is less trauma-focused, so more treatment sessions or additional components may be required to achieve the best possible results.

An alternative approach is to combine multiple disorder-specific models sequentially, based on a formulation of each problem's relative importance, alongside the client's goals and informed treatment choice (Whittington, 2014). Each disorder is formulated separately, with the links between them mapped out showing interactions and maintaining cycles. Sequencing is decided by identifying a primary problem to which to 'tether' the treatment, based on which is the most severe, most affects functioning, is the greatest priority for the client, and which developed first and/or is driving the other problems (Barton et al., 2017). To avoid 'diluting' the treatment, therapists work with one disorder-specific model at a time but shift to address secondary comorbidities where they present an obstacle to the treatment, or where there are residual symptoms. Zayfert and Becker's (2019) CBT case conceptualisation approach to PTSD is an excellent example of this.

A third approach is to deliver separate disorder-specific treatments concurrently, either combined into an integrated package or by dividing the therapeutic time between different disorders. This may be helpful where the disorders are either mutually maintaining or operate antagonistically (i.e. when one is targeted in treatment, the other gets worse). Examples in the PTSD literature include treatments for PTSD and BPD (Harned, 2014) where a skills training component, such as a DBT, precedes trauma-focused work. However, the necessity of a phased approach has been challenged. De Jongh et al. (2020) found that intensive prolonged exposure therapy led to improvement in both PTSD and BPD symptoms, and argue that interventions for BPD, such as emotion regulation training, may be more effective after PTSD treatment, rather than before.

Finally, transdiagnostic treatment models address the problem of comorbidity in emotional disorders by targeting themes and processes that are common to, and operate across, disorders. They may be most helpful when the relationships between disorders appear unclear, unstable, or do not clearly fit any disorder-specific model. These approaches also aim to simplify treatment delivery for therapists, who otherwise have a plethora of models and protocols to learn. Probably the best known transdiagnostic treatment is Barlow's 'Unified Protocol' (Barlow et al., 2017) which aims to target a suggested underlying factor common to emotional disorders: a propensity toward heightened emotional reactivity, combined with an increased tendency to view emotional experiences as aversive and attempts to alter, avoid, or control emotional responding. The protocol targets these factors using CBT principles and techniques, with a particular emphasis on emotional regulation skills (Ellard et al., 2010).

A recent approach, the 'Shaping Healthy Minds' programme (Black et al., 2018) has extended Barlow's treatment to incorporate elements of disorder-specific CBT treatments, combined in a flexible, modular approach to treat clients with multiple diagnoses. This treatment reflects the approach many therapists take when encountering multiple comorbid problems in their clinical practice, by selecting matching treatment techniques from different models. These types of personalised transdiagnostic treatments (e.g. Craske, 2012) allow therapists to target specific features of a disorder (such as using imaginal reliving to address intrusive memories in PTSD), while also working on common elements which run across multiple disorders (such as avoidance). However, once again, we would caution against delivering interventions in the absence of a clear formulation of their target, and its functional relationship to other problems.

When and how to adjust treatment

Personalised transdiagnostic treatments are not dissimilar to our approach when working with clients with comorbid problems. If the client's goals relate to PTSD and this is the main problem, our preference is for a disorder-specific treatment for PTSD. Where this is not possible due to considerable comorbidity which interferes with treatment, or the client's goals relate to various disorders, we take a more flexible approach, addressing the most important transdiagnostic processes. Since all our clients have PTSD, we do not want to miss out highly effective components of treatment for this problem, particularly working on the distressing meanings associated with their trauma memories. So, although we advise flexibility, where possible trauma-focused formulations and techniques should be prioritised. Here are some top tips.

DO A THOROUGH DIAGNOSTIC ASSESSMENT AND TIMELINE OF EACH PROBLEM

At initial assessment, we use brief screening interview questions (e.g. QuickSCID-5) and/or self-report measures (e.g. Brief Symptom Inventory). Where comorbidity is flagged, we follow up with relevant diagnostic modules from the SCID-5-CV, alongside disorder-specific self-report measures, to further explore the matching diagnoses or disorders. We also ask about the timeline of symptom onset for each disorder, and points at which they worsened or improved, to help map their relationships to each other and potential causal events.

EXPLORE HOW EACH DIAGNOSIS RELATES TO THE CLIENT'S GOALS

We collaboratively determine how and where to focus, by comparing the potential diagnoses with information from our client about:

- Which problems they identify as causing most distress or impairment
- Their treatment goals
- Whether any of the problems contribute to risk
- Whether any of the problems would interfere with treatment as a whole, or of another problem.

MAP THE COMORBIDITIES AND THEIR RELATIONSHIPS

We draw out a visual map of the longitudinal (which emerged when) and cross-sectional relationships between the diagnoses/problems (primary, secondary, co-occurring/mutually maintaining, unclear/unstable, or unrelated). We identify any obvious shared causal factors and maintenance processes.

For each diagnosis, we identify the relevant disorder-specific CBT treatment models. To decide which one(s) to use, we consider how the different problems relate to the client's goals, which are the primary sources of impairment, and the client's preferences for intervention type.

When PTSD is the main problem, treat it first

If the client goals/preferences and functional impairment relate primarily to PTSD symptoms, whenever possible we treat this first using CT-PTSD. Where other disorders have arisen at the same time as PTSD, or appear secondary to its impact, we formulate these as post-traumatic manifestations and assume they will resolve alongside. Treatment is, therefore, 'tethered' to the PTSD symptoms and we integrate the processes underlying the other disorders within the CT-PTSD formulation. For example, beliefs about permanent change which are common in PTSD may also underlie depression, as might the withdrawal associated with PTSD via a lack of positive and rewarding activities. Beliefs around PTSD symptoms as dangerous, e.g. 'when I have a flashback, I might lose my mind' can drive panic symptoms and be maintained via safety-seeking behaviours. A trauma-related auditory hallucination such as hearing the voice of an abuser can be formulated as a re-experiencing symptom that has been externally attributed and fuelled by a belief such as 'they can still control me'.

Here we only use a separate CBT model to target secondary disorders where we cannot integrate the maintenance processes into the CT-PTSD formulation, or where they strongly interfere with the CT-PTSD treatment, and then only until that obstacle is cleared sufficiently to return to a trauma-focused intervention. This may happen several times during a course of treatment, so we move back and forth as necessary, but as much as possible we stick to CT-PTSD treatment to avoid diluting it.

Farida developed PTSD following a sexual assault at her workplace. She resigned and was too frightened to seek a different job. In the weeks that followed, Farida also became depressed. She didn't want to tell her family about the sexual assault so avoided spending time with them and became very withdrawn. When she started therapy, Farida was extremely low in mood and reporting suicidal thoughts as well as experiencing flashbacks and nightmares of the assault. Her goals were to go back to work, sleep through the night without nightmares, and reconnect with her family. Farida did not attend her second session, saying that she was too low to come to the session. At her third session, she struggled to remember what had been discussed in session one and had not done the agreed homework of reading the psychoeducational leaflet on PTSD and doing a 'reclaiming your life' task. Although Farida's depression had developed secondarily to her PTSD, it was severe and was impacting on her ability to engage with therapy, so her therapist decided to spend a few sessions trying to stabilise Farida's mood before returning to PTSD work.

Another comorbidity that can be approached as a post-traumatic manifestation is where clients have experienced early life traumas which led to them developing both PTSD and features of a personality disorder. Here, a CT-PTSD approach can incorporate both problems. We like the approach described by Davidson (2014), where the formulation develops from an extended, detailed assessment of the client's early experiences and personality development, and is then written as a narrative or therapeutic letter. This allows for an empathic, normalising, and collaborative way of understanding the impact of both traumatic and developmentally adverse experiences on their core beliefs, emotion regulation, and coping styles. Memory-focused interventions targeting parts of the traumas which are re-experienced can follow, alongside experiential techniques such as imagery rescripting of those memories which were influential in core belief development, drawing on conceptualisations and techniques from schema-focused therapy (Arntz & Van Genderen, 2020).

TJ grew up in a refugee camp where his family was in constant danger. TJ's younger sister died as a baby, and his mother became severely depressed and struggled to care for her other children. TJ's father was also emotionally distant and was violent towards TJ's mother and the children. As a teenager, TJ travelled across Europe to the UK where he was eventually granted asylum. When he came to therapy a few years later, TJ met criteria for BPD and PTSD.

TJ and his therapist worked together to understand the impact of his childhood experiences on his re-experiencing symptoms of PTSD, his intense fears of abandonment, and his difficulties regulating strong feelings. TJ re-experienced three events from his childhood: finding his mother unconscious after a suicide attempt, a severe assault by his father, and an attempted sexual assault while TJ was travelling across Europe. TJ and his therapist worked on stimulus discrimination and a safe place image to help manage the distress that the memories invoked before addressing them, as the memories were sometimes a trigger to self-harm. They talked about the meanings of loss, betrayal, and shame associated with these events, which linked closely to TJ's core beliefs, and used imagery rescripting to bring new meanings into the memories.

Where problems relate to multiple disorders, target shared processes

Where it is not immediately clear how comorbid disorders interrelate with PTSD, or the client's goals encompass multiple problems, we draw out separate disorder-specific models for each condition and identify possible shared maintaining processes to target. These can often be brought back into a CT-PTSD formulation, or instead drawn out as an idiosyncratic/transdiagnostic formulation of the key causal factors and processes.

Arthur had a serious accident on his farm that led to the loss of his arm and meant he had to give up farming. Arthur had previously experienced several depressive episodes and reported lifelong excessive worry. Both problems worsened after the accident, and Arthur also developed PTSD symptoms. Arthur's goals related to various problems: he wanted to adjust to life without his arm, 'feel less useless', worry less, and sleep better. Arthur's formulation (Figure 20.1) mapped the crossover between his PTSD and depression symptoms and identified the key areas for intervention. Arthur's distress stemmed from post-traumatic appraisals such as 'I'm not the person I used to be', 'I've got no future', and 'I'm useless'. Arthur dwelled on these issues, further worsening his mood, fuelling his worry about the future, and affecting his sleep. Arthur and his therapist agreed to work on these appraisals, focus on reducing rumination, and introduce 'reclaiming your life' activities to help Arthur find meaning and direction. Although Arthur had occasional re-experiencing symptoms of the accident, they were rare and did not cause much distress, so they agreed to monitor these, and address them at a later point in therapy if they persisted.

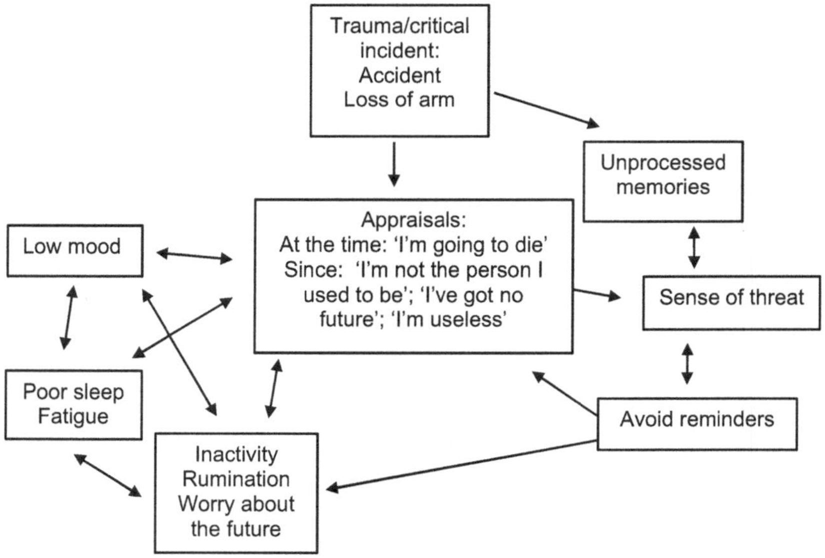

Figure 20.1 Arthur's idiosyncratic formulation

Many of the processes at the core of PTSD development and maintenance are also important in other disorders. CBT models often include life events or a 'critical incident' in the longitudinal formulation of the problem's development (e.g. Beck, 1987). Overestimation of threat is central to all anxiety disorders (and arguably many other disorders too); the main difference between them is the content of the threat. Clark (1999) outlined six processes that maintain anxiety-related negative beliefs across all anxiety disorders, namely safety-seeking behaviours, attentional deployment, spontaneous imagery, emotional reasoning, memory processes, and the nature of the threat representation. Even trauma memories, once considered a unique feature of PTSD, occur in many disorders; and techniques to address them, such as imagery rescripting, have been incorporated into CBT approaches for various problems, such as social anxiety disorder (Wild, & Clark, 2011) and depression (Wheatley et al., 2007).

Sharon developed PTSD after she heard that her old music teacher had been arrested, and recovered memories of him sexually abusing her in childhood. As well as flashbacks, Sharon began hearing a voice saying 'shut your mouth' and 'stop spreading lies'. Sharon and her therapist used imagery rescripting to address the abuse memories and the feelings of guilt and shame which related both to Sharon's intrusive memories of the abuse, and the voices that she heard. They used behavioural experiments to test the effects of answering back to the voices.

Recognising that processes overlap does not, in our opinion, mean that transdiagnostic treatments which apply the same approach to all disorders are the best approach. We still need to be specific about the role of any given process for an individual, then formulate idiosyncratic beliefs, behaviours, and memories. However, it does mean that we can 'borrow' techniques from treatment protocols for other disorders, and emphasise areas of crossover when they occur. Figure 20.2 illustrates some of the processes that PTSD shares with some commonly comorbid axis I disorders.

Jean-Luc developed PTSD after an assault. He became preoccupied with his safety and began to check the doors and windows were locked, and the oven and electrical devices were turned off multiple times before he went to bed or left the house. Jean-Luc was aware that his checking was obsessive, but he worried that something bad would happen again if he stopped. Jean-Luc's therapist helped him to examine these thoughts using the 'Theory A/Theory B' technique, commonly used in CBT for OCD. Theory A was that Jean-Luc and his family would be harmed if he didn't check everything properly and it would be all his fault as he hadn't protected them. Theory B was that Jean-Luc was understandably worried about harm coming to him or his family because of his trauma and because he cared about them so much, but that this level of checking wasn't needed or making them any safer. Instead, it was harming him by maintaining his emotional distress and stopping him finding out his fears of harm were inflated. They calculated the risk of another trauma occurring using the conditional probabilities technique and used behavioural experiments in reducing his checking to test his fears, thereby gathering evidence for Theory B.

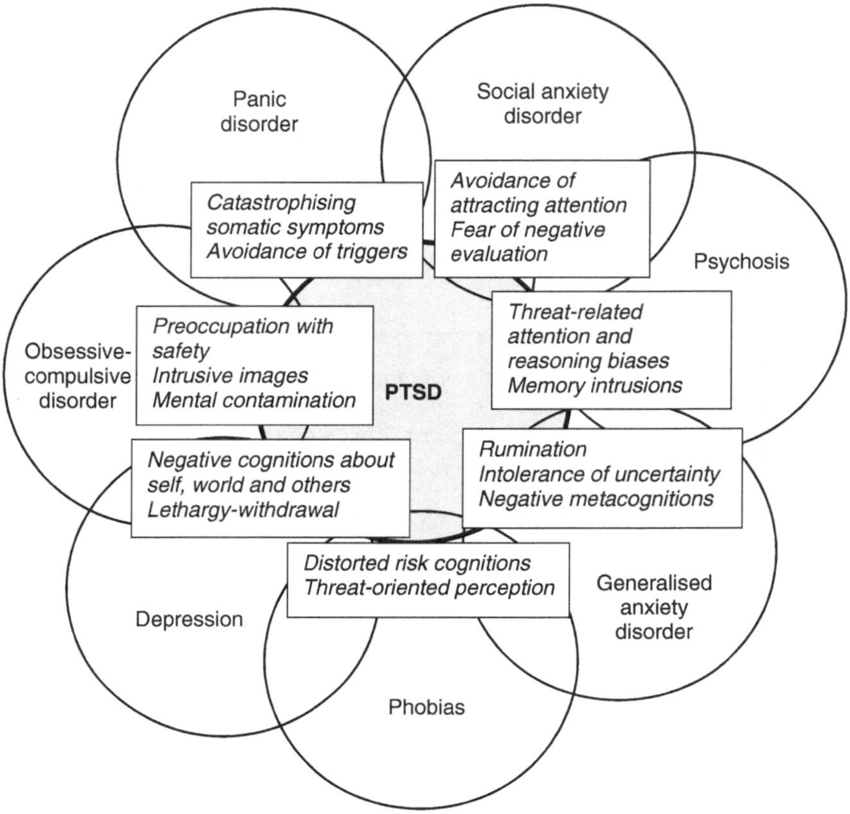

Figure 20.2 Venn diagram of overlapping processes between disorders

FAQ: Is borderline personality disorder the same as complex PTSD?

It has been suggested that BPD is a form of complex PTSD (Kulkarni, 2017) and there are certainly areas of overlap. One possibility is that there is a continuum of trauma-related disorders from classic PTSD towards a subtype of BPD, with complex PTSD an 'intermediate' manifestation (Giourou et al., 2018). Chronic PTSD, whether from childhood or adult traumas, may also eventually lead to personality change, particularly where it interferes with important developmental stages. However, at least according to current classification systems, there are differences in the symptom profiles of PTSD, complex PTSD, and BPD (Cloitre et al., 2014).

Figure 20.3 conceptualises the overlap and distinctive features of the three disorders. Complex PTSD includes the symptoms of PTSD, plus some additional features which overlap with, but do not fully encompass, the symptoms of BPD. Interestingly, the broader PTSD diagnosis in DSM-5 envelops several symptoms which are considered part of complex PTSD in ICD-11 such as 'reckless or self-destructive behaviour', the new 'negative alterations in cognitions and mood' cluster, and the dissociative subtype.

Distinguishing PTSD/complex PTSD from BPD is important because the recommended treatments differ with an emphasis on team approaches, longer duration of treatment, and different therapeutic interventions, such as DBT (NICE, 2009) for BPD. It is also important to note that, although the majority of people with BPD report a trauma history, a significant minority do not. Although complex PTSD is a potentially less stigmatising way of understanding BPD, this runs the risk of adding to the stigma for people with no trauma history. Instead, we seek to understand with our clients the multiple factors that impact personality disorder development, including earlier life experiences, in an individualised formulation. As before, where clients do not find the label helpful, we focus instead on their goals.

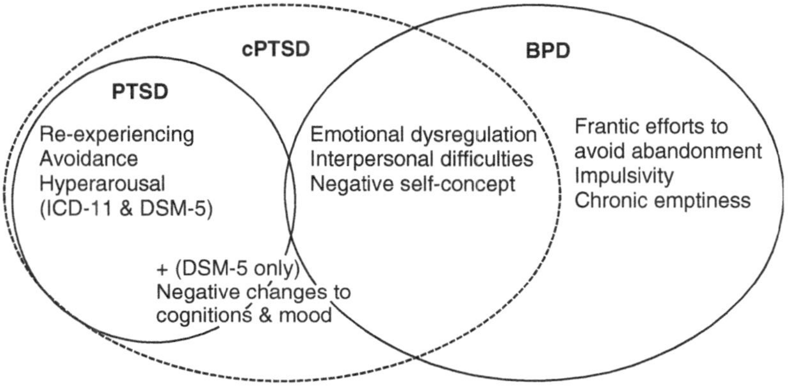

Figure 20.3 Venn diagram of symptomatic overlap between PTSD, cPTSD, and BPD

Where disorders are antagonistic or mutually maintaining, treat them concurrently

This requires switching between treatment models within or between sessions, or using a specific model designed for concurrent treatment. For example, alcohol use disorder and PTSD commonly co-occur and often maintain each other: excessive alcohol use blocks processing of trauma memories and contributes to self-blame and permanent change appraisals, while PTSD leads to distress which can be numbed with alcohol, and symptoms such as poor sleep which alcohol may (in the short term) relieve. Treatment may encompass an alcohol intervention concurrently with PTSD treatment; developing alternative means of coping with PTSD symptoms while also processing the memories which underlie PTSD (Chapter 17).

Where the relationship between disorders is unclear or unstable, collect more data

Here we proceed primarily based on the client's preferences and goals. We agree to 'tether' the treatment to one disorder for a fixed time, or to a provisional idiosyncratic formulation, while closely tracking progress, including the symptoms of other disorders. This can be presented as a form of 'extended assessment' or a treatment trial that aims to clarify how each comorbidity might interact, or respond to a given intervention. We regularly review progress on both the 'tethered' disorder and a broader index of symptoms, re-formulating as we obtain greater clarity about how the problems interact, and what may be obstacles to treatment. If there has been a lack of any progress or even deterioration, we revisit the formulation to consider if anything is missing and whether one problem may be interfering with progress on another. If so, we target the second disorder for a few sessions and review again.

Hot cognitions

- I have to drink/withdraw/ruminate to cope with my PTSD
- The trauma set off a chain of events that has made everything worse for me
- My previous problems have made the trauma even harder to deal with
- My problems are too complicated/varied – treatment only addresses one part of them

Offer sequential treatment modules for secondary disorders or residual symptoms

When PTSD treatment is complete, symptom-specific CBT treatments can be offered for residual problems such as sleep (e.g. Zayfert, & DeViva, 2004), or full interventions for secondary disorders which have not resolved.

Many clients have disorders that pre-date their PTSD. Where these have interacted with PTSD development or maintenance, they can be formulated within the CT-PTSD model (Figure 20.4). For example, prior beliefs and coping styles may have been confirmed/shattered or activated by the traumatic event. If pre-existing disorders do not interfere with PTSD treatment, they may be targeted sequentially after PTSD.

Lulu had suffered from trichotillomania since she was a teenager. She developed PTSD after the traumatic birth of her twin daughters and her trichotillomania also worsened. Most of Lulu's treatment goals were associated with PTSD, but she did find the consequences of her trichotillomania distressing. Lulu and her therapist formulated the different problems. Lulu's trichotillomania often worsened during periods of stress, so it made sense that her hair-pulling had increased since the trauma, given her PTSD and the stress of caring for two babies. It seemed likely that, if Lulu's PTSD symptoms improved, the trichotillomania would too, but may not fully resolve as it had pre-dated the trauma. Lulu agreed that PTSD should be the primary focus of treatment and this would be reviewed regularly. They agreed to reassess the trichotillomania once her PTSD had improved, to see if further intervention was required.

Where a personality disorder pre-dates an adult trauma and subsequent PTSD development, we review the client's goals to decide treatment priorities. If PTSD is the main target for treatment, we proceed with CT-PTSD as usual, although adaptations may be needed, such as focusing on safety (if required) or the therapeutic relationship if interpersonal difficulties emerge. Relevant aspects of the pre-existing personality disorder can be added to the CT-PTSD formulation.

Tumi sought treatment for PTSD following her boyfriend's sudden death. She reported a history of intense relationships and a sense of complete dependence on others. Her therapist noticed that she seemed helpless and passive in her interactions, and suspected dependent personality disorder pre-dating her PTSD. This impacted treatment in several ways. Tumi expressed appraisals of abandonment and devastation associated with the loss of her boyfriend, and struggled to engage with aspects of treatment like 'reclaiming your life'. She also quickly expressed a sense of reliance on her therapist and struggled with boundaries in therapy, particularly when her therapist took leave.

Tumi's therapist encouraged her to recognise her relationship patterns, and they discussed how these had developed. Tumi had often been told that she was 'clingy' and 'needy' in relationships and friendships and expressed a desire to be more independent. She agreed to give her therapist permission to gently point out these behaviours when they occurred so she could experiment with alternatives. They also agreed to address appraisals which linked to both her PTSD and her tendency to dependence in relationships, such as 'I am inadequate' and 'I cannot care for myself'.

Notes from the therapy room: Jason

Jason was injured in an accident at the garage where he worked, suffering burns to his hands and arms. At assessment, he reported PTSD symptoms related to the accident and social anxiety disorder (SAD) which had started in adolescence when he was bullied at school for being mixed-race. He described intense anxiety in group situations and avoided most socialising except for with a few close friends.

Jason's SAD, and his pre-existing beliefs about himself and others, influenced how the trauma was processed and how he coped. He described feeling very anxious when his injuries made him the centre of attention, including when he returned to work. Although people were generally sympathetic and supportive, Jason worried that others would judge him as 'attention seeking' for having PTSD, and would think the accident was his fault. He was self-conscious about his scars and covered his hands and arms when possible. Jason also worried about appearing jumpy in public and took beta-blockers to manage this. His formulation is in Figure 20.4.

Jason's treatment goals related to both his PTSD and SAD. He wanted to stop having nightmares, feel less anxious at work when he was dealing with fuel, go to the pub with his workmates and feel relaxed, 'accept' his scars, and stop taking beta-blockers. To address the first goal, they worked initially on the trauma memories, using imaginal reliving and updating. Some of Jason's peri-traumatic appraisals were fear-related, but he had also experienced an immediate sense of guilt that he had caused the accident. Reviewing the evidence revealed that this was not the case but Jason reported a 'head–heart gap' in accepting the updated appraisal. Jason had a longstanding tendency to blame himself, which was linked to core beliefs that had developed in childhood when he was bullied. These beliefs were also related to Jason's SAD, and several sessions of therapy were spent addressing them using continua techniques and writing a compassionate letter to Jason's younger self.

Jason's nightmares and intrusions were reducing, and he also began to use stimulus discrimination to help with triggers he encountered at work. However, he continued to feel anxious that he might make a fool of himself by becoming upset or having a strong startle reaction in public. To address this, Jason's therapist helped him to devise an anonymous survey. This revealed that people would be sympathetic rather than negatively judgemental if they saw someone upset or suddenly startled in public. They used behavioural experiments where Jason's therapist modelled jumping and also crying in public while Jason observed the response of passersby. To his surprise, most people ignored the reaction, or looked briefly and then kept walking. On one occasion, a member of the public stopped to offer help and appeared kind rather than critical. Jason agreed to an experiment of going for a drink with his workmates

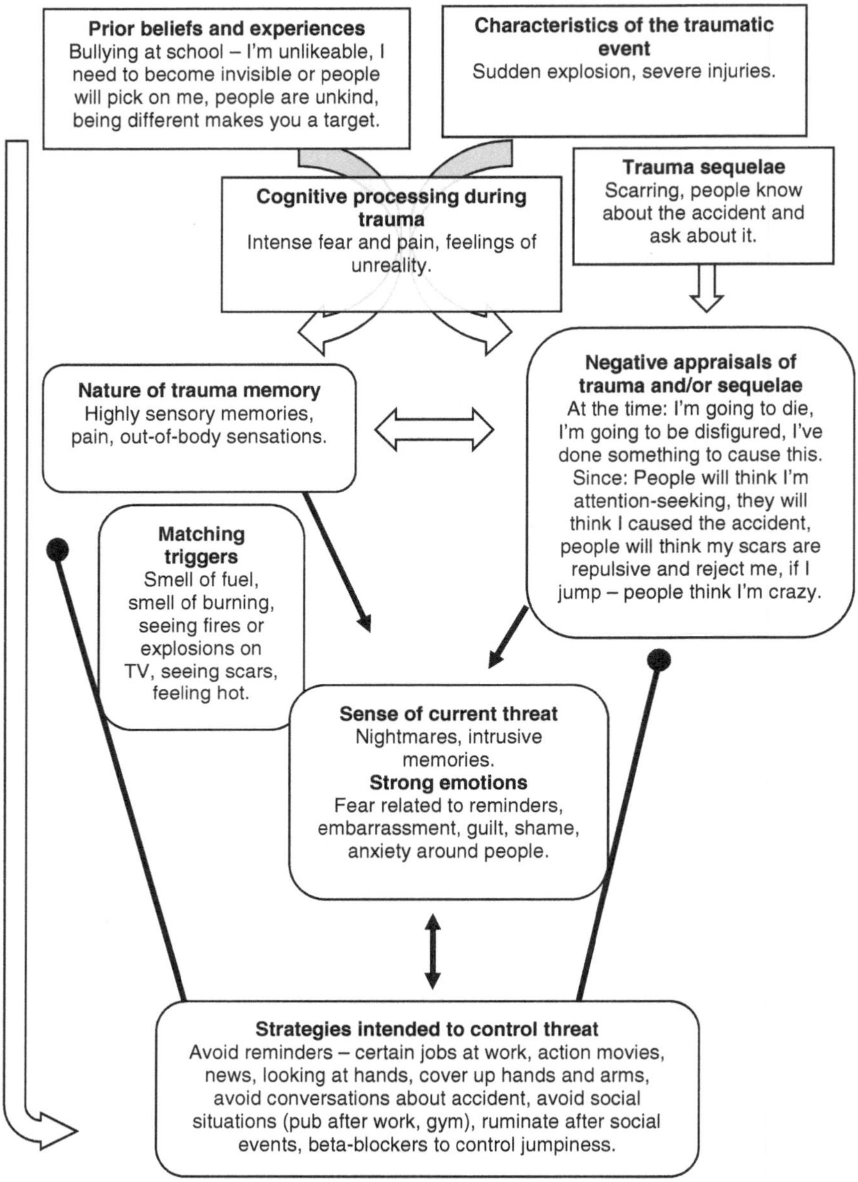

Figure 20.4 Jason's formulation

and, although he didn't feel relaxed, was pleased that he didn't become upset or make a fool of himself.

To address concerns about his scars, Jason's therapist encouraged him to reduce his avoidance by using hand cream and looking at them every day. They conducted another survey using photos of Jason's scars and asking people what they thought of them. Again, responses were mainly sympathetic. People commented that they may notice and be curious about scars but would not think anything negative. Jason conducted further behavioural experiments in deliberately revealing his hands, and even drawing attention to them by pointing to items on a menu when he ordered food in a café.

As his confidence grew in social situations, Jason felt able to test his beliefs further. He deliberately initiated a conversation about the accident with his workmates and asked them whether they thought it was his fault, or whether he was attention-seeking. This revealed that his boss actually felt very guilty about the accident, and apologised to Jason, becoming emotional himself. Reflecting on this experience, Jason realised that he had never considered that others would blame themselves, and also realised that his boss's display of emotion had not been judged negatively by his workmates.

In the final stages of therapy, Jason reduced and eventually stopped taking beta-blockers. He also used experiments where he deliberately jumped in public to show that, even if this symptom returned, no one seemed to notice.

FURTHER READING

Barton, S., Armstrong, P., Wicks, L., Freeman, E., & Meyer, T. D. (2017). Treating complex depression with cognitive behavioural therapy. *The Cognitive Behaviour Therapist*, *10*, E17.

Whittington, A., (2014). Working with co-morbid depression and anxiety disorders. In Whittington, A., & Grey, N. (Eds.). (2014). *How to become a more effective CBT therapist: Mastering metacompetence in clinical practice*. John Wiley & Sons.

Zayfert, C., & Becker, C. B. (2019). *Cognitive-behavioral therapy for PTSD: A case formulation approach*. Guilford Press.

CHAPTER TWENTY ONE
Physical comorbidity

Following a car accident, Dana experienced a range of physical and psychological symptoms, including pain, muscle weakness, and PTSD. Exploring her symptoms revealed some interactions between Dana's physical health and her PTSD, and these mutual maintenance cycles were addressed in treatment.

Early descriptions of PTSD such as 'railway spine' and 'soldier's heart' viewed it primarily as a physical disease. More recently, a substantial body of research has confirmed that PTSD is strongly associated with a wide range of physical and somatic comorbidities. This has prompted some to suggest thinking of PTSD as much a physical and systemic illness as a mental disorder (McFarlane, 2017).

People with PTSD experience poorer physical health and worse health-related quality of life than the general population (Pacella et al., 2013). Many of our clients present with comorbid health conditions, both diagnosed and 'medically unexplained'. Traumatic stress reactions often manifest as physical symptoms, such as startle responses and physiological reactivity to triggers which are part of the PTSD diagnosis. They may also be associated with a broad range of symptoms falling under the umbrella of 'conversion' or 'functional neurological' disorders (Karatzias et al., 2017).

The co-occurrence of physical and psychological symptoms often mean that these clients experience complicated treatment pathways, through healthcare systems that are structured to separate physical and mental health. Multiple referrals, assessments, and failed attempts at treatment can understandably erode trust in services and contribute to negative beliefs like 'I can't be helped' and 'others don't care'. In this chapter, we explore how to understand and address the ways that physical and emotional symptoms after trauma interact.

Understanding relationships between physical and psychological symptoms

There are numerous pathways between PTSD and physical health, which can also interact with each other, including:

- Physical damage caused by the trauma, such as pain, traumatic brain injury, scarring, disability, and disfigurement (see also Chapter 15).
- PTSD that results from catastrophic physical health problems such as heart attacks or strokes, complicated childbirth, or following invasive medical treatment, such as intensive care unit admissions.

DOI: 10.4324/9781003288329-26

- PTSD, especially when chronic, increases the risk (by up to four times) of developing a broad range of medical conditions including neurological, cardiovascular, gastrointestinal, respiratory, skin, bone, and joint diseases (Pacella et al., 2013; Schry et al., 2015). There are several potential reasons for this. Firstly, long-term activation and dysfunction of the body's stress response pathways affects immune responses, making people more susceptible to both infection and systemic illness (Dougall, & Baum, 2004). Also, people with PTSD are more likely to engage in unhealthy behaviours such as smoking and substance use, poor diet, lack of exercise, and avoidant coping like missing health appointments (van den Berk-Clark et al., 2018).
- Contextual factors may predispose people to both PTSD and physical health problems, including environmental, social, and economic deprivation. Shared genetic vulnerability factors may underlie diverse traits such as anxiety sensitivity and joint hypermobility and are associated with a wide range of psychological and physical difficulties including anxiety disorders, dissociation, postural tachycardia, vasovagal syncope fibromyalgia, and chronic fatigue (Eccles et al., 2015).
- Physical symptoms for which a medical explanation is not found (sometimes labelled 'functional' or 'somatic' symptoms) can arise after trauma, including chronic pain, fatigue, and neurological symptoms. Although still poorly understood, current models emphasise biopsychosocial frameworks (e.g. Deary et al., 2007; Espay et al., 2018).
- Medications can have physical and psychological side effects which interact with PTSD. For example, medication prescribed for an underactive thyroid can lead to anxiety, sweating, and an increased heart rate. These interactions can be complicated and difficult to tease apart from the underlying illness.
- People with PTSD may experience physical symptoms more acutely. For example, anxiety can increase pain sensitivity and lower pain tolerance.

> Emma reported recurrent urinary tract infections which she found embarrassing and upsetting. In therapy, Emma disclosed that she washed her vagina several times a day with antiseptic to combat feelings of contamination associated with flashbacks of childhood sexual abuse. She avoided visiting her GP until the infections were severe as she feared an intimate physical examination. Emma felt generally run-down, and was susceptible to infections, probably due to lack of sleep and chronic stress caused by her long-standing PTSD. This interacted with coping strategies she used to manage her PTSD symptoms, including excessive washing, which affected the healthy balance of bacteria in her vagina, and avoiding medical examinations, leading to frequent and severe infections. In turn, the infections contributed to her feelings of contamination, maintaining the problem.

GATHERING DATA

Understanding how these different processes operate for our clients first involves some 'detective work' – gathering information about how their physical and psychological symptoms interact. We need a thorough assessment of how and when the different symptoms started, how they have progressed (e.g. points at which they worsened or improved), perceptions and beliefs about them, coping strategies used, and how different symptoms affect them in terms of their mood, interference with activities, and relationships. It often helps to use individualised diaries to monitor and track different symptoms and to understand how they interact with behaviours, trauma reminders, and activity levels. This data will inform our formulations and highlight potential targets for intervention.

We also gather data by liaising with medical professionals involved in the client's care. When starting treatment with someone with physical health problems, we request a medical review, including blood tests. We have occasionally assessed clients where symptoms were assumed to be psychological due to their trauma history, but have never been properly medically investigated; for example, people with severe depression and fatigue who, when investigated, are found to have an underactive thyroid. Attributing physical symptoms to psychological processes is only appropriate if medical explanations have been explored and ruled out. We also find it helpful to research confirmed medical conditions alongside our clients. This information is often invaluable for both the therapist and client to understand the problem better and so share the 'detective work'.

FORMULATION

Although formulations are idiosyncratic, we generally find it easiest to start with our usual cognitive model of PTSD and add information about physical health problems within that framework, or by adding some additional boxes and possible maintenance cycles. Alternatively, different problems can be formulated separately, before looking for areas of cross-over. Typically these are shared maladaptive coping strategies or appraisals. We build these formulations up gradually through discussions and 'detective work' with the client, drawing out and testing possible feedback cycles as we go.

When considering functional symptoms, we have found approaches such as Deary et al.'s (2007) CBT model helpful, as it dovetails well with the cognitive model of PTSD. In brief, this model suggests that a variety of factors (both genetic and environmental, including early-life trauma) predispose certain people to become sensitised to, and distressed by, physical symptoms. Physical symptoms triggered by a life event, injury, or illness, become chronic due to various interacting processes including attentional and attributional processes, illness appraisals, behaviours such as avoidance, physiological changes, and social factors. The experience of the physical symptoms and accompanying 'current threat' maps well into the 'current threat' box of the CT-PTSD model, with similar processes of distressing appraisals and unhelpful coping acting to maintain them.

Deary et al. (2007) highlight the importance of creating a detailed explanation with the client for symptoms that may have felt (and been externally judged) to be unfathomable, and in so doing create a credible rationale for treatment targets. This includes challenging the notion of mind–body dualism and introducing the idea that physical symptoms interact with psychological ones and manifest as 'stress', both a physical and psychological experience. Information on the defence cascade (Kozlowska et al., 2015; Schauer, & Elbert, 2010) is also useful in explaining dissociative reactions which underlie many functional neurological symptoms such as paralysis and dissociative seizures (see also Chapter 6).

Formulations are by their nature hypothetical, and we are particularly aware of this when working with physical symptoms which have a range of possible causes and maintenance cycles. Some clients may be sceptical about the possibility that physically experienced symptoms may have, at least in part, a psychological explanation. If so, we treat psychological therapy as an experiment. If the physical symptom(s) improve alongside the PTSD symptoms, then this is a good result! If PTSD symptoms improve, and other symptoms do not, or even worsen, then further investigation is required. It also helps to suggest that, whatever causes physical symptoms, it may be possible to improve their impact on quality of life via behavioural change.

Hussain was referred for treatment of PTSD following experiences of torture in Yemen. As well as PTSD symptoms, Hussain experienced fainting episodes, for which doctors could not find a medical cause. Hussain believed he had suffered brain damage when he was beaten around the head. This idea made him feel hopeless about the chance of recovery. In therapy, Hussain agreed to keep a fainting diary for a few weeks and noticed that they often happened when he felt stressed or following a flashback. His therapist explained there can be a range of explanations for fainting and introduced Hussain to the 'defence cascade' model of dissociation. This explains fainting as the final stage of an automatic defence cascade which has evolved to protect us from inescapable threat when active defence responses have failed. They explored this idea and Hussain recalled passing out during some of the torture episodes. Hussain agreed this new explanation was a possibility and agreed to use PTSD therapy as an experiment to test it out further: if Hussain felt less stressed following treatment and his fainting episodes became less frequent, it was likely they were related. If Hussain's other symptoms improved but he continued to faint as often, they would refer him back to neurology for further investigations as the two processes would have proved to be unrelated.

Top tips: Physical comorbidities and the therapist's stance

Some clients have had multiple unsatisfactory healthcare experiences and may feel their physical problems have been dismissed, misunderstood, or inadequately treated. For others, a psychological approach to physical health problems is perceived as implying 'it's all in your head' or 'you're making it up'. For these reasons, a compassionate, validating, and curious therapist stance is particularly important. Here are our top tips:

- *Take physical symptoms seriously*: Allow time in sessions for physical health problems to be discussed. Make it clear that you view them as important, relevant, and real. Where the client is preoccupied with their health or tends to express their distress by talking about physical symptoms, add them to the agenda with an agreed time limit.
- *Collaborative empiricism*: Understanding the problem is a shared task. We do not have all the answers, so we remain curious and model actively seeking information. Your client will need to feel their physical concerns are given priority and heard before considering psychological explanations and interventions. You can help them link the two by exploring their emotional impact, and cognitive and behavioural efforts to cope with physical symptoms.
- *Sensitivity to language*: Many clients do not like the term 'medically unexplained symptoms', but 'functional' or 'persistent physical symptoms' may be preferred (Marks, & Hunter, 2015). Use and reflect the specific language and turns of phrase your client uses rather than imposing your own language. (e.g. 'pain' or 'tiredness' rather than 'somatic symptoms' or 'lethargy').
- *Liaise with other disciplines*: Several clinical teams may be involved, so it can become important to facilitate effective interdisciplinary communication. As well as seeking advice and opinions from medical specialists, we sometimes try to coordinate between different specialities to 'join up' our client's care, for example, arranging joint reviews and planning meetings.
- *Be flexible in delivery while staying close to your treatment model*: You may need to adapt how PTSD treatment is delivered to accommodate physical health issues. We discuss this further in the next section.

Treatment adaptations

SEQUENTIAL, CONCURRENT, OR INTEGRATIVE TREATMENTS

As with psychological comorbidity, there are different treatment options where physical symptoms occur alongside PTSD. Firstly, we can try to deliver CT-PTSD as usual, making only the adaptations necessary to complete the treatment. After the PTSD is treated, we reassess whether other problems require additional treatment. There is some (albeit limited) evidence that some physical health problems improve if PTSD is successfully treated (Beck et al., 2009; Galovski et al., 2009), which we would expect if PTSD symptoms exacerbate the physical health problem.

Assuming this fits with the client's goals, focusing on PTSD in treatment is usually our preferred option. However, there is also evidence that clients with physical problems have poorer outcomes in psychological therapy (Taylor et al., 2001). There may also be situations where focusing on PTSD is impossible, for example where physical health problems are so severe that they continually become the primary focus in sessions or interfere with therapy tasks, where reducing physical symptoms is the client's main goal, or where attempts at trauma-focused CBT have previously proved ineffective (this latter example is a good source of information for identifying future obstacles). In these scenarios, we can refer the client elsewhere for treatment of their physical health problem either before, or concurrently with PTSD treatment, or we can attempt an integrated treatment.

As we described in Chapter 20, integrated treatment does not mean abandoning the principles and techniques of CT-PTSD. Instead, we try to formulate both problems and understand the overlapping processes. We then use techniques from both CT-PTSD and other relevant CBT models (e.g. for chronic pain) to address the key maintenance processes.

ADAPTING THERAPY DELIVERY

For our clients with physical health problems, we need to discuss what adaptations they need to access and benefit from therapy. These could include:

- *Pacing therapy* to manage fatigue, concentration, and pain. Consider shorter sessions, and negotiate achievable homework tasks and 'reclaiming your life' activities.
- *Discussing optimal delivery modalities* such as phone or video sessions if clients struggle with attendance. Choose the best time of day for appointments, for example, afternoons if they are fatigued in the mornings.
- *Using memory aids* such as appointment reminders, written summaries of sessions, and asking the client to record sessions on their phone, especially for those with cognitive impairments or conditions which impair concentration. Offer email or automated text check-ins and reminders between sessions to support engagement.
- *Optimising communication* (both written and verbal) to suit the individual, particularly if there are barriers such as sensory impairments or learning difficulties.
- *Addressing ways to manage the client's physical symptoms for sessions*, such as making sure they have eaten, rested, and appropriately used their medication.
- *Liaising with medical professionals* if required around medication management, including promoting adherence to a regular schedule (to avoid overuse or rebound effects) and ideally reducing opiate-based pain medication to create a window of cognitive processing for sessions (page 198).
- *Where symptoms occur during sessions*, agree how these will be managed and encourage self-management. For physical symptoms that appear dissociative, work early in treatment on identifying triggers and early signs, then developing grounding skills and stimulus discrimination.

FAQ: Is it safe to do reliving with someone with a physical health problem?

Some clients have been told to avoid stress, have beliefs that stress is dangerous, or are concerned that becoming upset or anxious will exacerbate an illness. With a diagnosed condition, it is appropriate to consult a medical expert, explaining that imaginal reliving (and some other therapy tasks) can temporarily increase emotionality and therefore physiological arousal, and asking their views on what risks this may present.

This is sometimes a concern for pregnant women but, assuming the pregnancy is normal, psychological therapy is usually considered safe for the mother and baby (Baas et al., 2020), especially considering that the alternative, not treating PTSD, has potential negative effects of chronically raised stress hormones on foetal development, and interfering with maternal bonding.

Indeed, for most people, the longer-term health and quality of life risks of chronic PTSD and the physiological impact of chronic stress are often more damaging than a temporary increase in distress and symptoms in PTSD treatment. Re-experiencing symptoms will already be increasing physiological arousal and conversely depleting their cognitive resources for coping with medical problems. Addressing traumatic memories in a well-managed therapy session is generally less upsetting than living with unpredictable PTSD re-experiencing symptoms.

Clients' concerns may also arise from inflated risk perceptions typical of PTSD, which can be addressed in treatment. We also need to be mindful of our own unevidenced beliefs about treatment which support collusion in avoidance. However, we always want our clients to feel that PTSD interventions are tolerable, predictable, and controllable, so work with them to adapt and adjust as necessary to stay in the therapeutic window of tolerance. This will itself be determined by both their physical and psychological discomfort.

IMPROVING ILLNESS MANAGEMENT

Another important focus of treatment can include supporting clients to manage their physical health as effectively as possible. Symptoms of PTSD, and other problems such as depression, sometimes interfere with clients accessing check-ups, physical health treatment, or adequately managing chronic medical problems (for example, cervical screening, Cadman et al., 2012; diabetes, Egede, & Osborn, 2010; respiratory conditions, Waszczuk et al., 2019). In collaboration with medical professionals, we clarify the appropriate management of their health issues and support our clients to develop action plans to overcome any barriers, such as identifying and sharing personalised 'dos and don'ts' with their healthcare team.

Treatments for persistent physical symptoms such as chronic fatigue, pain, and irritable bowel syndrome often emphasise consistency rather than the 'boom or bust' patterns that can develop. We may need to focus on ensuring paced regular activity, appropriate nutrition, and sleep.

Some clients experience barriers to illness management that are closely related to their PTSD symptoms. These should be identified and addressed early in therapy, particularly where they pose substantial or immediate risks, such as from hypoglycaemia in diabetes or non-adherence to a chemotherapy regime. Here are some examples:

- *Trauma reminders*: If physical health problems were directly caused by the trauma, or a client's trauma occurred in a medical setting, appointments and treatment can trigger re-experiencing symptoms. Medical procedures which include lying down or being restricted (e.g. MRI scans), being touched by a stranger, removing clothing, or simply feeling vulnerable or intruded upon can be triggers for a wide range of traumas. Oral, gynaecological, or rectal examinations are often particularly difficult following sexual assaults. In these cases, we prioritise stimulus discrimination and behavioural experiments, alongside developing shared plans for making the procedure as predictable and controllable as possible.

- *Low self-worth*: For some clients, self-care is difficult because of feelings of self-hatred and/or low self-esteem, often fuelled by shame-filled traumatic memories. Related beliefs, such as 'I deserve to suffer', are likely to be important to other aspects of their clinical presentation, so should be addressed. Additionally, it can help to broaden the concept of 'reclaiming your life' to also reclaiming your body and wellbeing from the trauma, and potentially back from a perpetrator who intended to control and defile their body (e.g. after torture or abuse).
- *Recklessness*: As discussed in Chapter 18, various processes can motivate reckless or risky behaviours, and some illness management behaviours can be formulated similarly. For example, physical symptoms may be intentionally exacerbated or neglected to 'affect match' or control emotional states, like food deprivation to increase alertness, or over-using pain medication to manage emotional distress.

If necessary, we set minimum criteria for adequate illness management before agreeing to proceed with treatment. For example, if a client's illness is so poorly managed that they are placed at risk (for example, through regular episodes of hypoglycaemia due to poorly managed diabetes, dangerous weight loss, or frequent epileptic seizures and falls due to non-compliance with medication) or symptoms consistently prevent them from engaging with therapy tasks, we do not proceed with PTSD treatment and focus instead on stabilising the illness, and supporting them to access appropriate specialist interventions (e.g. regular reviews by a diabetic nurse).

TARGETING SHARED PROCESSES

Research has highlighted several shared processes between PTSD and physical health conditions, particularly chronic pain (Beck, & Clapp, 2011; Sharp, & Harvey, 2001). Understanding these allows us to work concurrently with both problems, to target both cognitive content (shared meanings) and cognitive-behavioural processes which may drive or maintain them. This both maximises the impact of our interventions and helps avoid problems of 'interlock', where attempting to treat one problem on its own is hindered by or exacerbates another. Here are some shared processes, and ways of targeting them:

Physical symptoms as re-experiencing symptoms

Where a trauma involved intense physical sensations, like pain, these may be re-experienced as somatic flashbacks (Salomons et al., 2004). This link may or may not be immediately obvious to clients or indeed medical practitioners. Traumas involving intense somatosensory input and/or other conditions affecting cognitive processing like partial consciousness, blindfolding/darkness, drugs, or alcohol, often lead to particularly fragmented memories and re-experiencing may be primarily somatic and visceral without any verbal or visual memory component.

To assess this, we ask clients to describe their current physical symptoms in detail and look for any matches with their peri-traumatic experiences. Bringing the memories to mind may trigger physical sensations, and sometimes physical or physiological changes reminiscent of the trauma (like flushing or swelling of injured parts of the body). If so, we formulate the link and reattribute the cause of the physical symptoms to the traumatic memories. These should typically resolve as the memories are processed during treatment by fully contextualising the physiological aspects of the relevant hotspots (page 92) and using updates in physical modalities (e.g. page 175).

Yasmin developed PTSD after experiencing a major postpartum haemorrhage. She described a range of current physical symptoms including pain during sex, feelings of weakness, and fatigue. Yasmin's memories of the trauma were very unclear, fragmentary, and accompanied by strong affect and physical symptoms. She and her therapist developed a timeline of the trauma with the help of her partner, who was with her during the trauma and had a clearer recollection of events. They were able to identify the moments where she had experienced the physical symptoms which were now re-experienced, such as feeling intensely weak and fatigued just before she lost consciousness, and updated these with new cognitive information, accompanied by physical movements that gave a feeling of strength, such as muscle clenching. Yasmin also learned to recognise the triggers to her symptoms during sex and, with her partner's help, how to discriminate the memories of the haemorrhage alongside paced intimacy tasks.

Physical symptoms as memory triggers

Physical symptoms may trigger re-experiencing symptoms. For example, clients may feel terrified or helpless when they experience pain because it is a reminder of their trauma. This can interact with the previous process if the triggered memories contain somatic information, leading to a 'folding over' where physical pain in the present and memories of pain in the past synergistically interact. If re-experiencing leads to increased arousal, this physiological change can exacerbate physical sensations, for example, muscle tension may worsen pain.

As with other triggers, we help clients to recognise them and use stimulus discrimination to differentiate them from trauma memories. It also helps to map out the process in a diagram, to help the client understand how the experience may move from subtle internal or external triggers through escalating cascades of sensations, intrusive memories, and appraisals.

Amir developed PTSD after a severe anaphylactic shock when his airways narrowed, making it difficult to breathe. Amir also suffered from asthma, which sometimes caused breathlessness. This sensation was a trigger to the anaphylactic shock memories, making Amir feel highly anxious and start hyperventilating, worsening his asthma symptoms. Amir and his therapist discussed recent examples of this cycle, mapping the interaction between Amir's memories, emotions, behaviours, and physical symptoms, and identifying targets for treatment. They used the 'then versus now' technique to discriminate asthma symptoms from anaphylactic symptoms and worked on reducing hyperventilation and replacing it with an appropriate asthma attack treatment plan, which Amir was given by his asthma nurse.

Hypervigilance/attentional bias towards threat

People with PTSD tend to be hypervigilant towards threat, whether internal or external. The same response is common in people with physical illness symptoms, particularly where the symptoms are appraised negatively or catastrophically. Where both PTSD and physical symptoms are present, this tendency can generalise and a mutual maintenance cycle emerges, where people who already feel under threat and are vigilant to one set of cues, are sensitised to the experience and attend to the other with excessive vigilance and checking.

In CT-PTSD, behavioural experiments are used to demonstrate the effect of hypervigilance on anxiety and related threat appraisals, and we can do the same with physical symptoms, drawing on techniques used to treat health anxiety (e.g. Bennett-Levy et al., 2004) that demonstrate how focusing attention on a particular part of the body can amplify normal sensations and makes them feel like threatening symptoms. Similarly, we use experiments to help clients test out, by first increasing then decreasing, attentional responses that maintain a threat focus, such as over-checking or 'provoking' the physical symptom (e.g. poking or rubbing the affected area), or worrying about it.

Threat appraisals

Over-estimation of the likelihood of further trauma, or the consequences of PTSD symptoms, are hallmarks of PTSD. Similarly, fear of re-injuring oneself, worsening physical symptoms, or stigma associated with them are common appraisals with physical health problems. Other shared appraisals can include beliefs about being unable to change or improve the symptom, being useless, powerless, or unsupported to cope with it, being permanently damaged, or life having been destroyed. Anxiety sensitivity, the tendency to misinterpret anxiety arousal symptoms as threatening, is thought to underlie both PTSD and physical health problems. Beliefs about health, coping, and the meaning of illness often have foundations in earlier life and cultural viewpoints; for example how caregivers dealt with illness in the family, or previous experiences of living with or witnessing others with illnesses in their community.

The same cognitive techniques that we use to address trauma-related appraisals are used to address beliefs about physical symptoms, including sourcing and reviewing evidence and behavioural experiments. In both cases, we discuss the possibility that our feelings are not good sources of information to assess objective risk. For example, PTSD can make us feel under threat when we are not. Pain can send a message that our body is physically damaged, but these signals can persist even once the body has healed.

Hot cognitions

- People think I'm making this up
- I'm seen as an invalid and worthless to society
- I can't be helped
- I'll never get my old self back

Avoidance

Understandably, clients will attempt to avoid triggers to both their trauma memories and their physical symptoms. The consequences of avoidance can also become interlinked, preventing the disproval of threatening appraisals, the processing of somatic trauma memories, and the re-evaluation of internal and external triggers. Where a client is depressed, their lethargy and fatigue may also lead to inactivity. Avoidance and inactivity can exacerbate some symptoms further. For example, avoiding movement can lead to disuse syndrome and physical deconditioning, contributing to worsening pain and stiffness, and appraisals of hopelessness that drive lethargy and withdrawal (Vlaeyen, & Linton, 2000).

Replacing avoidance with gradual approach and activation is a major part of most CBT interventions, including for PTSD, chronic pain, and chronic fatigue syndrome (e.g. Nijs et al., 2013). Behavioural experiments in dropping avoidance can therefore be used to target both PTSD and physical health symptoms.

Charlie suffered a serious injury to his hand when it became trapped in a printing press at work. His hand was reconstructed surgically but remained painful. As a result, Charlie kept his hand immobilised against his chest the whole time. Physiotherapists had advised Charlie to exercise his hand and arm but he found this too painful.

Charlie experienced spikes of pain related to re-experiencing symptoms. During imaginal reliving in therapy, his hand throbbed. It appeared that at least some of the pain was caused by the memories, so Charlie's therapist helped him update the relevant hotspots with new information including looking at his hand and wiggling his fingers to show himself how well it had healed. They used stimulus discrimination while Charlie did his physiotherapy exercises to separate the trauma memory-related pain from the pain he felt in movement. They tested and restructured his beliefs about needing to protect his hand and practised holding it differently, to see if the unnatural posture increased his pain and awareness of his hand as 'damaged', as well as his self-conscious beliefs that others saw him as 'disabled'.

Systemic issues

Experiencing an illness, injury, or trauma often results in unwanted changes to social networks including valued relationships, social, and occupational roles, contributing to distress. Equally, there may be inadvertent positive outcomes, such as receiving more care and being relieved of stressful responsibilities. Clients' fears of losing these if they recover can generate ambivalence around wanting to change and create tensions in relationships.

In therapy, we discuss and normalise potential barriers to change, validating the person's experiences of 'primary losses' as well as their understandable fears about losing their 'secondary gains' (see also Chapter 19). We help our client explore the pros and cons, both short- and long-term, of resuming activities and roles and consider how their role may change if they recover from PTSD and/or become less impaired by physical health problems. We also address ambivalence by supporting our clients to identify and address their legitimate emotional and physical needs, and to make plans for protecting or maintaining their gains whilst reclaiming the losses as best they can. Sometimes, when we explore the historical origins of their fears of recovery, it appears that PTSD and/or illness has arisen on a background of pre-existing negative schema, and compensatory coping behaviours relating to emotional deprivation or self-sacrifice. Usually, these have origins in experiences of childhood trauma or neglect, which may be helpful targets for intervention.

Notes from the therapy room: Dana

Dana reported a range of physical symptoms, alongside long-standing PTSD, which developed after a serious car accident a decade earlier. Dana had lost consciousness during the accident and experienced headaches, dizziness, and nausea in the weeks afterwards. Scans revealed no visible brain injury and she was diagnosed with post-concussion syndrome. Her symptoms improved after a few months but recurred periodically, and Dana also experienced diffuse body pains and fatigue. She gradually found herself unable to sustain her job as a teacher and became isolated and depressed.

Over the years following the accident, Dana was assessed and treated by several different services, including a pain clinic, neurology, neuropsychiatry, and a sleep clinic. A range of diagnoses was offered by different specialists, including fibromyalgia, chronic fatigue syndrome, bulimia nervosa (as she often vomited after meals), narcolepsy (as she often fell asleep suddenly), and central vestibular disorder (associated with recurrent dizziness). This was the first time she had been offered psychological therapy, and she was not hopeful that it could be effective.

Her therapist expressed empathy and compassion for her symptoms, and her understandable pessimism, and obtained Dana's agreement for them to learn more, together, about how her symptoms may be understood.

Dana's therapist asked her to keep a record of her various symptoms and they discovered that some were related to trauma reminders. For example, Dana felt nauseous and often vomited when she ate or brushed her teeth. She had also felt nauseous when she regained consciousness after the accident and had vomited in the ambulance when the paramedic had asked her to swallow a pill, so it was possible that having something in her mouth was a reminder, and that Dana had become sensitised to gagging. Her PTSD symptoms also seemed to interact with some physical symptoms. Dana's sleepiness and dizziness were worse when her sleep was disrupted by nightmares, and her difficulties with eating had led to vitamin deficiencies which were hypothesised to contribute to fatigue and light-headedness. Dana and her therapist drew out provisional maintenance cycles together and agreed possible treatment targets. Her overall formulation is in Figure 21.1.

The diaries also helped them decide how to schedule therapy sessions. Dana found that her energy levels were highest at mid-morning, especially if she had a small snack beforehand. They agreed to have video sessions on days when Dana was too unwell to travel. As reading could make her dizzy, they agreed to record brief voice notes on her phone at the end of each session that Dana could listen to afterwards as 'audio flashcards'.

The first steps in therapy included improving and stabilising Dana's nutritional intake through regular small meals and vitamin supplements, with advice from Dana's GP. They used stimulus discrimination to address the feelings of nausea that Dana experienced when she ate. Dana experimented with eating small amounts of new foods and found that concentrating on new flavours and textures helped her feel more present in the here and now and less nauseous. They also introduced more structure to Dana's day, with regular times for sleep, exercise, and enjoyable activities.

Dana's therapist next introduced the idea of rebuilding your life. Dana's life had changed completely since the accident and she felt unable to engage with previously enjoyed activities due to her physical problems. Dana agreed to experiment with gradual increases in activity and measured the outcomes against a range of individualised parameters: mood, energy levels, pain, and dizziness. She started with light physical exercise such as short walks, as well as home-based activities such as calling a friend, cooking a new recipe, and sketching. Although Dana found exercise tiring, it had a positive effect on her mood and proved less painful than predicted.

Dana was reluctant to go out in public due to fears that she would be knocked over and injured again, and believing her head was now too fragile to withstand another blow. Her therapist helped her review evidence for and against these beliefs. Dana had experienced occasional knocks over the previous decade, including banging her head on a door frame once, but had not been seriously hurt again, and the pain was only fleeting. Dana was hypervigilant to possible collisions with other people when she walked, so her therapist helped her do a behavioural experiment where she attended to all the possible collision hazards in the therapy room, to show that she felt more unsafe the more she looked for danger. They generalised the learning from this experiment to internal hypervigilance. Dana found that when she focused her attention on her elbow (which wasn't usually painful), it began to throb, and they discussed the effect of attention on heightening physical sensations and practised moving attention around the body and switching between internal and external focus. Dana and her therapist also practised lightly tapping their own, then each other's, heads with a wooden spoon, to test her fears about the safety of small knocks to her head.

Dana's memories of the accident were blurry and disjointed. With her therapist, she constructed a written narrative, incorporating information from other sources such as eye-witness reports

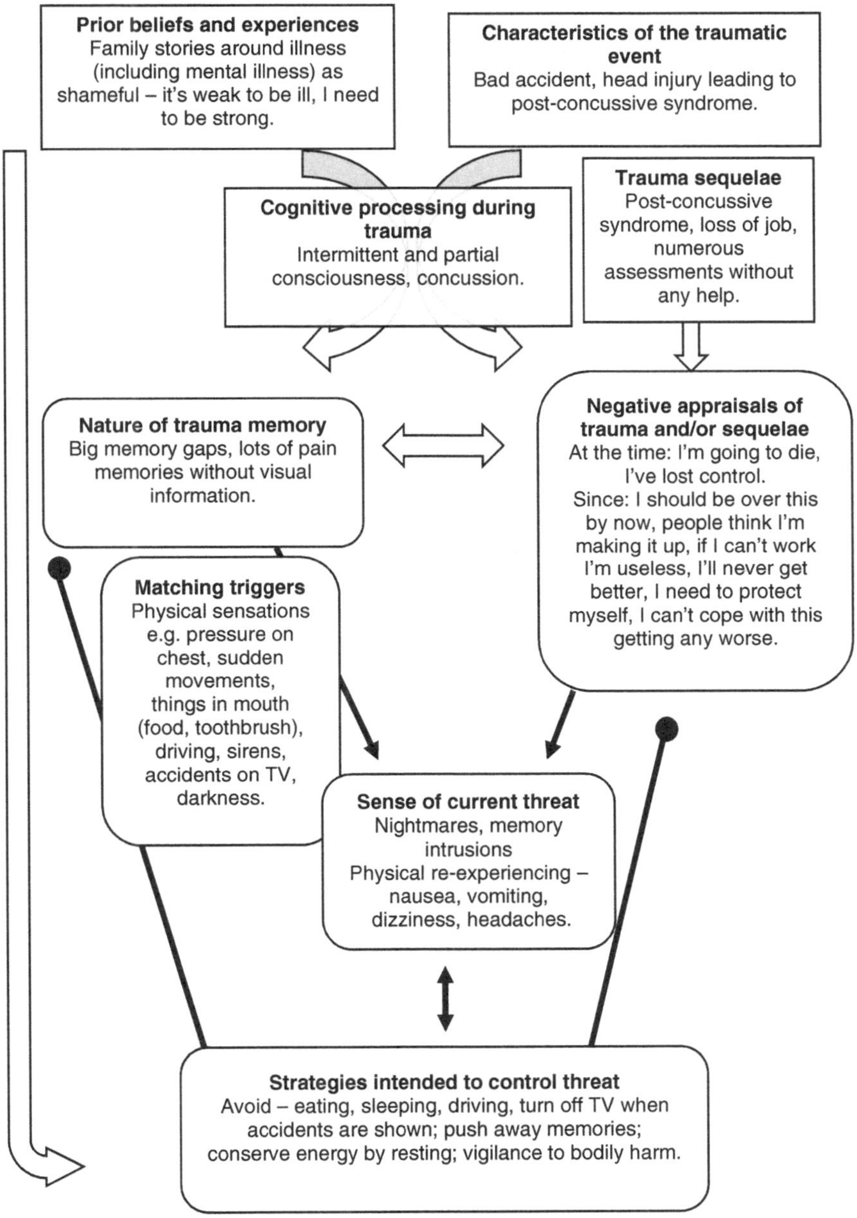

Figure 21.1 Dana's formulation

and her hospital records to fill in the gaps where possible. They then relived the specific hotspots that Dana could remember. Many of the memories comprised strong sensory and somatic fragments with few visual details to tie them together, so they tried to include information about what Dana now knew had happened to contextualise the memories. For example, Dana remembered regaining consciousness momentarily in her car, in darkness, and feeling sick, dizzy, and in pain. They added the information that Dana's car had rolled and she had been upside down, held by a seatbelt, having knocked her head, which explained her physical sensations. As they updated the memories, Dana's therapist asked her to open her eyes and stand up to show that she could see and move, and tap her body and head to show that she was no longer injured, that there was no blood, and that her skull was intact.

Dana's nightmares reduced following work on the trauma memories and she noticed reductions in anxiety, nausea, and dizziness. She was able to increase her range of activities and, although she continued to tire easily, could spend more time with friends and family and exercise more. Dana reported self-critical thoughts that 'I should've pulled myself together before now' and 'I let my life slip away because I was scared'. Dana revealed that, as a child, she had been taught that it was possible to 'push through' illness and that it was a sign of weakness. This belief had been strengthened by her physical symptoms not being taken seriously by medical professionals. Her therapist helped Dana construct a survey to gather other opinions on whether her symptoms were 'justified', given her serious accident, and Dana was surprised to discover that most responses were compassionate and supportive. Dana felt encouraged by this to practise talking to herself with kindness. This led to a shift in how Dana viewed her rebuilding your life activities. Rather than criticising herself for what she couldn't do, she praised and rewarded herself for everything she achieved. She began to take photos on her phone of every reclaiming task and saved them in an album that she could use to remind herself of her progress and successes.

At the end of treatment, Dana's PTSD symptoms were much improved, and she reported reductions in, but not complete recovery from, her physical health symptoms. Importantly, she noted a marked improvement in how much her physical symptoms distressed her, and how much they interfered in her life.

Recommended reading

Beck, J. G., & Clapp, J. D. (2011). A different kind of comorbidity: Understanding posttraumatic stress disorder and chronic pain. *Psychological Trauma: Theory, Research, Practice, and Policy*, 3(2), 101–108.

Deary, V., Chalder, T., & Sharpe, M. (2007). The cognitive behavioural model of medically unexplained symptoms: A theoretical and empirical review. *Clinical Psychology Review*, 27(7), 781–797.

CHAPTER TWENTY TWO
Social comorbidity

Suresh was claiming asylum in the UK and lived in difficult circumstances, separated from his family, with little money and poor housing. These factors interacted with Suresh's symptoms of PTSD and depression, exacerbating his hopelessness and increasing his risk of suicide. In the early stages of therapy, Suresh's therapist worked with him to improve his social situation within the limits of what was possible, and to address the impact of these factors on his mental health.

Many clients are affected by external stressors, such as financial, legal, housing, immigration, and employment problems. They may also describe significant relationship issues, such as conflict within their family, lack of social support, and parenting problems. Some of these issues are closely linked to PTSD, for example, when an ongoing court case relates to the traumatic event, or where symptoms of PTSD such as irritability are causing relationship problems. Other social issues are unrelated to PTSD but add to the emotional burden on an individual, and PTSD symptoms can make it harder to think through and respond effectively to practical and social challenges.

As with other forms of comorbidity, social problems can increase over time when PTSD remains untreated. Clients who have been unable to work because of their difficulties, for example, often end up in financial difficulty, placing strain on relationships, and raising additional challenges such as navigating the welfare benefits system. These struggles, understandably, add extra stress and place additional demands on already stretched personal resources, make recovery from PTSD more difficult, and the development of further psychological and physical problems more likely.

Since our expertise is in psychological therapy, not social work, ideally our focus in sessions should be on PTSD treatment. However, it is impractical and unsupportive to ignore social problems that our clients face, or expect them to be 'left at the door' during therapy. In this chapter, we describe how to support and help clients facing difficult life circumstances, while still progressing their PTSD treatment where possible. Different types of social comorbidity will affect individuals in different ways so, as usual, we personalise the approach to suit the needs of each client.

Assessing and formulating

Where clients are facing external stressors, we devote time early in treatment to explicitly discuss the nature and impact of these issues, and to validate our client's emotional reactions. Validation can also offer a mini-formulation to help our client draw links between their environment, thoughts, feelings, and behaviours: 'it's understandable you feel so angry and fed up, living in such bad conditions and believing that no one listens to you or helps' or 'it's no wonder you can't sleep, with all these very real worries turning over in your mind' or 'given the terrible losses you have had, it makes sense you are struggling to rebuild your life, and that you feel so

DOI: 10.4324/9781003288329-27

hopeless about the future'. Each validation also potentially orients our clients towards possible solutions. In the CT-PTSD formulation, these stressors will often be located in the box for trauma sequelae and will feed appraisals that link to feelings of hopelessness, helplessness, and injustice.

It can sometimes be hard to judge the extent to which a client's experience of social problems is affected by their psychological symptoms or cognitive distortions, including the heightened perception of threat which is inherent to PTSD. Often the external stressor and some cognitive distortion will overlap, making these judgements even more complicated. Additionally, clients who are from disadvantaged communities are disproportionately affected by issues such as poverty, discrimination, and harassment (see also Chapter 25). As therapists, we occupy positions of privilege so we need to be especially cautious about making judgements using our own experiences, as they may not match our client's. Instead, we ask for details of specific examples of external stressors, and then consider with the client how the stressor, their interpretations, and reactions to it might affect each other, and whether there are any 'vicious' maintaining cycles. This can also help decide whether to take a problem-solving approach, to help the client find ways to change the reality of the situation, a reappraisal/behavioural experiment approach to address appraisals about the situation, or a combination of the two.

Sinead was desperate to move out of her council flat, saying the flat was in a dangerous area, but the council had repeatedly denied her request. Sinead's ex-partner had previously shared the flat and was now in prison having been convicted of assaulting her. To assess the risks, Sinead's therapist asked for specific examples of the dangers present in her living environment. Sinead's main concern was her neighbours: they were noisy, often slamming doors and yelling. She found this very distressing, as sudden noises and shouting made her jump, and triggered memories of her ex-partner breaking down the door. There seemed to be a vicious cycle whereby Sinead's PTSD symptoms were triggered by the noise, and also made her more sensitive to perceiving the excessive noise as threatening and targeted at her.

Sinead and her therapist decided to take both a problem and emotion-focused approach. Her therapist wrote a letter to support Sinead's request to be moved and they also problem-solved alternative strategies to minimise the effects of the noise, including Sinead keeping a record of incidents that she fed back to the council through the complaints system, and using earplugs to help her sleep. They also agreed to focus some therapy sessions on helping Sinead feel safer in her flat, by working on trigger discrimination and risk appraisals.

The impacts of social circumstances are dynamic, and treatment decisions are sometimes simply about timing. For example, treatment may need to be delayed due to stressful upcoming events, such as a court case or impending eviction. Conversely, there may be a window of time we can capitalise on, when the client is in a position of relative stability while still anticipating a future stressor. Where it is unclear if social issues play a role in maintaining psychological problems, or are an obstacle to treatment, we build in regular review points to assess how treatment is progressing, and whether the focus needs to shift temporarily to address these problems and their impact.

FAQ: In what social circumstances is PTSD treatment unhelpful?

There are some social circumstances where PTSD treatment is contraindicated. In Maslow's (1943) hierarchy of needs, basic physiological needs critical to survival must be met before people can move on to addressing their psychological needs. If our client lacks food and a place to live, they will be unable to engage with psychological therapy for PTSD, as all of their energy will, understandably, be focused on fulfilling their basic needs. In these situations, our priority is to provide practical help, and/or signpost them appropriately, at least until these needs are fulfilled.

Another example is where clients face obstacles to attending and engagement with therapy, such that an appropriate 'dose' cannot be delivered. This may happen because of practical constraints, such as not having childcare to support attending sessions, or money to pay for travel to appointments. Here, we try to problem-solve these obstacles and also flex our modes of delivery to make treatment as accessible as possible, for example delivering sessions remotely if needed, offering time-intensive interventions to capitalise on windows of opportunity, or setting between-session self-study modules to support sporadic attendance.

Sometimes clients are so preoccupied with an external stressor that they struggle with the structure of CBT treatment and maintaining focus on the trauma. The strategies described in the next section may reduce the impact of social problems and resulting preoccupation sufficiently for effective treatment to take place, but this is not always possible. As circumstances change over time, we may instead discuss whether the issue is currently limiting their ability to benefit from treatment, agree minimum change criteria, and offer to reassess and reconsider psychological therapy in the future once the issues have been addressed.

How to help

SIGNPOSTING AND PROBLEM-SOLVING

Our most common intervention with social comorbidity is to help clients find appropriate organisations and resources to support them. These will vary depending on the problem but may include community organisations, charities, legal advisors, and support workers. We will often try to help where we can, for example by providing a report to support a client's asylum claim or housing application, or by offering to speak to relevant people within their network to explain their difficulties or advocate for their needs. Beyond this, we do not intervene too much on our client's behalf for various reasons: we are often not the best people to do so, it risks therapeutic drift away from a trauma-focus, and because our preference is to teach problem-solving skills to empower clients to solve their own problems. However, deploying our professional power to advocate on a client's behalf, or alongside them, can help model problem-solving skills and build trust within the therapeutic alliance. Clients can often also achieve more for themselves when supported by someone with some experience of the systems they are navigating.

Often our clients feel despondent in the face of social problems and chronic adversity. People in disempowered groups may understandably learn to expect discrimination, mistreatment, and injustice from others, including the police and the state, and feel powerless, distrustful, and pessimistic about their ability to influence their situation. Growing up and living in disadvantaged and persecutory contexts naturally engenders an external locus of control. This 'learned helplessness' can be protective against experiencing repeated failure when the odds are stacked against you, and also potentially inhibits adaptive efforts at problem-focused coping where stressors can be influenced. We believe it is important to validate prior experiences of mistreatment, and the understandable cognitive and behavioural consequences, and then help our clients develop adaptive problem-solving for those challenges they now face (see also Chapter 25).

Billy had experienced repeated discrimination because he was a member of the Traveller community. After his wife died in an accident, Billy contacted a local pub to use their function room for a wake. When they found out that Billy and his family were Travellers, the pub refused to rent them the room. Billy did not challenge it at the time, but he continued to ruminate about the incident and, in therapy, he expressed anger and distress about the situation, which had fuelled his beliefs about being mistreated by others. Rather than attempt to challenge these beliefs, his therapist asked Billy how they could address the issues of discrimination that he and his family faced. Together, they researched equality and discrimination legislation, and Billy decided to contact the UK government's 'Equality Advisory Support Service' (EASS) and to write a formal letter of complaint to the pub landlord, quoting the relevant legislation and asking for an apology. Knowing his rights made Billy feel more empowered to deal with such situations in the future, and his therapist also helped him reflect on the benefits of taking action in response to mistreatment, compared to brooding about it.

ADDRESSING BARRIERS TO TREATMENT

Some obstacles may complicate PTSD treatment by restricting the client's ability to access therapy or engage with specific treatment elements. For example, some 'reclaiming your life' activities may be impossible because of financial hardship, and creativity may be required to find free or cheap alternatives. Homework tasks like reviewing session recordings can be difficult for those who have little privacy or free time. Making time to get to appointments may be a struggle for those who work long hours, and have limited support from employers to attend appointments, or who have caring responsibilities. These types of difficulties can lead to treatment drop-out, so require attention early in treatment. It is a good idea to ask about potential obstacles in the assessment, to plan for these constraints.

Another useful approach is to harness an individual's existing strengths, by asking them 'what personal qualities have helped you overcome problems previously?' or 'where have you drawn strength from in the past?'. Our clients have often faced enormous adversity and have reserves of resilience which we can help them draw upon to overcome, or tolerate, challenges in their social situation. We can also help identify resources within their network to support them in achieving maximum benefit from treatment. Using the metaphor of a sports team that has supporters or cheerleaders to spur them on when things get difficult, we also routinely ask our clients to identify one person who may be willing to support them through their treatment. This person can be enlisted, for example, to offer a 'check-in' after sessions, accompany them on behavioural experiments or reclaiming tasks, listen to them explain a formulation, prompt coping or stimulus discrimination skills, or arrange enjoyable activities with them after memory-focused work.

Jo had previously been discharged from services for failing to attend appointments. She was the sole carer for her two sons, the younger of whom had a learning disability, and she had little family support. Jo identified early on that barriers to attending appointments arose when one of her sons was ill and during school holidays. She also struggled with homework tasks as she had little free time. Jo's therapist helped her problem-solve how she could attend sessions. They agreed to begin treatment at the start of the school term and arranged appointment times for after school drop-off. Jo worked part-time, so her therapist wrote to her employer requesting a morning off every week for ten weeks to attend therapy appointments. They also researched low-cost childcare options and found an 'after-school club' that both her sons could attend once a week, so that Jo could have a couple of hours to herself to do a 'reclaiming your life' activity. Jo also joined a Facebook group for local mums in her area, that gave both emotional and practical support.

MANAGING UNCERTAINTY

Some of our clients live with uncertainty about the future, for example regarding unresolved police investigations, compensation or criminal cases, asylum claims, or employment tribunals. Preoccupation with these stressors and worry about feared outcomes can exacerbate other psychological symptoms and make it difficult to maintain a trauma-focus in therapy. Where they are linked to trauma memories, stressors also act as triggers, multiplying their emotional impact. This may make it difficult for people to feel sufficient 'psychological distance' to put trauma memories into the past through treatment, particularly if the uncertainty also fuels important personal meanings, for example, about future threat or injustice. Some clients choose to postpone treatment until after stressors resolve, but this may be impractical, particularly where no clear end is in sight. Their ability to manage the stressors may itself be impaired by PTSD symptoms and create mutually maintaining cycles that prevent progress. Postponing treatment also presents risks, in terms of the distress and impact of chronic PTSD on wellbeing and functioning, and gives the message that the individual's life must be put on hold.

In these situations, we first help clients evaluate the costs and benefits of proceeding versus postponing treatment. We may offer a limited number of sessions and then review, sometimes as an 'extended assessment', to establish whether the client can work within the CBT structure and maintain a PTSD treatment focus. We also draw on techniques used in treatment of generalised anxiety disorder to target unhelpful coping that may be fuelling the disruptive impact of the stressors, including helping clients accept and tolerate uncertainty, and manage the unconstructive worry these situations provoke (e.g. Robichaud et al., 2019). We validate how difficult living with an unknown future is, help clients learn to notice worry, consider its intended function in this context, and evaluate its usefulness. This typically reveals maintaining beliefs about worry such as 'it helps me prepare for a bad outcome', which can be addressed using cognitive techniques. We encourage use of simple worry delay strategies such as 'worry trees' and 'worry time'. Where there are required actions, or steps can be taken to address the stressor, we may agree to devote a small amount of time each session, usually at the end, to briefly review and problem-solve. Practical steps can be reframed as 'reclaiming your life' activities, even if it involves unenjoyable activities such as filling in forms, as it encourages clients to replace rumination about their situation with a sense of progress and agency.

AVOIDING THERAPIST DRIFT

Where a client is facing considerable external stressors, it is easy for therapy sessions to be consumed by discussing them. It can be difficult to strike a balance between empathic and productive work on social problems, without drifting too far from the primary goals of treatment. We need to monitor this, for ourselves, with the client, and through supervision. A useful question to ask ourselves before devoting therapy time to social issues is 'how does this task move trauma-focused therapy forward?'.

If we do notice drift, we jointly review the client's goals and discuss the focus of therapy, e.g. 'I've noticed that we often plan in the session to work together on the memories of what happened, but we end up talking about your work situation. Have you noticed that?' and 'these [social] problems are really important and distressing for you at the moment, and of course the PTSD is as well. I want to make sure we make the most of these sessions to help reduce your PTSD symptoms. How do you think we can best do that when you also have these other areas on your mind?'.

Legal processes

Police investigations and legal cases can complicate therapy in various ways. They can last a long time, with sudden flurries of activity against long periods of anxious waiting. They usually have significant practical and emotional implications for the person's future, adding to the sense of current and future threat. Correspondence and meetings with police and lawyers can be stressful and often trigger PTSD symptoms. Clients usually have to repeatedly narrate their traumatic experiences in great detail, may undergo forensic interviews or hostile cross-examinations, and potentially have to face the perpetrator in court. There may also be concerns about what might happen if the perpetrator is not convicted, including fears of reprisals.

These factors can reduce the benefits clients can achieve through therapy and some clients may feel it would overwhelm them, or are deterred by how it may interact with legal processes (see top tips), so choose to wait until the case is resolved before undertaking treatment. Other clients are less preoccupied with the case or wish to prioritise their recovery. The decision to proceed must therefore be made collaboratively, based on clients' informed consent and full transparency of the limits to privacy, and weighing the relative costs and benefits of moving forward with PTSD treatment.

An alternative can be to offer a shorter course of therapy before the court case, including some elements of CT-PTSD to help clients prepare psychologically, but delaying the memory-focused treatment elements until after completion. Aspects of preparation can include learning stimulus discrimination and grounding tools to cope with memory triggers, managing worry and uncertainty while waiting, activating appropriate support networks, present-focused coping including behavioural activation, planning for coping with the trial including accessing support as a vulnerable witness, and problem-solving potential outcomes.

Top tips: Conducting treatment when clients will be going to court

Clients may have been advised against psychological therapy before giving witness statements or evidence in court, due to concerns from investigators and prosecutors that detailed re-telling of the trauma narrative in therapy can be portrayed as 'coaching the witness' or 'elaborating false memories', thereby discrediting the evidence and jeopardising the prosecution. Clients may also feel deterred when told that information from their therapy sessions may be sought by the police or the court even without their consent. Medical records including materials from therapy sessions can be subpoenaed, therapists can be asked to give a witness statement, and details from the records may sometimes be used to challenge the client's evidence or their reliability. However, recent guidelines (under consultation at the time of writing; Crime Prosecution Service, 2020) now place a greater focus on prioritising the wellbeing of the 'victim', including not delaying treatment if it is in their best interest, and only obtaining their records without consent where there is a legitimate line of enquiry. Here is our approach:

- *Allow the client to make informed choices about treatment*: Our policy is not to withhold treatment if someone wants it and could benefit from it. We explain the CPS guidance and different treatment options and allow the client to choose how they wish to proceed.
- *Keep detailed records*: Make sure all your records are clear, detailed, and up-to-date. Concerns about coaching are based on the possibility that therapists may inadvertently implant false memories or suggest interpretations of events to clients. Recording sessions can therefore be helpful, to demonstrate if needed that the client's account of the trauma has not been altered by your therapy sessions.
- *Liaise with experts*: We often contact the client's solicitor (with their permission) and the CPS, to inform them of our involvement, and to check any areas of concern. We can also check our clients are being supported as vulnerable witnesses, for example, given the option to give evidence via video link.

A further issue can arise when a medico-legal claim is being assessed, or damages sought for psychological injuries. This can work against a client's motivation to engage with treatment, for example, through blocking beliefs like 'if I recover now, I will be disbelieved or my injuries won't be properly compensated'. Where our role is providing psychological therapy, we are generally neither in a position, nor required, to assess the reliability of our client's account or their entitlement for damages. However, as a professional witness, we may be asked to give details about their diagnosis, treatment, functional impairment, and prognosis to Criminal Injuries Compensation Authority (CICA), to their insurer, or the court. In our experience, most clients are primarily motivated to recover from their PTSD symptoms but, as with all treatment obstacles, if progress seems limited in the context of an ongoing compensation claim, we discuss the option to delay treatment until it is resolved, and document the reasons for doing so in the discharge plan.

Relationship and other interpersonal issues

PTSD can both cause, and be maintained by, relationship difficulties, and the quality of social support is one of the most important predictors of recovery. For most clients, PTSD symptoms have a detrimental impact on their interpersonal functioning and are a common cause of conflicts (Whisman, 1999). Indeed, the secondary impact of PTSD symptoms can sometimes be the reason for seeking treatment. Frequent arguments, problems with intimacy, unsupportive or critical partners, or loved ones struggling with their own mental health can exacerbate PTSD symptoms, reinforce negative appraisals of themselves and others, and maintain unhelpful coping including withdrawal. As before, we need to strike a balance between validating and supporting our clients to manage such problems, while maintaining a trauma-focus during therapy. Here are some ways to help.

INVOLVE SIGNIFICANT OTHERS

We have mentioned already the importance of involving significant others in the client's network as 'cheerleaders' and supporters, but it is even more important where aspects of the relationship are interacting with the maintenance of a client's PTSD (e.g. reinforcing avoidance) or where the client's PTSD is impacting on their relationship.

A good starting point is to share psychoeducational information about PTSD symptoms and the reciprocal influence of relationship problems, alongside a rationale and overview of trauma-focused therapy. The goal is to stimulate dialogue and promote a shared understanding of problematic symptoms such as irritability or withdrawal, validate the experience on both sides, and identify potential maintenance cycles within their interactions. Externalising the problem, and giving it an identity of its own, helps reduce stigma and blame by encouraging loved ones to separate their feelings about the PTSD symptoms from those toward the client and, rather than divide, join them in resisting the problem (White, 1998). We generally offer the client to invite important people in their life to attend an early therapy session where they can share the formulation and treatment plan. This is particularly important where other people hold beliefs about PTSD which may create obstacles to the therapy process (e.g. 'talking about the trauma makes it worse'). We also facilitate a discussion about how they may best support the client (e.g. 'I might feel upset after a session, and that's normal. I need you to remind me that it is part of the process and to prompt me to do a pleasant activity. I might not want to talk much.').

If interpersonal issues significantly interfere with trauma-focused therapy, or PTSD symptoms cause unmanaged risks within the family, such as aggressive outbursts around children, our intervention may extend to several sessions to address the obstacle, drawing on modules from conjoint CBT for PTSD (Monson, & Fredman, 2012). However, our aim is not to provide relationship therapy *per se*, but rather to help our client engage with CT-PTSD treatment. As PTSD symptoms improve, often so do relationship difficulties or, at least, clients are in a better position to address them. If relationship problems do not improve following successful treatment of PTSD symptoms, we would generally consider either onward referrals or offer an additional treatment module.

Hot cognitions

- I can't put my trauma behind me until my housing/court case/asylum claim/financial problems have resolved
- I'm in a deep financial hole and there's nothing I can do about it
- My partner/family don't support me or understand what I am going through
- I have been treated badly all my life and I probably deserve it/there is no justice
- The whole system is stacked against me

TOXIC AND ABUSIVE RELATIONSHIPS

Where clients disclose ongoing abuse in their relationships, our priority is to manage this risk through safeguarding rather than proceed with trauma-focused therapy. Where a relationship is not overtly abusive or coercive, but is emotionally 'toxic', this can exacerbate PTSD symptoms and interfere with recovery. For example, when a partner or family frequently makes critical or demeaning comments, blames the client for traumatic events, or are themselves emotionally volatile and behave unpredictably.

Intervening in these cases can be challenging, as the other party may be hostile to the process of therapy, and our client understandably ambivalent about addressing the issues. They may feel disloyal for disclosing their experience, fearful of safeguarding processes being triggered, and of losing any practical and emotional support, despite the toxicity. There is also a risk that, as a client recovers, or attempts to express their needs more assertively within a relationship, the abusive behaviour escalates as a means to re-establish control. We therefore proceed cautiously, adhering to principles of maximising our client's control and choice-making, alongside the therapist's predictability and transparency. We encourage open, non-judgemental discussions about their safety and wellbeing, and validate their feelings, including ambivalence. We also insist that reviewing risk incidents remains a standing agenda item and collaboratively agree the threshold for shifting into safeguarding.

When clients are in long-term toxic relationships or have prior experiences of domestic abuse, they may not recognise other people's behaviour as coercive or abusive, or may hold deeply held beliefs about themselves as deserving of mistreatment. We may use Socratic techniques, for example, to ask what the client would say to someone else who described their relationship or arrange a survey to obtain a range of opinions. Through this process, a client may recognise and acknowledge emotional toxicity or coercive behaviours in others and this can increase their motivation to take steps to address the issues.

Again, we may offer to include the other person in some therapy sessions, if both parties are willing. If not, we discuss with the client how they can more effectively communicate their needs and wishes within the relationship. This may include practising ways to ask for support or to explain the impact of the other person's behaviour; and supporting the client to begin placing boundaries around mistreatment, such as practising how to assertively respond to critical and demanding comments, and developing 'zero tolerance' to mistreatment (Kubany, & Ralston, 2008). This may lead to the relationship improving. Equally, as clients become more aware of mistreatment and address negative beliefs about themselves as deserving, they may decide to renegotiate or end a relationship, enforce boundaries, or distance themselves from the other person. Here, we support the client to manage this both practically and emotionally, signpost them to external resources as needed, and monitor risks carefully.

IMPACT OF RECOVERY

Relationships often change to accommodate PTSD symptoms or have formed after PTSD has developed. While recovery might seem in everyone's best interests, it can also put pressure on relationships and affect their dynamics. For example, partners of people with PTSD who have taken a caregiving role, and found value in supporting the person, may fear that changes will lead to the person no longer needing, or 'outgrowing', them.

Often this process becomes more apparent as therapy progresses and symptoms start to improve. This can be confusing for the client, so it can be helpful to discuss how relationships may be changing both for the better and worse. Sometimes, as the client's needs are met, other people in the system feel more able to safely express their own needs, for example, their resentment about living with someone who has been irritable or having lost their social life. If other people in the system are struggling to adjust to changes, we encourage an open discussion, normalise, and validate everyone's struggle to adjust. We may use the metaphor of 'ripple effects' spreading out from the client, and affecting everyone's 'balance'. Often it is enough for others to feel that the client has heard and recognised their concerns, so we encourage clients to listen and acknowledge rather than become defensive.

Craig and his partner Lois had been experiencing relationship problems since Craig left the army. Lois wanted them to spend more time as a family, while Craig wanted space away from her and their three children. As Craig's PTSD and depression symptoms began to improve, their relationship deteriorated further.

Craig's therapist invited Lois to join a therapy session so they could talk it through. They both agreed that they had blamed all of their relationship difficulties on Craig's PTSD, but actually some issues had been there much longer and needed to be addressed. Lois interpreted Craig's need for space as a rejection of her and the children, while Craig saw it as essential for managing his stress levels. Craig shared that he was glad he had left the army and could spend more time with the family, but he was still adjusting to the change. They agreed to talk more often about their feelings and made a plan for each week to include some family time all together, and some time for both Craig and Lois to spend alone.

NOTES FROM THE THERAPY ROOM: SURESH

Suresh escaped persecution in Sri Lanka and claimed asylum in the UK. His asylum application had been rejected and he was appealing the decision. While he waited, Suresh was not allowed to work, lived in dirty hostel accommodation, and received a small weekly payment from the National Asylum Support Service (NASS). Suresh had been tortured and was terrified of being deported to Sri Lanka, where he was certain he would be killed. His family there were frequently visited by police asking about his whereabouts, so he also feared for their safety. Suresh was required to attend and sign at the UK Border Agency (UKBA) every fortnight, and his PTSD symptoms always increased around this time as he feared the border authorities might detain him. At assessment, Suresh described strong feelings of hopelessness and thoughts of suicide, as he believed that his family would be safer if he was dead and that he had no future either there or in the UK. His formulation is in Figure 22.1.

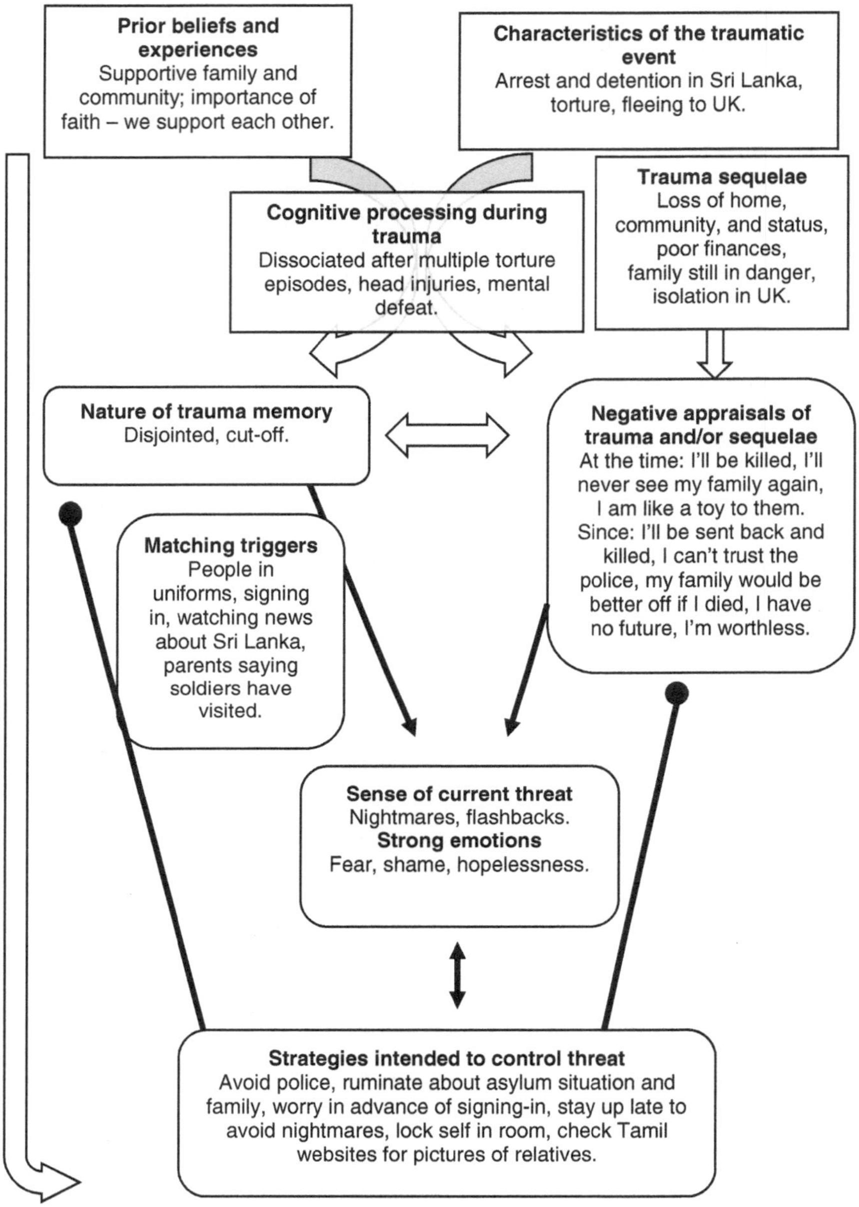

Figure 22.1 Suresh's formulation

The early sessions in therapy were spent addressing Suresh's suicide risk. Through discussion with his therapist, Suresh realised that, regardless of the risks to them, his family would want him alive rather than dead, so they wrote this on a flashcard, along with Suresh's other reasons for living and goals for the future if he was given asylum. Suresh's therapist was also worried his risk may increase if his social circumstances worsened, such as his asylum application being rejected again or hearing bad news about his family, so they agreed a risk management plan for these situations.

They also discussed ways to improve Suresh's social circumstances within the limits of his situation. His therapist wrote to the UKBA explaining that Suresh was suffering from PTSD and requesting that he sign in monthly rather than fortnightly, which was agreed. They also wrote a letter highlighting that Suresh was an 'adult at risk' according to UKBA's 'Rule 35' guidance, so should not be detained for immigration reasons on three grounds: that he had a mental health disorder, was at suicide risk, and was a torture survivor. Suresh took the letter with him whenever he went to sign in, and in case he was arrested by the police, which made him feel slightly safer. Learning stimulus discrimination also helped Suresh to cope with his interactions with UK authorities. People in uniforms, including UKBA staff, triggered memories of his arrest and detention. This sometimes led to him dissociating and acting in a suspicious manner, such as running away when he saw police officers. He learnt to pay attention to the differences between the uniforms of British Police and UKBA staff compared to Sri Lankan Police, to remind himself they were different. His therapist helped him write a note on his phone to show police officers in case he was stopped, which read 'I'm an asylum-seeker and I don't speak English. I have PTSD. If I run away, it is because I am scared. I don't have a criminal record. If you need to know more about me please call my cousin [who spoke English well]'.

Next, they identified possible 'reclaiming your life' tasks. Suresh didn't know if he would be allowed to stay in the UK, and was limited by lack of money and opportunity, but wanted to feel more settled and at home. They agreed to add decorations to his sparse hostel room, including a union jack flag on the wall to remind him he was in the UK and some posters of his favourite cricket stars. This helped him discriminate the hostel room from the prison cell when he woke up from nightmares of torture. Suresh also developed a daily routine, where he slept at night rather than staying up late, and exercised by running in his local park every day. Using a map from his therapist, he also joined a local library where he would spend time improving his English by reading the newspapers and use the internet to look at things that interested him rather than Tamil news sites. Suresh had identified that in prison and during his escape to the UK he had drawn strength from his faith. His therapist helped him find a nearby Tamil temple where he could pray, join a meditation session, and attend regular meetings with other Tamils where they also shared a meal. They also contacted a local refugee charity that offered weekly English lessons, free meals, legal advice, and occasional social events.

As Suresh began to feel safer, more settled in a routine, and more hopeful for the future, therapy moved on to addressing his torture memories. They made a timeline of Suresh's six months in prison with key events either side, including the lead up to his arrest, and his escape and arrival in the UK. They matched the events on the timeline to his flashbacks and nightmares, and used imaginal reliving for the main memories that he re-experienced. They noticed links between Suresh's trauma experiences and thoughts he had during them, and how he perceived his current life difficulties. For example, Suresh had felt powerless and like a worthless object when in prison and believed he would never see his family again, and he had similar thoughts and feelings about the hopelessness of his current situation as an asylum-seeker, and about future threats. He and his therapist worked to update these meanings within the trauma memories, often using the things he was doing day to day now as updates. The therapist also encouraged Suresh to reflect on what he had achieved each week, and how that helped him rethink his beliefs about being worthless and powerless.

Recommended reading

Grey, N., & Young, K. (2008). Cognitive behaviour therapy with refugees and asylum-seekers experiencing traumatic stress symptoms. *Behavioural and Cognitive Psychotherapy*, 36(1), 3–19.

Monson, C. M., & Fredman, S. J. (2012). *Cognitive-behavioral conjoint therapy for PTSD: Harnessing the healing power of relationships*. Guilford Press.

CHAPTER TWENTY THREE

Risk

Joao reported frequent suicidal thoughts, past suicide attempts, and thoughts of harming others in the context of PTSD and depression. Careful risk assessment and management was a central aspect of his treatment. His therapist targeted the cognitive, emotional, and systemic mechanisms underlying the association between his PTSD symptoms and risk factors.

The vast majority of people with PTSD do not harm themselves or others. However, PTSD symptoms, particularly in combination with depression, increase the risk of various types of harm: non-suicidal self-injury (NSSI, Zlotnick et al., 1999), suicidal thoughts and behaviours (Panagioti et al., 2009), death by suicide (Gradus et al., 2010), experiencing further trauma, including being harmed by others (Jaffe et al., 2019), and aggression towards others (Elbogen et al., 2014).

Treating PTSD alongside clinically important risk presents a challenge as, for some clients, therapy temporarily increases PTSD symptoms, associated strong emotions, and coping behaviours that are functionally related to risk. While caution is therefore required, delaying or withholding treatment also confers risks; of untreated PTSD, and its associated longer-term risks of harm, aggression, and non-accidental death, as well as the secondary psychological, physical, and social consequences. The challenge is therefore walking the fine line between managing potential short-term risks while working towards longer-term benefits.

In this chapter, we only briefly describe fundamental aspects of risk assessment and management; many texts are available which cover this in more depth. Instead, we focus on the risks commonly associated with PTSD and how to approach treatment in the context of ongoing risk.

Basic principles

When assessing and managing risk, we start with some basic principles.

- *Use facts, not feelings*: Most psychological therapists are familiar with assessing factors known to predict risk, such as concrete plans to harm oneself or others, a history of suicide attempts/violence, preparation, rehearsal, and access to means. In forensic settings, 'actuarial' risk assessment tools are often employed, evaluating risk based on the cumulative impact and interaction of known predictors, both proximal and distal (e.g. social support, previous suicide attempts, current chronic pain, recent losses). Hence, we base our clinical judgements on observable risk factors rather than intuition. The principle also holds when we are assessing risk to our clients from others. We need to seek details and examples of the risk. For example, when did they last have contact with the perpetrator, in what context, and what exactly happened?

DOI: 10.4324/9781003288329-28

- *Risk is dynamic*: We always assess risk at the start of treatment, but situations change, so regular reviews are important. Risk also changes moment-to-moment for some people. In a session, someone may not feel suicidal or angry, but an upsetting phone call later that day, or a nightmare that night, may increase risk substantially. We need to ask about risk when it is at its worst. Our risk plans must be dynamic and responsive to changing situations.
- *Personalise assessments and safety plans*: The use of actuarial risk tools can mask individual variability in risk factors and should not be used in isolation. Indeed, most tools developed to measure suicidal behaviour have insufficient predictive accuracy to be relied upon (Runeson et al., 2017). Understanding an individual's personal risk factors, the functional 'chains' of events and responses, and the underlying psychological mechanisms can improve the accuracy of our assessments, and also help us design effective, individualised safety plans (Zortea et al., 2020).
- *Managing risk is a shared task*: From the start of therapy, we aim to create a collaborative and transparent approach to monitoring and managing risk. This includes discussing how therapy can feel safe for both the client and us, including how and when we will monitor risk, what we will do if risk increases, and giving our clients responsibility for following mutually agreed plans. A commitment to transparency and shared responsibility is a necessary precursor to any therapeutic work. A strong therapeutic relationship is important in determining our client's willingness to disclose and seek help for risk issues, and our ability to ask 'tough questions' of them. We acknowledge and validate our client's struggles with risk, whilst modelling hopefulness and a relentless determination to find solutions together.
- *The 'good enough' rule*: It is unrealistic to eliminate all risks for all clients before starting treatment. Many clients have lived for a long time with suicidal thoughts which they have not acted upon, and do not intend to, or with anger control problems that have never escalated into violence. Similarly, some clients live with a degree of ongoing risk in their personal circumstances, such as the risk of being re-traumatised due to the nature of their job, or living with the possibility of threat due to being a member of a marginalised group or living in poverty (for example, living in a high crime area). We aim to minimise these risks but also deliver treatment in less-than-ideal circumstances to mitigate against the longer-term risk of untreated PTSD. Risk may fluctuate during treatment and may move from a 'good enough' position into a situation where trauma-focused treatment is unsafe. If so, we pause our intervention to prioritise managing the risk and continue again when possible.
- *Minimise risks and maximise protective factors*: We aim to both reduce risk factors where possible and enhance protective factors, resilience, and adaptive coping to help our clients manage challenges they face.
- *Involve others*: Risk cannot be managed alone. We share, discuss, and manage risk alongside our colleagues and supervisors, within teams, and with relevant agencies. This provides the best support for our clients, helps us to double-check our thinking, and to manage what can be anxiety-provoking work for us as therapists.
- *Document*: Keeping detailed records of risk assessments and safety plans ensures we adhere to professional practice standards, and helps us think through our clinical decision making in a systematic way, which is particularly important when we feel anxious. It also enables us to demonstrate our decision-making process in the event of a risk incident.

For more detailed discussions of core risk assessment principles, see Granello (2010).

FAQ: When is it too risky to use trauma-focused treatment?

There are some situations where trauma-focused treatment is inappropriate and risk must be prioritised in therapy, and relevant safeguarding procedures followed. Some risks can be mitigated, as we will discuss in the next section but we do not proceed with trauma-focused therapy where our assessment indicates a high risk, as defined by:

- A strong wish, specific plan, and/or intent to die or harm someone else
- A recent episode of serious self-harm (high-risk NSSI or suicide attempt), or violent behaviour causing injury
- Current high-risk reckless or self-destructive behaviour
- Current objective threat of serious harm from others.

Or unmanaged moderate risks, as defined by:

- Non-specific suicidal or violent thoughts in the context of a significant risk history, limited access to crisis support between sessions, and an absence of (or unwillingness to implement) a safety plan
- Historical or current self-harm, suicidal or violent behaviour, where there is no explicit agreement for transparency and disclosure of risk incidents
- Imminent objective future risk, such as a violent ex-partner who has made threats and is about to be released from prison, in the absence of an appropriate multi-agency risk management plan.

Risk to self

Many of our clients report common clinical indicators of risk to themselves, such as suicidal ideation, feeling a burden, and/or NSSI behaviour. We understand suicidality and self-harm as essentially an avoidance strategy intended to resolve or escape painful psychological states, and linked to deficits in problem-solving, emotion regulation, and cognitive reappraisal (Bryan, 2016). Approximately one third of people progress from thinking about to attempting suicide, and the transition is not strongly related to the severity of their ideation. Rather, unbearable pain (both physical and psychological) alongside hopelessness and lack of connectedness appears to most strongly motivate suicide. What then distinguishes those whose motivation turns into attempting suicide is the acquired capability to cause oneself lethal harm, both through having the knowledge and means to do so (e.g. acquiring helium or hoarding tablets); and through experiences of overcoming natural barriers of fear and pain, such as exposure to violence and death (common amongst combat veterans, refugees, emergency service workers), or previous experiences of self-harm, e.g. suicide attempts, NSSI, or restricted eating (Klonsky et al., 2018).

Bryan (2016) offers a practical framework for managing suicide risk in PTSD based on assessing severity (see FAQ box above). Where risk is high, we do not offer a trauma-focused approach and instead deliver suicide-focused treatments. This may comprise targeted modules or a full package of evidence-based treatment, most commonly DBT skills training (Linehan, 2014) or CBT for suicide prevention (Bryan, & Rudd, 2018). If high risk emerges during trauma-focused treatment, we similarly switch to suicide-focused treatment until the risk reduces.

We do deliver trauma-focused treatment where clients present with moderate risks, such as suicidal thoughts without clear plans or NSSI without serious injury or potential lethality. We enhance the safety of our treatment by collaboratively developing a safety plan that helps clients 'ride out' a crisis. The plan includes a list of our client's 'red flag' situations and personal warning signs (including PTSD triggers), problem and emotion-focused coping skills they can use to manage a crisis, and personal and professional sources of support. We keep safety on our agenda each session, regularly reviewing risk and whether/how the plan is working, and encourage our client to be open with us about changes in their risk signs, so we can work together to manage them.

As part of developing a safety plan, we formulate and prioritise the psychological mechanisms that trigger or worsen suicidal thoughts and NSSI. Here are some examples:

- *Re-experiencing symptoms*: Where flashbacks or nightmares are a trigger to suicidal thoughts or NSSI (e.g. feeling so distressed by a nightmare that they want to die), we first provide psychoeducation to foster hope that these symptoms can improve. We help clients increase their control over symptoms with intrusions diaries to understand triggers and grounding/self-soothing strategies, stimulus discrimination, and updating (including with imagery) to manage flashbacks and their aftermath.
- *Mental rehearsal and suicide 'flash-forwards'*: When feeling suicidal, people often 'daydream' about suicide. They may imagine preparing or going through with the act, or imagine themselves dead. These images contribute to suicidality both by fuelling distress and providing comfort, and may increase preoccupation, focus, and action. We encourage our clients to instead rehearse imagery of implementing their coping skills, or rescript the imagery to lessen its strength, for example, imagining having a loved one comfort them and help them throw their stockpiled pills away (Carey, & Wells, 2019).
- *Dissociation*: Where clients dissociate in response to triggers, we prioritise grounding strategies. Clients may be more vulnerable to self-harm when they are dissociated, and some use NSSI as a means of grounding themselves, so effective and safe alternatives are developed and practised.
- *Heightened emotions*: Suicidal ideation can happen when clients feel overwhelmed with strong emotions, and NSSI can also operate as a way of releasing strong feelings (see Chapter 18). We draw on DBT distress tolerance skills to help our clients discover ways of accepting, tolerating, and changing strong emotions (page 45). This includes helping clients recognise that strong emotions and suicidal thoughts usually pass if they 'sit' with them.
- *Guilt and shame*: Guilt and shame, driven by self-blame and self-attack alongside negative self-concept, have been linked to suicidal ideation and NSSI, and may mediate the relationship between PTSD and self-harm (Sheehy et al., 2019). We carefully assess for these emotions during a crisis, addressing the related appraisals and maintaining processes including rumination and withdrawal. Promoting compassionate self-soothing through self-statements and imagery can also be helpful (Chapter 13).
- *Hopelessness/defeat*: Hopelessness and defeat often motivate suicidal thinking and may be driven by appraisals characteristic of PTSD, e.g. 'my life is over' or 'I'm damaged goods'. These appraisals are addressed through psychoeducation, 'reclaiming your life' tasks, and cognitive restructuring. We help clients access alternative perspectives in a crisis with flashcards, photos of reclaiming activities, and videos or letters to themselves. Hopeless feelings can also arise when peri-traumatic hotspots related to mental defeat are triggered, so we work to update these hotspots as soon as possible.
- *Drugs and alcohol*: Using alcohol or drugs can significantly increase suicide risk and lower the threshold for acting on suicidal or NSSI thoughts. Poly-substance use, particularly mixing alcohol and cocaine, confers the highest risk (Conner et al., 2017). We target substance misuse early in treatment, working toward harm minimisation and ideally abstinence, and continually monitor use where it is implicated in risk incidents (Chapter 17).
- *Life events*: Risk may rapidly increase in response to life events, both predictable (e.g. trauma anniversaries) and unpredictable (e.g. sudden bereavements). Where possible, our safety plan

considers predictable future triggers, with contingencies for a range of eventualities (e.g. 'if *x* happens, I will do *y*'), as well as unexpected events (e.g. 'any time I feel bad, I can call *z*'). Interpersonal difficulties including arguments and relationship breakdowns are common triggers of sudden risk escalation. Teaching DBT interpersonal effectiveness skills may be helpful in these situations.

- *Social issues*: Social stressors including homelessness, financial problems, and struggling to meet basic needs may be important factors contributing to dysphoric mood and hopelessness, particularly where our client lacks the knowledge, skills, or support to find solutions. We address these issues through advocacy, problem-solving, and signposting (Chapter 22).

> Mieko developed PTSD after the death of her husband Kenji. She experienced suicidal thoughts which were strongest when she woke from a nightmare of Kenji's death and were related to feelings of guilt that she should have been able to prevent the pain he suffered before he died. Mieko's therapist decided to address her guilt beliefs before working on other aspects of Mieko's trauma memories. They also developed a plan for how Mieko could calm herself quickly when she woke from a nightmare. Most of Mieko's family lived in Japan and she felt too ashamed to tell them how much she was struggling or to ask for support. However, Mieko's sister was very supportive and was often awake when Mieko woke from a nightmare due to the time difference, so Mieko planned to call her if she felt upset.

Risk from others

People with PTSD have often been severely harmed by other people and are not always safe when they seek treatment. An abusive partner, spouse, associate, or family member may still be living with or near them, have contact with them or their family, or be harassing or stalking them. Certain jobs (e.g. police officers), associations (e.g. gang membership), adverse social contexts (e.g. homelessness), and activities (e.g. sex work) can also increase risks of experiencing harm.

RISK ASSESSMENT

Accurately assessing risk from others can be challenging. The sense of current threat characteristic of PTSD can skew our clients' judgements of safety. They may interpret ambiguous, or mildly threatening stimuli and situations, such as briefly seeing someone resembling their perpetrator, as highly dangerous. Other clients underestimate risks, having lived under severe threat for so long that it feels normal. Early life traumas may mean people have never learnt what it means to feel safe, or how to accurately assess risks from others. Equally, as therapists we may struggle to objectively appraise risks in situations outside of our direct experiences; we will have 'blind spots' leading us to over- or underestimate risks (Chapter 25). Lacking an objective means of evaluating risks could have significant consequences for how we approach threat-related treatment tasks with our clients, not least establishing what are reasonable safety precautions rather than excessive vigilance behaviours.

Assessing risk from others, therefore, needs a systematic approach. We gather detailed examples from our clients of both historic and recent risk events, when and in what contexts they occurred, and any protective or mitigating factors. Where possible, we also gather information from other sources (such as people in their social network, police, or social services), to help put their experiences and perceptions of threat in context. Structured risk assessment tools for intimate partner violence are very helpful in assessing the full range of types of domestic abuse, including psychological, emotional, financial, sexual, and physical abuse, some of which the client may not spontaneously report if they have normalised them within the relationship. A good example is the domestic abuse, stalking, and harassment (DASH) checklist (Richards, 2009), which we use as a comprehensive risk assessment tool, and for evaluating whether risks are severe enough to require a referral to a Multi-Agency Risk Assessment Conference (MARAC, see next section) for UK-based clients.

When assessing risk from others, we also need to check if perpetrators pose a risk to anyone else. For example, a perpetrator of childhood sexual abuse may no longer be a risk to our adult client but may be a risk to other children in their network. A violent ex-partner may be a risk to a new romantic partner, or children that they share with our client.

MANAGING RISK FROM OTHERS

Where we identify significant risks, we follow local and national safeguarding policies and involve other agencies including the police and social services. We discuss our concerns and intended actions transparently with our client and offer information about the processes. In the UK this may include referral to a MARAC for adults, and the local Multi-Agency Safeguarding Hub (MASH) if there are concerns about children. Wherever possible, we prioritise our clients' autonomy and self-determination by supporting them to involve others, especially where they have previously had negative experiences with services.

Where there are no immediate risks, but concerns or future risks, we create a safety plan. This includes detailing what the risks are, in what contexts, ways to minimise or manage them, and 'trigger points' for escalating or reviewing the safety plan.

> Bilal had previously been assaulted by his son Jas, who had a drug addiction and sometimes came to Bilal for money. At the time of the assessment, Bilal hadn't seen Jas for several months, but he had received text messages asking for money. Bilal felt very conflicted about how to help Jas; he didn't want to turn his back on him but was also frightened that Jas could become violent when he was desperate for drugs. Bilal and his therapist came up with a safety plan to minimise risks, including not letting Jas into the flat if he turned up, and contacting the police if he became threatening or mentioned carrying a weapon. They also researched resources for family members of those with addictions about how to best support Jas and identified supportive people in Bilal's network who could help. Bilal decided to respond to Jas's messages only to give him information about where to seek help.

Planning for treatment may also include finding a 'window' where the client is less likely to be exposed to risk; for example, for someone in a high-risk occupation, this might be while they are on sick leave or reduced duties. Sometimes clients in high-risk jobs are uncertain about whether they wish to continue in an occupation which likely exposes them to further trauma. We often encourage clients to delay their decision until they have completed treatment and consider any adjustments that might help them to return to their role.

> Kirsty developed PTSD after attending a serious fire in a high-rise building. She was on sick leave from her job as a firefighter but told her therapist she was planning to resign. Kirsty feared her PTSD would interfere with her ability to do her job; that she might freeze up or have a flashback and put her crew at risk. With the support of her manager and union, Kirsty agreed to wait until completing PTSD treatment to consider her career options. Her therapist also helped her negotiate a phased return to work, with reduced duties until she felt able to consider returning to her full role and to explicitly use this to test out her fears by gradually increasing her involvement in fire-fighting incidents.

RISK OF RE-VICTIMISATION

As well as immediate risks, there are also more chronic risks of re-victimisation associated with PTSD (Orcutt et al., 2002). Certain coping strategies can place people with PTSD at risk of re-victimisation, such as substance use and risky sexual behaviour. Chronic exposure to threat also interferes with people's ability to recognise risky situations, and PTSD symptoms such as dissociation may prevent them from responding effectively. Those with histories of interpersonal trauma may struggle to know how or when to assertively lay boundaries in relationships, and guilt and shame can lead people to believe they deserve mistreatment. As well as individual factors, external variables are also important, such as the behaviour of perpetrators (who may specifically target vulnerable people), and social factors which place people at risk (Messman-Moore, & Long, 2003).

Addressing these issues with our clients involves assessing variables that may place them at risk of future harm, then working to reduce them and build resilience. For example, when people have experienced abuse in multiple relationships, we look together at patterns in those relationships or situations, to identify any factors which might place them at risk in the future (Chapter 18). We discuss how to identify signs of potential perpetrators, place boundaries assertively on unwanted demands, and respond effectively to mistreatment or controlling behaviour. For example, Kubany and Ralston (2008) list 20 'red flags' for identifying potential abusers in relationships such as possessiveness, jealousy, disliking your friends and family, lying, secrecy, and belittling your opinions. For clients who have repeatedly been re-victimised in relationships, discussing these warning signs can be empowering. However, we are explicit that it is not the client's fault that they might struggle to recognise warning signs or respond effectively. Instead, we normalise how hard it is to spot these signs without knowing what to look for, especially as perpetrators attempt to actively charm, deceive, and conceal their controlling behaviours at the start of relationships.

Hot cognitions

- The future is hopeless, my life is ruined
- I/others would be better off if I was dead, rather than being like this
- Cutting myself is the only way to relieve my pain/feel anything
- I deserve to be mistreated
- I attract people who will hurt me
- If you show any weakness people take advantage

RISK TO OTHERS

Some of our clients have histories of violence or other perpetration and may remain a risk to others. PTSD is associated with an increased risk of violence, but this link disappears when controlling for other risk factors also elevated in people with PTSD, particularly alcohol misuse and anger severity (Blakey et al., 2018). Additionally, people who have lived in circumstances where violence is commonplace or glamorised are more likely to perpetrate violence, and PTSD may increase this risk (Nandi et al., 2015). Hence, when assessing a client's risk of violence in the context of PTSD, we also investigate known risk factors including sleep problems, pain, financial instability, homelessness, combat experience, alcohol use, anger, and forensic history; and protective factors including social support, spirituality, work, and ability to meet basic needs (Elbogen et al., 2010).

Where there is an immediate or serious threat to others, for example, a concrete plan and access to the victim, or physical punishment of children, our priority is safeguarding and we share our concerns with relevant agencies, disclosing information against our client's wishes if necessary. Where the threat is less severe, we collaboratively develop a safety plan, continuously review risk, adapt the delivery of therapy to prioritise working on anger and aggression, and incorporate skills-based anger management interventions into treatment (e.g. Chemtob et al., 1997). Successful treatment for PTSD should reduce anger if the two are related, so we also progress trauma-focused treatment either sequentially or concurrently.

To help guide our interventions, we review recent incidents of aggression in detail to establish the chain of antecedents, responses, and other psychological mechanisms. We offer psychoeducation on anger and PTSD, for example, reframing it as an understandable survival mechanism given their experiences. We also emphasise that while PTSD may partly explain aggression and that it may be triggered by other people's behaviour, our clients remain entirely responsible for controlling it and accountable for the consequences of aggression.

Here are some common mechanisms and how we address them:

- *Anger in response to memory triggers*: Some of our clients respond aggressively in situations reminiscent of their traumatic experiences. For example, someone who was held captive may feel trapped in a crowded space and 'fight' their way out. Re-experiencing symptoms make everyday situations feel like 'life or death', triggering a fight/flight response. We help clients predict and prepare for these triggers and reassess the objective threat of the situation by using stimulus discrimination. We combine this with teaching skills for managing physiological arousal and practising assertive verbal communication.
- *Aggression to change feelings*: For some of our clients, aggression has a rewarding effect. It may cut through feelings of numbness, help them feel powerful rather than humiliated or helpless, and provide a release from frustration and pain. If so, we identify the need that aggression fulfils through functional analysis, help the client weigh up the costs and benefits of this behaviour, and find alternative, less 'costly', ways of meeting their needs (Chapter 18).
- *Revenge fixation*: Some of our clients feel (often accurately) that they have been wronged, and develop a fixation with revenge. Peri-traumatic memory hotspots of powerlessness, humiliation, and rage may fuel subsequent brooding on revenge when memories are triggered, so both processes may be targeted early in treatment. The wish for revenge may be fuelled by violent mental imagery, with an underlying function of seeking justice and/or communicating to the perpetrator the harm they have caused them. Exploring the function, costs, and benefits of seeking revenge, and possible alternatives (including using imagery interventions to meet the need for justice) can be useful, particularly where there are beliefs such as 'I won't get over this until I get my own back'.
- *Hostile attribution bias*: Biases in reading social cues have been associated with PTSD. For example, people who feel shame may be more likely to interpret other people's behaviour as rejecting (Sippel, & Marshall, 2011). Veterans with PTSD who perceive 'hidden hostile intent' in others are more likely to respond with aggression (van Voorhees et al., 2016). In the context of a supportive therapeutic relationship, we can help normalise and understand this pattern, recognise when it is triggered, and look for ways to test appraisals.
- *Aggression as learnt behaviour*: Some of our clients have been exposed to, repeatedly perpetrated, and become skilled in aggressive behaviour and instrumental violence. Often aggression is effective in meeting short-term needs and resolving disputes, albeit with high longer-term costs. Aggression may be part of a valued identity within a cultural group, where there are strong beliefs about honour or respect that frame aggression as an acceptable response to slights. It may also relate to a learnt strategy in certain groups, such as learning to dehumanise the enemy in the military (Grossman, 1996). Here, we need to bring greater awareness to

these processes. We explore our client's relationship to aggression as a 'way of life', and help them consider if and when to give it up. It can be useful to also work on developing skills to cope differently with conflict, such as problem-solving, assertiveness, and communication, and focus on developing other valued aspects of their identity.

Theo had been shot by members of a gang in revenge for a crime that a friend had committed. Theo's friend was in prison and, along with other members of his community, urged Theo to take revenge for the shooting. Theo felt that he would lose face amongst his friends and family if he didn't act and often fantasised about violent revenge. Theo's therapist helped him to consider the pros and cons of taking revenge. Theo had previously spent time in a young offenders institution and did not want to go to prison, particularly as he had a young child. He was also aware that acting would continue the pattern of revenge attacks that could lead to further deaths. These reasons were compelling and Theo's therapist asked him to make a note of them on his phone, along with a picture of his baby daughter. Theo's therapist helped him think through how to talk to others in his community about his reasons for not acting, and to identify people who would support his decision. They discussed different ways of thinking about respect and strength. The urge for revenge also seemed linked to re-experiencing symptoms as Theo had felt helpless during the attack, so they agreed to update these hotspots with new meanings.

Notes from the therapy room: Joao

Joao was born in the UK but, after his parents divorced when he was five, he moved to Brazil with his mother. In his twenties, Joao was imprisoned for helping an armed gang rob the bank where he worked. Conditions in prison were terrible and violence was commonplace. Joao was beaten up multiple times and on one occasion raped by another prisoner.

After his release, Joao was deported to the UK, where he had no friends and only distant relatives. He was experiencing nightmares and flashbacks of the assaults in prison and was referred for PTSD treatment. At assessment, he reported feeling suicidal, and his therapist also had concerns about his risk to others, as he was having frequent confrontations with residents of the hostel where he lived.

Joao's therapist reviewed recent risk episodes. Joao reported feeling hopeless about the future and frustrated with his current circumstances. He had attempted suicide twice in prison but not in the year since his release, although he reported frequent ideation and struggled to identify any protective factors, other than not wanting to cause his mother further pain. Triggers to his suicidal thoughts included flashbacks of the rape, which made Joao feel deeply ashamed.

Regarding risk to others, Joao reported conflicts with others in the hostel, especially when they were noisy or tried to approach him. Joao explained that he had learnt in prison that you needed to be aggressive to prevent becoming a target, and he believed that others would attack him if they saw him as weak. Joao also reported a recent incident where two men speaking in Portuguese had triggered a flashback where he felt he was back in the prison and was 'ready to attack' the men. Joao's formulation is in Figure 23.1.

Joao's therapist normalised these experiences and provided psychoeducation about PTSD symptoms and how treatment would work. They agreed to do a risk check every session and made a personalised assessment tool. They also worked on a safety plan including ways to cope if Joao experienced suicidal or violent thoughts. He agreed to save a photo of his mother on his

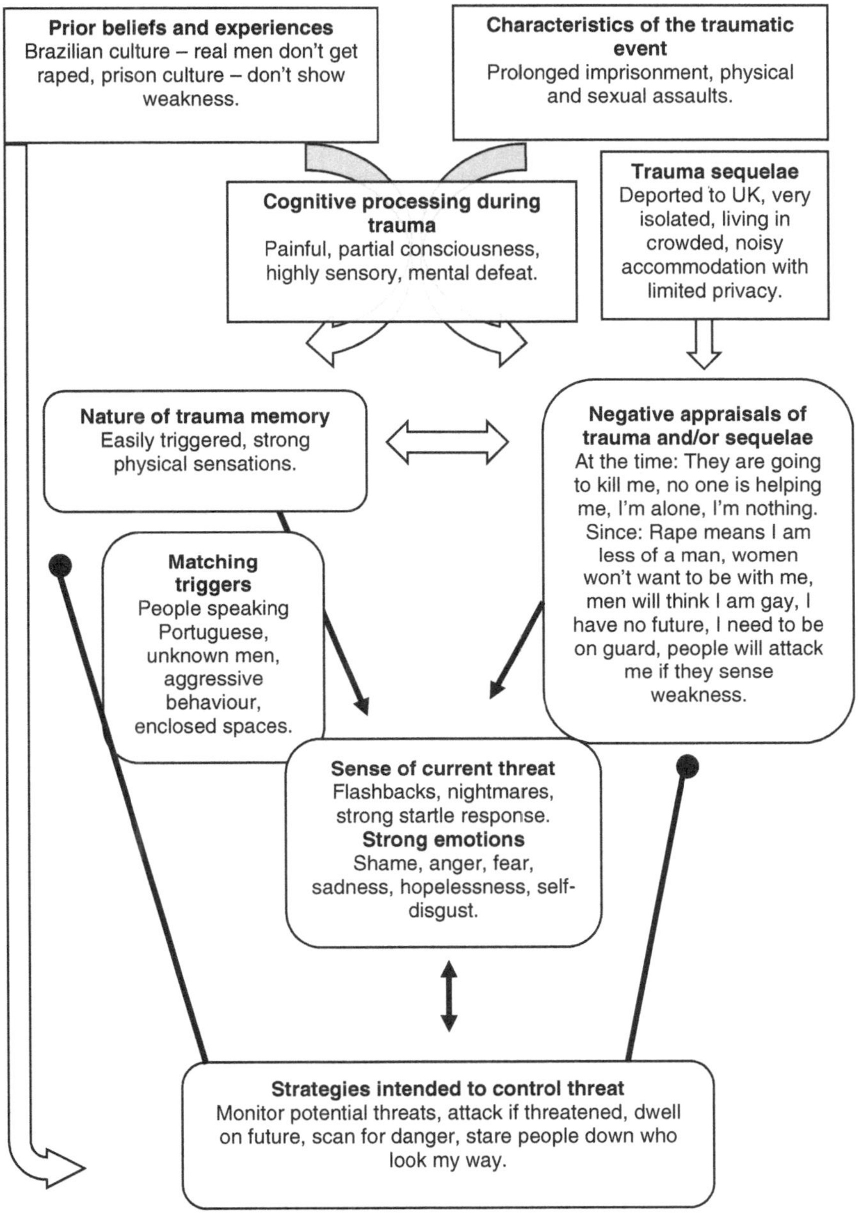

Figure 23.1 Joao's formulation

phone lock screen as a reminder of his reason for living. They worked on treatment goals to give Joao a sense of hope and agreed to keep monitoring and adding to these.

Joao and his therapist agreed to prioritise the triggers to suicidal and violent thoughts. Joao kept an intrusions diary to identify his main triggers, and they practised stimulus discrimination and grounding in session. They addressed Joao's belief that people would attack him; Joao acknowledged that no one in the UK knew him or had reason to harm him. Joao tended to scan for danger when he was out of his room and would 'stare down' people who looked his way, which led to confrontations. They used behavioural experiments to test what would happen if Joao dropped this behaviour. Although he initially felt more vulnerable, Joao realised that people didn't approach or attack him.

Joao's living circumstances were a trigger for suicidal thoughts, and he tended to ruminate about the hopelessness of his situation and his future. He believed that no one would employ him because of his prison record. Joao had been helped by the charity 'Prisoners Abroad' to find housing when he arrived in the UK so contacted them again for advice on finding work. They enrolled him on a work preparation programme and gave him information about voluntary work to build his CV for future paid employment. Joao also began attending a church with a largely Brazilian congregation and a bible study group they ran. He felt safe in this setting and spent less time at the hostel.

Joao's feelings of shame triggered suicidal thoughts, so were addressed next in therapy. Joao explained that male rape was never discussed in Brazil and there was a huge stigma attached to it, although he knew it had been common in prison. He believed that having been raped made him 'less of a man' and that no women would want a relationship with him. His therapist helped him research different perspectives on male rape. Together they read some survivor stories on the 'Survivors UK' website, a charity dedicated to men who have experienced sexual assault. They also composed a survey on views about male rape, asking whether it made you 'less of a man' and whether people would have a relationship with someone they knew had been raped. Joao was surprised by the compassionate responses he received and it gave him more hope that he would not be rejected by others because of his experiences.

When Joao felt ready to talk about his experiences in prison, they made a timeline to identify key memories. Joao continued to monitor risky thoughts or behaviours with his therapist, and they agreed to pause memory work if needed.

Recommended reading

Messman-Moore, T. L., & Long, P. J. (2003). The role of childhood sexual abuse sequelae in the sexual revictimization of women: An empirical review and theoretical reformulation. *Clinical Psychology Review*, 23(4), 537–571.

Taft, C. T., Creech, S. K., & Murphy, C. M. (2017). Anger and aggression in PTSD. *Current Opinion in Psychology*, 14, 67–71.

Zortea, T. C., Cleare, S., Melson, A. J., Wetherall, K., & O'Connor, R. C. (2020). Understanding and managing suicide risk. *British Medical Bulletin*, 134, 73–84.

PART SIX
Complexities for the therapist

CHAPTER TWENTY FOUR

The therapeutic relationship

Danny experienced an accident that ended his career as a paramedic. In therapy, he spoke repeatedly about his anger at his employers and seemed irritated by the therapist's attempts to structure sessions. His therapist formulated their interactions to better understand this obstacle in their therapeutic relationship and how to address it with Danny.

Establishing a strong therapeutic relationship has long been considered the foundation for delivering effective psychological therapy. The working alliance, the most studied aspect of the therapeutic relationship, is usually thought to comprise the emotional bond that forms between the client and therapist, alongside the tasks and goals of therapy (Bordin, 1979). It may be especially important in PTSD treatment, where our clients are disclosing intensely personal, painful, and humiliating experiences. They may have also suffered interpersonal trauma, betrayal, rejection, or lack of support from trusted others, which naturally impedes the development of a trusting therapeutic alliance (Keller et al., 2010). Research has generally supported a link between alliance and therapy outcome in PTSD, with clients who rate the working relationship more positively tending to do better in treatment (Ellis et al., 2018).

One of the biggest differences between CBT and psychodynamic therapies is the role of the therapeutic relationship, considered 'necessary but not sufficient' to effect change in CBT (Beck, 1979), but the central vehicle of change in psychoanalysis and related therapies. This distinction may not be so clear-cut; in CT-PTSD, the therapeutic relationship can be a tool, for example, to model how other people can be trusted, that hearing about terrible experiences can be tolerated, and expressions of strong emotions are acceptable. Furthermore, when a client's interpersonal style affects the therapeutic alliance, it becomes an important focus of treatment, both to keep therapy on track and to tackle the negative impact on other areas of the client's life (Moorey, & Lavender, 2018).

What therapists as individuals bring to the therapeutic relationship is important too; how our unique experiences, personalities, differences, and communication styles interact with those of each client. Some aspects of PTSD treatment can be particularly challenging for therapists. Particular clients, or certain types of trauma, may strike a personal chord with us (Chapter 26). We may find ourselves feeling as if we are the only ones who can really understand a client's experience, or that we need to 'save' them; or the opposite, feeling disconnected, annoyed, or even mistreated by them. These experiences are normal. Nonetheless, 'counter-transference' should not be ignored; we need to be mindful of our reactions, and reflect on them rather than be pushed and pulled by them.

In this chapter, we first consider the qualities that underpin a strong therapeutic relationship, before discussing potential difficulties. Resolving impasses is an important aspect of treatment; when unresolved they can lead to worse outcomes and dropout (McLaughlin et al., 2014). A significant minority of clients do not complete, or do not benefit from, PTSD treatment (Schottenbauer et al., 2008). As therapists, we need to be alert for ruptures in the alliance and indicators that our clients are disengaging. These issues are relevant more broadly, but we focus here on those commonly encountered when treating PTSD.

DOI: 10.4324/9781003288329-30

Basic principles

SOLID FOUNDATIONS

A client's engagement in early treatment sessions is predictive of outcome (Brady et al., 2015), so we build the foundations of a strong alliance from the first therapeutic encounter.

Some clients will be wary of the therapist and the demands of therapy, and may easily interpret ambiguous interpersonal cues (such as silence) as threatening or judgemental. In our early interactions, we express warmth and empathy clearly in our words, tone, and body language. This is especially important when working remotely or through an interpreter, as subtle cues may be 'lost in translation'. We give lots of positive feedback, and praise the client's courage for attending and contributing to the session, while acknowledging how intimidating and challenging this may have been.

Making early gains is also predictive of successful outcomes. We want every client to leave their first session feeling they have gained something useful. To achieve this, we use 'easy win' interventions such as teaching grounding skills or doing a behavioural experiment with a high chance of a useful or engaging outcome. We also agree small but meaningful 'reclaiming your life' tasks from the first session, choosing enjoyable tasks over those that require approaching trauma reminders. We try to be practically useful to our clients too; providing information, answering questions, directing them to resources, offering to write letters, or speaking to relevant people in their network. Going the extra mile for our clients is a good way of demonstrating our commitment to their recovery and helps build trust.

SAFETY

We discuss and model safety from the start of treatment. This starts with discussing our client's needs in the physical environment, such as where they want to sit, if they need water, or the door left open, and offering to change aspects of the space to suit them. Safety is also important within the therapeutic relationship, for example, thoroughly discussing confidentiality and its limits, giving information about treatment, the service, and ourselves. Where possible, we give clients choices around their therapist, for example, if they prefer to see a man or woman, and around their interpreter if present. At every stage, we want to maximise our client's sense of control and predictability over the therapeutic process, as a distinct contrast to experiences of helplessness during trauma.

This is especially important when it comes to discussing trauma memories. We offer a rationale for the importance of talking about memories and take time to address specific concerns. We explicitly give our client full control over what they say and when, including the choice to stop at any time. For those who have experienced sexual assault and abuse, we agree which words to use to describe acts of sexual violence and parts of the body; equally, we ask about words not to use, for example, that may relate to PTSD triggers or were spoken by the perpetrator.

Clients sometimes worry about how we might react to hearing about their traumatic experiences (see also page 53–6). We always acknowledge that we are human beings, not 'therapy robots', and we may feel shocked or upset by things we hear; that it is normal and healthy, and that we can cope with whatever they wish to share with us. It can also help to offer information about our experience and training in working with PTSD, as well as the networks of support and supervision in our team. We sometimes use the metaphor of therapy being 'like a laboratory', where we have all the necessary personal protective equipment for handling toxic memories safely together.

Safety is a shared task within therapy. When our client has a risk history, we explain that, to be effective therapists, we need to feel safe too, so we can 'think straight', and that feeling safe for us comes from knowing, evaluating, and planning for any risks as well as agreeing a policy of openness and transparency about risk issues.

ACTIVE COLLABORATION

Collaboration is central to the therapeutic relationship and, from the outset, we emphasise and model working as equal and active partners. We sketch formulations jointly, carry out behavioural experiments together, and share between-session or information-gathering tasks. We demonstrate our confidence and expertise in treating PTSD, but are curious and defer to our patient's expertise on their experiences, positioning therapy as a shared learning endeavour.

Clients who have expectations of more directive, or less active, therapy may find collaboration initially alien and even uncomfortable, and may repeat 'I don't know' or 'you tell me!' when we try to engage them collaboratively. At these times, we are careful not to put them on the spot or 'think for them'. Using closed rather than open questions and drawing on a client's past achievements, areas of specialist knowledge, and skills are good ways of encouraging their active involvement. We may be more didactic in earlier sessions and gradually shift the balance of collaboration during therapy as our client becomes more confident and knowledgeable about the process of treatment.

AUTHENTICITY AND TRANSPARENCY

Our clients need to trust us with very personal information, and will understandably be reluctant to do so if we come across as false or disingenuous. Clients who have been harmed interpersonally may be particularly good at picking up these signs. We try to be transparent about everything we do in treatment, even if it necessitates awkward conversations. Part of being genuine is also showing that we are human. Without taking the focus from the client, or breaching professional boundaries, we try to let our personality come across and express genuine emotions. We accept when we get things wrong, apologise, and offer redress. We reflect on our mistakes or assumptions, admit when we don't have all the answers, and commit to learning alongside our clients.

We also promote transparency through the getting and giving of feedback. We may ask 'how will you let me know if something feels too uncomfortable to discuss?', 'what can I do more, or less of, next time to be a better therapist in working with you?' and 'what can we do in our sessions to make sure we stay on the right track?'.

Resolving impasses

Resolving impasses and ruptures in the therapeutic relationship is essential to keeping treatment on track. Read the 'top tips' box for ways to move forward when you are feeling stuck, and below we consider some common impasses in more detail.

Top tips: What to do when you are feeling stuck

We all feel stuck at times, when it feels like therapy is not progressing, or we and our client seem to be on different pages. Whole books have been written about client 'resistance' but blaming lack of progress on the client, or indeed ourselves, is generally counter-productive. Instead, try to understand what is going on and how to get back on track.

- *Go public with your data*: In concrete terms, offer your observations of the behaviours that are hindering progress, ask if your client has also noticed and what they make of it. Be curious, not critical.

- *Validate and formulate*: If you feel like you are pulling in different directions, stop and explore what is happening. Use validating statements and draw these into mini-formulations, e.g. 'It sounds as if the homework task we agreed felt too much for you. It makes sense that if you believed you'd get overwhelmed, you would naturally want to avoid it.'
- *Accept responsibility*: When you have identified a sticking point in therapy, ask yourself and your client 'what am I doing that contributes to this?'. Check you are delivering the best treatment you can.
- *Get back on the same page*: If therapy feels like a tug-of-war, try to reset the balance of responsibility for change. Review treatment goals and formulations together, and ensure you are really listening to the obstacles the client faces.
- *Stay empathic*: If you feel frustrated with apparently 'resistant' or therapy-interfering behaviours, formulate the beliefs and schemas which drive them. Often the client is trying to protect themselves or is responding in a way that has been adaptive in the past.
- *Be firm and flexible*: Rigidly pushing ahead is unhelpful if your client is struggling. Don't abandon the model, but be flexible and creative. If your client understands and accepts the rationale for an intervention, you can better work out how to achieve it together. However, if they want to adapt or exclude important elements of treatment, be clear about the limits of flexing the treatment while remaining effective. Remind them that having CT-PTSD treatment is their choice, and may not suit everyone.

AVOIDANCE

Chapter 19 focuses primarily on the client's avoidance but, as therapists, we may also avoid difficult parts of treatment, such as discussing the most distressing or embarrassing details of traumas, specific therapeutic tasks where we lack confidence, awkward conversations, or unsatisfactory endings. We try to spot and acknowledge our natural inclinations towards avoidance, discuss them in supervision, and test out our beliefs.

Anya, a CBT therapist, was working with her client Meg, who had been sexually assaulted. Anya and Meg spent the first six sessions of treatment focusing on psychoeducation and stabilisation to help Meg cope with her constant feelings of anxiety alongside intrusive memories. When Anya's supervisor suggested moving on to trauma-focused work, Anya realised she felt anxious about the prospect and had been avoiding asking Meg for details of the trauma. Anya's supervisor normalised this understandable reaction and encouraged Anya to reflect on her appraisals about working with Meg's trauma memories. Anya expressed anxiety about 're-traumatising' Meg, who seemed fragile, and also about hearing details of a violent sexual assault. Anya's therapist helped her think through the pros and cons of memory work with Meg and explored the concept of 're-traumatisation'. Anya realised that Meg was already traumatised and the therapy had a greater potential to help her than to harm her. She agreed to a behavioural experiment where she discussed the rationale behind memory work with Meg and sought a brief account of the trauma, to test how Meg responded, and better understand her own experience of hearing about a difficult trauma.

DIFFICULTIES WITH TRUST

Naturally, clients with a history of abuse or mistreatment may find it difficult to trust a new person, especially where feelings of shame, guilt, and/or humiliation are involved. We need to validate and normalise this experience and take time to nurture trust in the therapeutic relationship by being open, consistent, and sensitive to concerns.

As with other possible impasses, we find it helpful to discuss the process of establishing trust and frame it as a shared task of therapy. For example, we ask our clients 'what can we do in therapy to build the trust between us?' and take ratings on a percentage scale of trust in the relationship. This allows us to monitor it, identify factors that influence levels of trust as we proceed through treatment, and include them in our formulation.

Jay was a Royal Marine who developed PTSD after a series of combat traumas. In his first therapy session, he said 'I don't trust anyone'. He appeared uncomfortable in the session and avoided eye contact. His therapist was concerned he may drop out, so decided to raise the concern.

THERAPIST: Can I ask – how did it feel, coming here today?
JAY: It's been okay.
T: Did you have any worries about it beforehand?
J: Not worried, but I didn't know what to expect.
T: Well that's understandable because you said you haven't done anything like this before?
J: No.
T: Is there anything I can do to help it feel easier? Is there any more you want to know about the treatment or the work that we do here?
J: No, it's fine.
T: I wanted to check something in particular. You said earlier that it is difficult for you to trust people, and I appreciate that coming here and talking to me is probably quite a big step and that it might be quite hard to trust me too.
J: I don't really trust anybody.
T: No, and based on everything you have told me that has happened in your life, I can absolutely understand why. You've been let down and badly treated many times.
J: Yeah, I don't feel sorry for myself though. But I've learnt to just not expect anything from anyone. I just rely on myself.
T: That's really interesting. Shall I write that on the board, where we've been drawing up these cycles? It makes total sense that, given everything that's happened, you've learnt not to expect anything from other people, and just rely on yourself.
J: Yeah, okay.
T: I'm so impressed and pleased that you came here today. It can't have been easy to come and meet a total stranger who is asking lots of nosy questions about your life.
J: Well, you've got to know stuff to help me.
T: Yes, that's true. But I want you to be in control of the process. You can tell me as much as you want, but if I ask you something that you don't want to talk about just yet, you can tell me to leave it alone, okay? I give you permission [smiling].
J: There's some stuff … I can't say everything that's happened.
T: That's fine. You've been through a lot, and I imagine some of the memories are really difficult to think about, let alone talk about. Are there things that you haven't told anyone?
J: Ummm … yeah.
T: Okay, well we can leave them until you feel ready. It's really common that people who come here have had some awful experiences, and may have seen or done things that make them feel bad about themselves.
J: Does that get better?
T: It can do, yeah. I can't make promises and I don't have a magic wand. But PTSD is something that we can treat and people often feel a lot better after treatment. You won't forget what happened, and we can't change the past, but the symptoms you've told me about, the flashbacks and nightmares and all that, they can absolutely improve.

J: I want to just take my brain and wipe it clean.
T: Yes, I can imagine. You just want all those bad memories to go away?
J: Yeah.
T: Well, if you're willing to work with me, we can do our best to at least make them less powerful and less upsetting. And, just so you know, I don't expect you to completely trust me right away. It's something we can work on, and hopefully it might get stronger over time.
J: You're not so bad. It's not you, I just don't trust anyone.
T: Yes, that's understandable. Is there anything I can do in therapy, or we can do together, that will make it easier to build a bit more trust?

ANGER

Irritability is a common symptom of PTSD, and many clients feel understandably angry and bitter about their traumatic experiences and the devastating impact on their lives. Anger has been associated with worse outcomes in PTSD treatment (Forbes et al., 2008) and can impact the therapeutic relationship, especially when the client becomes angry with the therapist. Where anger is prominent, we prioritise it in treatment and move quickly to resolve any impasses in the therapeutic relationship.

Working with anger and hostility can be challenging, especially when it is directed at us. We acknowledge our emotional reactions and try to share them with our clients. Dalenberg (2004) interviewed clients about their therapists' responses to anger and found their least favoured reaction was the 'blank screen', i.e. showing no response to expressions of anger. The most favoured reaction was 'openly showed sadness or discomfort and discussing it'. The same study showed that clients highly value a genuine apology from their therapist for any errors; if we make a mistake or let our client down in some way, we apologise, validate the hurt caused, and offer redress where we can.

We can also address anger in sessions by working on a shared understanding of how and why it arises. Clients who are frequently aggressive often have experiences of needing to use anger to protect themselves or communicate their needs. Formulating this can help the client better understand their triggers to anger and also helps us to validate, not withdraw, in the face of their angry outbursts.

Saira had significant difficulties with anger, which was one of her reasons for seeking therapy for PTSD related to childhood abuse. In an early session, Saira became angry with her therapist, who had misunderstood something she said. Her therapist responded with genuine remorse for the misunderstanding and expressed his desire to understand their interaction better so that they could work together on Saira's therapy goal to reduce her anger responses. Saira explained that she felt dismissed and unimportant when she wasn't properly listened to, and her therapist validated how upsetting this felt. Saira was able to draw links between this feeling and her experience of not being cared for properly as a child. They added this to their formulation and agreed to address it as a priority in treatment. Saira's therapist also asked how they could make therapy a supportive, safe environment for her, and how they could best manage if Saira felt angry or dismissed by her therapist again.

Hot cognitions

- My therapist will think I'm crazy/disgusting if they know what happened
- My therapist can't cope with hearing what I've been through
- No one can truly understand me – there's no point trying
- I can't trust my therapist to keep this private

HOPELESSNESS

Many of our clients feel entirely hopeless about the potential for recovery, especially those who have had a lifetime of trauma, very chronic PTSD, or multiple unsuccessful treatment attempts. The experience of PTSD contributes to hopelessness; unpredictable nightmares and flashbacks give the feeling of being stuck in time. Rather than make plans, many people focus on just getting through each day. Hope is crucial because positive expectancy about treatment is a known predictor of outcome (Westra et al., 2007). It may be particularly important in PTSD treatment, as hope is associated with approach, rather than avoidant, coping (Glass et al., 2009).

We promote hope in the early phases of treatment by explaining how PTSD is a normal and understandable reaction, how effective treatment can be, and through planning achievable goals and milestones. We also share (with their consent) video and written testimonies from former clients talking about their experience of PTSD and treatment. Often, they describe their own hopelessness before starting treatment, as well as both the benefits and challenges of therapy. We find new clients value these accounts as they carry credibility and help them realise they are not alone in their experiences or problems.

We never oversell the potential benefits of treatment. Equally, where clients have had PTSD for many years, we are honest with them that they are very unlikely to recover without treatment. Clients who rate their chances of recovery from PTSD as very low may still be prepared to give therapy a try, so we frame it a 'no lose' experiment: if their symptoms improve even a little, then they have benefitted and, if not, at least they have tried.

Lastly, we are mindful that a client's hopelessness can be contagious for the therapist. We maintain a stance of 'relentless optimism' while remembering that not all clients make rapid progress or total recoveries and that it is possible to still live a good life with some PTSD symptoms. Above all, we persevere with treatment when we see small signs of progress, approach every setback as an opportunity, and overcome obstacles by applying 'rigorous creativity'.

FAQ: How do I cope when my client won't stop talking?

Some clients can be difficult to interrupt or keep on track during sessions. Perseverative thinking (repeatedly returning to the same issues, rumination without productive outcomes etc.) has been shown to predict worse outcomes in CT-PTSD (Brady et al., 2015), so we need to intervene when it occurs. Therapists often feel rude or awkward when interrupting and we need to find a way to do so sensitively so our client doesn't feel silenced.

We find this easiest by raising the topic and framing it as a shared issue to manage. For example, we say 'I've noticed that sometimes time gets away with us in the session, and we don't always get around to all the topics on our agenda. Have you noticed that?' or 'I've got a dilemma, because I really want to hear what you have to say, but I also know that we agreed to work on your next trauma hotspot'. We then seek agreement about how best to interrupt or manage time in the session by asking 'what do you think would be the best way of us keeping on track?' and 'I don't want to be rude and interrupt you when you are talking, and I don't want you to feel as if what you are saying isn't important or relevant, because it is. How should I best indicate if I need to ask you something or move the topic on?'.

Various issues can underlie perseveration. Some clients understand psychological therapy as simply a space for them to talk and be listened to, so psychoeducation about the active nature of CBT is helpful. Often perseveration reflects a client's internal rumination, so we label this and design interventions to target it. Lastly, perseveration may indicate an underlying cognitive impairment, such as traumatic brain injury or dementia. Treatment can be adapted for those with cognitive impairments, depending on their nature (page 244).

CLIENTS WHO ELICIT STRONG REACTIONS IN US

Some clients invoke strong reactions in us as therapists; we may feel anxious or notice we are dreading their session, we may feel emotionally involved with their story, or personally invested in their recovery. Some traumas may really get 'under our skin', while others may feel harder to relate to. These feelings are normal and, rather than suppress them, we notice and label, discuss in supervision, and formulate them.

A helpful tool is Stirling Moorey's (2013) 'cognitive interpersonal cycle' worksheet. This translates the traditionally psychotherapeutic concept of transference and countertransference into CBT terms (Moorey, 2014), by formulating how the thoughts and behaviours of the client and therapist can interact. It can be used in supervision, by the therapist alone, or alongside the client.

Anya realised she was dreading her sessions with her client Meg. Anya had raised the possibility of working with Meg's trauma memories, and Meg got upset at the prospect. For several weeks, Meg had brought day-to-day difficulties to the sessions and every week they had focused on these instead of the trauma memories. Anya's supervisor encouraged her to use the 'cognitive interpersonal cycle' worksheet to formulate what was happening (Figure 24.1).

Anya decided to talk to Meg about what was happening in therapy, to get a better understanding of her thoughts about working on the trauma memories. This revealed they were both avoiding conversations where Meg might become upset, thinking the other believed they weren't ready, although they agreed it was a necessary part of working on Meg's PTSD. They decided it was time to move forward with treatment and planned for how Meg could tell Anya if it felt too distressing. With these agreements in place, Meg felt safer to start writing a narrative of her trauma.

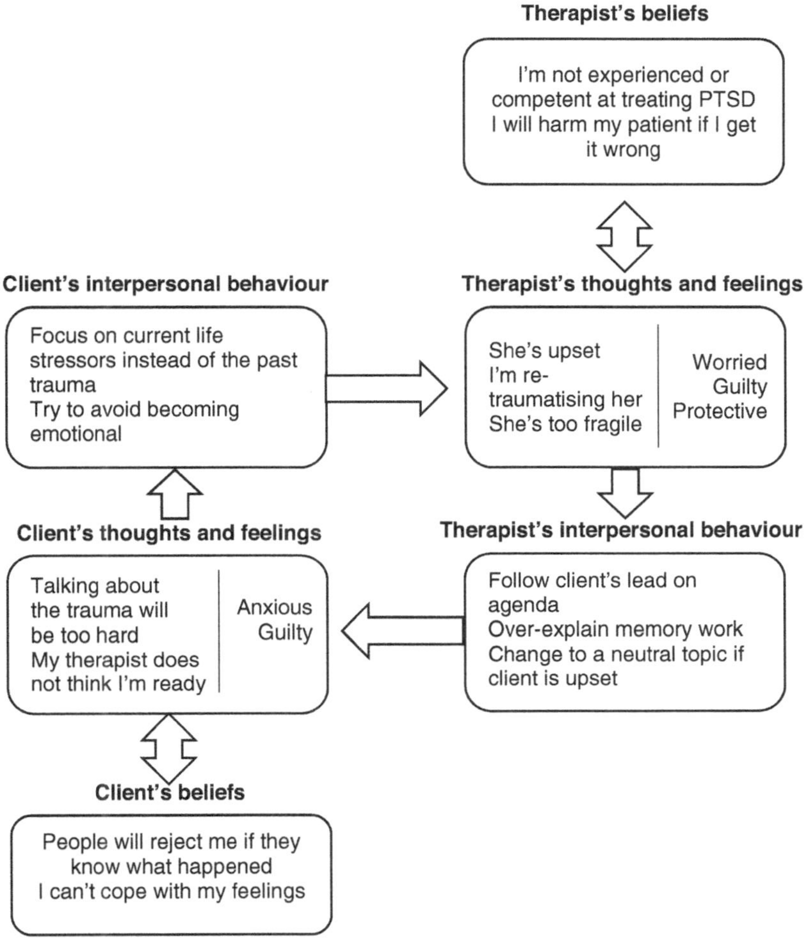

Figure 24.1 Anya and Meg's cognitive interpersonal cycle (based on Moorey (2007), reproduced with permission, available at www.cognitiveconnections.co.uk)

Notes from the therapy room: Danny

Danny began PTSD treatment after retiring from the ambulance service, having worked for over 20 years as a paramedic. He had taken retirement after a back injury caused by an accident while he was driving an ambulance. Danny was angry about the way his career had ended, feeling he had been badly mistreated by his employers, who he had unsuccessfully taken to an employment tribunal.

In his first session, Danny was openly sceptical about whether treatment could help. He had previously had a course of counselling arranged by his work which he hadn't found helpful. He spoke at length about his back pain and his anger at his employers. Danny found it difficult to identify any concrete goals for treatment. His therapist asked him to complete an intrusions diary before the next session, but he returned the next week without it, saying he'd forgotten it at home. When his therapist tried to set an agenda for the session, Danny seemed irritated, saying he didn't have anything to discuss. He then began speaking again about how his employers had betrayed him and how no one understood what it was like to be in constant pain.

Danny's therapist decided not to pursue the other agenda items and instead initiated a conversation about his thoughts and feelings about treatment. Danny said he had been reluctant to have treatment and didn't think it would work for him, and his therapist validated this concern and praised his courage and determination for attending two sessions even though he wasn't hopeful of any success.

His therapist gently observed that Danny appeared frustrated when they were setting the agenda. Danny agreed, saying he had never liked workplace meetings as they made him feel under pressure and reminded him of 'performance reviews'. His therapist apologised and agreed that she often found business meetings stressful too. She explained that, in therapy, there was no expectation of bringing items, rather the agenda was simply a way to make sure they didn't get side-tracked. They then discussed the differences between CBT and counselling. Danny had often felt frustrated that counselling 'didn't go anywhere' and agreed that a more active, structured treatment could suit him, as long as he didn't feel too 'judged and inspected'. He also said that he'd always hated paperwork and didn't want to fill in forms, but was happy with active homework tasks, so they planned a 'reclaiming your life' assignment.

After the session, Danny's therapist formulated the interaction between them. She had felt frustrated and anxious, thought that she wasn't structuring the session well, and wanted to move Danny's focus away from his repetitive verbal preoccupation with his employers onto treatment tasks. Danny may have interpreted this behaviour as not listening to, or wanting to hear, his concerns. In turn, he felt frustrated, not 'good enough', and dismissed, and his therapist wondered if this reflected Danny's previous experiences with his employer. Her increasing attempts to impose structure on the session may have therefore made Danny feel dismissed, so he 'pushed back' against the structure and focused on his anger. Danny's therapist also realised that her anxiety reflected her beliefs that, as she was much younger than Danny, he wouldn't take her seriously, which may have led to her being more rigid than usual about managing the session.

In the next session, Danny's therapist initiated a conversation about how his previous experiences with his employers had affected him, and Danny talked more about feeling betrayed and let down by them. They added this to the formulation (Figure 24.2) and Danny's therapist shared the dilemma of wanting their limited sessions to be effective, without cutting Danny off or making him feel as if his problems weren't significant. They also agreed to address Danny's anger with his former employers as a priority and composed a letter together expressing how he had been mistreated, which Danny agreed to read aloud and then tear up as a homework task. Empathising and validating Danny's anger at his employers seemed to help Danny feel better supported by his therapist, and their alliance improved.

They spent the next session discussing Danny's goals for treatment and used psychoeducation and micro-formulations to link these to specific therapy interventions. Danny described feeling more confident that treatment had the potential to be helpful although he still had doubts. His therapist suggested that they keep this under review as they continued.

Recommended reading

Grey, N., House, J., & Young, K. (2018). Posttraumatic stress disorder. In S. Moorey, & A. Lavender (Eds.). *The therapeutic relationship in cognitive behavioural therapy* (pp. 121–134). Sage.

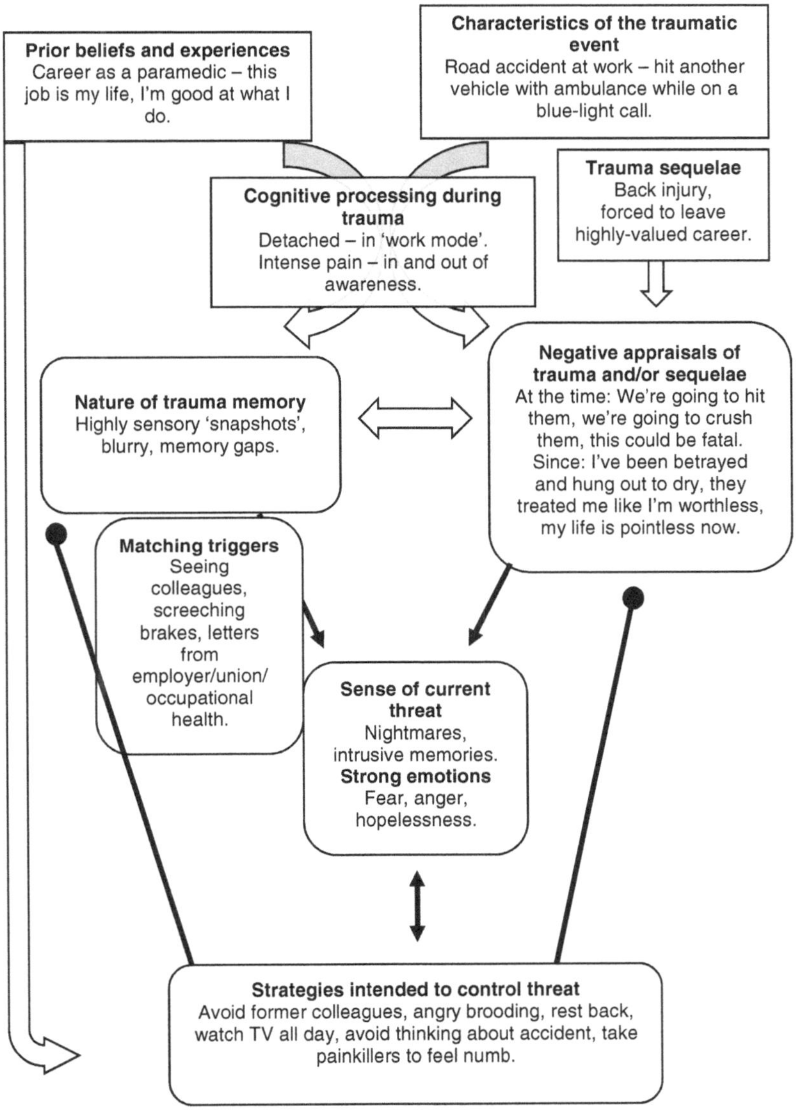

Figure 24.2 Danny's formulation

Moorey, S. (2014). 'Is it them or is it me?' transference and counter-transference. In A. Whittington, & N. Grey (Eds.). *How to become a more effective CBT therapist: Mastering metacompetence in clinical practice* (pp. 132–145). John Wiley & Sons.

Worrell, M. (2014). What to do when CBT isn't working. In A. Whittington, & N. Grey (Eds.). *How to become a more effective CBT therapist: Mastering metacompetence in clinical practice* (pp. 146–160). John Wiley & Sons.

CHAPTER TWENTY FIVE

Diversity

Col experienced racist bullying during his career in the British Army, culminating in a severe assault. He developed beliefs that all white people are racist and became hypervigilant to both threat and signs of discrimination. In treatment with a white therapist, they addressed how to build an effective therapeutic relationship, given Col's experiences.

Every one of us differs in a myriad of ways, both visible and invisible, important and irrelevant. These variations interact with our environment and context and, as therapists, our differences interact with those of our clients. For example, an Irish therapist working in England may often draw an interested remark without it impacting the therapeutic relationship, until working with a client affected by the Troubles in Northern Ireland.

The ways in which people are diverse can be encompassed in checklists such as Burnham's (2012) 'social GGRRAAACCEEESSS':

- Gender
- Geography
- Race
- Religion
- Age
- Ability
- Appearance
- Culture
- Class/caste
- Education
- Economics
- Ethnicity
- Sexual orientation
- Spirituality
- Sexuality

Checklists provide a helpful structure for us to identify our, and our client's, diversity characteristics and cultural/contextual influences. However, people are more than a checklist and grouping people into categories can obscure the heterogeneity within groups. For

DOI: 10.4324/9781003288329-31

example, two similarly-aged women of Jewish origin may have very different lifestyles and world views depending on their denomination (e.g. Haredi versus secular). We also need to consider intersectionality – how different characteristics interact. For example, a white transgender woman of lower socioeconomic status may have an entirely different experience of prejudice than someone of higher status, or a Black African transgender woman, or a transgender man.

A common criticism of CBT is that it was developed and tested predominantly with members of majority groups, i.e. white, English-speaking, able-bodied, cisgender, neurotypical adults under 65 years old. In the field of PTSD, there is some evidence of efficacy of trauma-focused psychological therapies with specific minority groups, such as refugees (Thompson et al., 2018) but little systematic data beyond case studies with other groups typically excluded from research trials, such as older adults (Clapp, & Beck, 2012), people with learning disabilities (Jones, & Banks, 2007), and autism (Carrigan, & Allez, 2017).

Reassuringly, CT-PTSD has not shown differential effects for ethnic minority clients (Ehlers et al., 2013), but other minority groups have not been studied. Given the well-acknowledged barriers to effective psychological treatments for ethnic minorities (Beck & Naz, 2019), some culturally adapted treatments for PTSD have been developed, which tailor existing protocols to fit the needs and belief systems of specific groups (e.g. Dixon et al., 2016; Hinton et al., 2012; O'Cleirigh et al., 2019; Zoellner et al., 2018). However, research is needed to establish the relative benefit of adapted versus non-adapted trauma-focused CBT and to answer the important questions of how much, and in what ways, treatments should be optimally adapted.

Chu and Leino (2017) describe a helpful framework for how psychological treatments may be culturally adapted:

- Core adaptations involve modifying core parts of treatment or adding additional modules/ components
- Peripheral adaptations promote treatment access, engagement, or retention
- Treatment delivery adaptations include using relevant language, materials, or cultural examples
- Therapy framework adaptations include modifying the session structure (number and length), interpersonal style of the therapist, location/medium, and involving others (such as family, physician, priest etc.) in treatment.

In our opinion, one of the strengths of a formulation rather than protocol-based treatment such as CT-PTSD is that it readily provides the flexibility needed to accommodate such adaptations. Throughout this book, we have used examples of clients from diverse groups with whom CT-PTSD has been effectively used. Our stance is always to individualise formulations and to flexibly apply treatment strategies to meet the needs of individuals. This enables the delivery of treatment which is personalised and culturally responsive but remains as close as possible to the evidence base (see El-Leithy, 2014).

In this chapter, we will provide further examples of working in this way. We also explore the relevance of diversity to PTSD and its treatment, plus how to tailor treatment and overcome potential obstacles to meet the needs of individuals.

Relevance of diversity to PTSD and its treatment

There are several ways that diversity issues may impact a person's experience of trauma, their PTSD symptoms, and their treatment. Here are some examples.

EXPOSURE TO TRAUMA

Some people are more likely to be exposed to traumatic experiences because they belong to a particular minority group, e.g. experiencing racist, homophobic, or gender-based violence; or indirectly because of risks arising from a characteristic, e.g. both poverty and disability are associated with an increased risk from violent crime (Focht-New et al., 2008; Webster & Kingston, 2014).

EXPRESSION OF SYMPTOMS AND DISTRESS

How people express their distress and psychological symptoms may tend to differ between groups. For example, people with learning disabilities may express PTSD symptoms differently (Tomasulo, & Razza, 2007) and some symptoms are reported more frequently in women when compared to men (Carragher et al., 2016). Cross-cultural studies have shown that, while there is good evidence for the validity of the PTSD diagnosis across cultural groups, there are also marked differences in how symptoms are expressed (Hinton, & Lewis-Fernández, 2011). For example, while re-experiencing and physiological hyperarousal symptoms are consistently reported, there is more variability in the avoidance symptom cluster (possibly because coping behaviours are more culturally bound than biologically determined). Several studies have found that somatic symptoms are reported more frequently in some cultural groups, perhaps linked to cultural 'idioms of distress', such as 'ataque de nervios' (attack of nerves) in Latino populations (Guarnaccia et al., 2003), 'khyal' (wind) attacks among Cambodian refugees (Hinton et al., 2002), and 'ihahmaku' (breathlessness) in Rwandans (Hagengimana, & Hinton, 2009). The meanings attached to psychological symptoms also differ between groups; hence, some PTSD symptoms may be perceived as more threatening because of culturally bound interpretations.

> Marwa developed nightmares and sleep problems after a sexual assault. She frequently woke with the feeling of pressure on her chest, as if someone was holding her down. Marwa's family took her to see a faith healer, who suggested she was possessed by a djinn. This was a common spiritual explanation of psychological symptoms in Marwa's country of origin, Egypt. An attempted exorcism was unsuccessful and Marwa was told that her faith was not strong enough, so she needed to pray more often. Marwa's therapist did not challenge the idea of djinn possession, but instead offered some information about PTSD nightmares, 'night hag syndrome', and sleep paralysis. They agreed a treatment plan which supplemented the traditional healing approaches and prayer with cognitive therapy techniques, and Marwa agreed this with her faith healer too.

MEANINGS OF TRAUMA

The ways different traumatic events are interpreted are often affected by diversity characteristics. For example, Tibetan refugees rated the destruction of religious objects as a more severe trauma than being tortured (Terheggen et al., 2001). The meanings given to sexual assault differ greatly across communities, with a greater likelihood of victim-blaming, stigmatisation, and rejection in some cultural contexts. Differing belief systems also interact with characteristics of the victim, creating even greater barriers to disclosure, support, or treatment. For example, in some countries, rape within marriage is legal or is legalised if the perpetrator marries the victim. In others, male rape is not acknowledged socially or legally, and rape of older people is often a taboo subject.

The meanings given to traumatic sequelae are also affected by cultural norms. In some religions, distress may be construed as 'punishment' for past sins. People from cultural contexts which place high value on the importance of families may be more likely to feel they have let family members down, or that they are no longer acceptable or attractive in the eyes of others, due to psychological or physical consequences of trauma. Men from some cultural backgrounds may be more likely to view themselves as weak for having psychological or emotional difficulties. Many of these appraisals relate to familiar cognitive themes and emotions in PTSD, such as shame, guilt, and anger; understanding the cultural lens through which trauma has been interpreted helps us, and the client, to better understand and address their idiosyncratic appraisals.

OVERARCHING CULTURAL FRAMEWORKS

Idiosyncratic meanings sit within broader culture-bound cognitive frameworks which shape appraisals and coping. These may differ between therapist and client, so we need to be aware of our implicit assumptions and influences. For example, one of the often-cited differences between eastern and western cultures is the collectivist versus individualistic lens. Therapists from western cultures may inadvertently miss important collective meanings by focusing exclusively on the experience of an individual, while clients see their experience as intrinsically linked with that of their family and community (Engelbrecht, & Jobson, 2016).

> Gil's home village in the Philippines was destroyed by a typhoon. He moved to the UK soon afterwards. Gil described a strong sense of guilt about leaving and struggled with some of the updates to his trauma memories that his therapist suggested, such as 'I survived, I'm alive'. He explained that his survival meant very little to him when so many others had died or had their homes destroyed, and if he could not help rebuild his community.

As therapists, we should be curious about, openly explore, and avoid directly challenging our clients' cultural frameworks. Typical overarching belief systems that might be important include fatalism, life after death, reincarnation and karma, ghosts and omens, determinism versus free will, and blood debts. Rather than attempting to restructure cultural beliefs, we work with and within them.

MINORITY STRESS

Longstanding experiences of stigma, discrimination, and victimisation that arise as a result of belonging to minority groups may be important elements in our PTSD formulations. Often termed 'minority stress', these experiences do not always represent 'criterion A' traumas, but the psychological consequences can nevertheless share many features with PTSD. For example, Livingston and colleagues (2020) write compellingly about the effect of chronic 'distal stressors' faced by members of the LGBTQ+ community, such as systemic and institutional oppression, discrimination, and microaggressions. These experiences can condition people to feel shame, anticipate rejection, conceal aspects of their identity, and isolate themselves. Similar response patterns can be experienced by people in other minority groups, such as ethnic minorities (sometimes termed 'racial trauma'), and groups who are persistently discriminated against in society (e.g. people with physical and learning disabilities). In combination with an increased risk of exposure to criterion A traumas such as violence and victimisation, it is easy to see how minority stress can increase vulnerability to PTSD development and complicate recovery, for example by reinforcing trauma-related appraisals.

The interactions between minority stress experiences and PTSD may represent independent treatment targets or, potentially, obstacles to recovery. When faced with persistent discrimination and harassment, it could be argued that some coping strategies usually considered unhelpful may be adaptive. For example, people may avoid holding hands with a same-sex partner in public to avoid negative attention; or confront or run from the police when stopped because of expectations of discriminatory treatment due to their ethnicity. Recognising which coping strategies are unhelpful will be difficult for people who have been chronically exposed to minority stress. Equally, therapists who have not had these experiences will have 'blind spots' where they struggle to appreciate the functional value of these coping strategies.

> Adrian suffered a head injury in a boating accident. The long-term effects included limb weakness that gave him an unusual gait, eyesight problems, and a slight slurring of speech. Adrian often felt that people stared at him and treated him rudely because of his disability. An alternative hypothesis was that Adrian's sense of current threat, arising from his PTSD symptoms and trauma-related appraisals of permanent change, was exacerbating this self-consciousness. To investigate this, Adrian's therapist followed him at a distance as he walked down a busy street and interacted with strangers, and observed that people did indeed stare at Adrian with one person calling out to him rudely. Adrian and his therapist agreed to learn more about how people perceived Adrian's disability using surveys and behavioural experiments. This revealed that most people did not perceive Adrian negatively, but some people did express discriminatory and stigmatising attitudes. They agreed to work on how Adrian could best identify and respond to circumstances when people were being rude or unpleasant, rather than curious about his differences.

Minority stress is associated with other vulnerability factors for ill-health, such as a lack of social capital: the capacity for social connections to act as resources to generate positive outcomes. Social and community resources that contribute to recovery from PTSD may be depleted or lacking for some of the people we work with, such as refugees. Fostering these resources and relationships may therefore form an important part of treatment.

TREATMENT PERCEPTIONS

The concept of psychological therapy and the structure and techniques of CBT can seem alien for some groups, and psychological therapists may be viewed with suspicion for various reasons. For example, some will be aware of psychology's historical links to pathologising homosexuality and developing 'conversion' therapy. Other clients may feel wary that therapists act as agents of the state, for example, those with strong political beliefs worrying about being reported to the 'Prevent' programme (a UK-based government programme developed to identify people at risk of radicalisation). Military or emergency services personnel may fear that a diagnosis of PTSD will affect their employment. Other clients may fear forced or compulsory psychiatric treatment, having had or heard about negative treatment experiences within mental health services. Aspects of CBT such as homework may be off-putting for people with literacy or developmental difficulties, or negative experiences of schooling, and the active collaborative style of therapy may feel uncomfortable to some. For example, in Japanese culture, asking questions is considered rude if someone is a higher status to yourself, or when the question makes the other person appear stupid.

WORKING WITH ISSUES RELATED TO DIVERSITY

When working with people from diverse groups, particularly those that differ from us in minority status, we must be responsive in our practice. This includes being mindful of the inevitable gaps in our knowledge and awareness of people's experiences when they arise from difference or cultural contexts. We would also argue that it is incumbent upon us to champion equality at a systemic level, by influencing service delivery within our organisations, and engaging local communities to shape and inform our practice (see the IAPT positive practice guidance; Beck et al., 2019 for example). Here are some specific recommendations.

LAYING THE GROUNDWORK

From our very first interactions with clients, we create a therapeutic frame that is accepting, respectful, and valuing of people's differences. This includes simple gestures like asking which name, title, and pronouns a person prefers, making sure written information is inclusively designed (e.g. regarding gender identity, available in different languages, adaptable for people with sensory impairments or reduced literacy), proactively checking access requirements to attend sessions, showing sensitivity to cultural differences in interactions (for example, orthodox Jewish people do not touch members of the opposite sex, so a handshake or other physical touch is inappropriate) and, where possible, offering choices of therapist (particularly regarding gender).

We also open conversations about differences to show awareness of, and sensitivity to, diversity issues. Beck (2019) suggests that therapists should routinely ask about culture, ethnicity, and faith, acknowledging differences where they are present, for example 'as I'm from a different culture to you, it would really help me understand you and your difficulties better if I could ask about your background'. Tasks such as taking a personal history, asking about social and community networks, and drawing a genogram can open up conversations about aspects of diversity. We also recommend routinely asking about experiences of discrimination, even if these do not appear related to the index traumas, and exploring and validating these experiences when they are mentioned.

ASSESSMENT

A comprehensive assessment encompasses not only the index traumas but also important life experiences, including those related to minority stress and their cognitive, affective, behavioural, physiological, and social impact. Some of these areas may overlap with or influence PTSD, but not all. We aim to establish what requires focus in treatment, whether methods of treatment delivery require adaptation, and to be aware of issues that may affect the therapeutic relationship.

Several assessment tools are available which measure minority stress including the 'Everyday Discrimination Scale' (Williams et al., 1997) as well as tools for specific minority groups, e.g. 'The Gender Minority Stress and Resilience measure' (Testa et al., 2015). These can form a useful starting point for conversations about discrimination and its impact.

FORMULATION

Diversity issues, and related experiences and contexts, may be relevant to an individual's formulation in many ways. They can shape belief systems, and therefore appraisals about traumatic events, symptoms, and ways of coping (see Figure 25.1 for an example). However, we avoid stereotyping or drawing generalisations based on group membership (e.g. all older male veterans see emotions as a sign of weakness). Instead, we use our understanding of common features of specific diversity groups as a provisional template, within which to curiously explore how an individual's experiences, beliefs, and systemic influences are relevant to the formulation (e.g. 'many veterans I have met tell me that showing emotion was seen by their colleagues as a sign of weakness – does that fit with your experience?').

TREATMENT

Difference does not inherently mean treatment needs to be adapted; rather adaptations are tailored to the individual. Some adaptations will be practical, such as using an interpreter if required (see 'top tips' box), or adapting the structure or delivery of treatment to make it more accessible for people with disabilities (page 244). Our choice of intervention technique and our emphasis in delivery will also vary. For example, for people who express their PTSD symptoms primarily in the somatic domain and prioritise physical symptoms in their treatment goals, we focus on these in early sessions, track them with idiographic measures, develop and test shared explanations for how they might interact with psychological process that we can target (such as rumination or self-focused attention), and focus on somatic elements of trauma memories during imaginal reliving and updating (see Chapter 21). Some clients struggle to work with imagery, for example, due to preferences, sensory deficits, or difficulties constructing images related to cognitive functioning, so we may work in a more concrete style, using written techniques, site visits or 'board game' reliving when working on trauma memories, or prioritising in vivo over imaginal methods.

Sean was a military veteran who was initially reluctant to engage in psychological therapy, joking in his first session that it was too 'airy-fairy' for him. His therapist asked him to give feedback on different therapy tasks and they agreed that Sean would try everything once, but could veto anything he found too 'airy-fairy'. He engaged well with imaginal reliving but found imagery rescripting too 'wafty' so they focused on written and physical updating instead. Sean also disliked homework, as it reminded him of negative experiences at school. However, he was prepared to do behavioural assignments between sessions, which they termed 'tactical ops'. They limited paperwork to small 'flashcards' that were similar to the 'standard operating procedure' cards Sean had carried on military manoeuvres.

Top tips: Working via interpreters

For clients who speak a different language to us, we routinely work with interpreters. Adding a third person into therapy raises several issues. Here are our top tips:

- *Always use a professional interpreter*, never a friend or family member.
- *Talk to your interpreter before you start*. If they aren't familiar with treating PTSD, explain the rationale for treatment, check how they feel about interpreting traumatic material, and how you can support them. Request exact translation.
- *Check your client's preference for the gender and ethnicity of the interpreter*. Although they speak the same language, there may be reasons why clients prefer not to have an interpreter of a particular ethnicity, e.g. regional dialects, if they were persecuted by members of that group, or concerns about privacy within local communities.
- If possible, *check with your client separately that they are comfortable* with the interpreter. If they are, try to keep the same one throughout treatment.
- *Allow more time*. Everything will move slower due to the time taken in back and forth interpreting so you will need longer and/or more sessions than usual. Ninety minutes with an interpreter is equivalent to 60 minutes without.
- *When you talk about confidentiality*, reassure the client that the same rules extend to the interpreter.
- *Speak directly to, and look at, your client* when speaking or listening (rather than the interpreter), even if you cannot understand each other. 'Turn up' your non-verbal signals indicating engagement.

- Don't forget to still use *validation, paraphrasing, summarising, and empathising* statements. These can get 'lost in translation' so make sure they are interpreted to your client.
- *Design your sentences to be concise*, speak in 'chunks', avoid jargon and vague analogies to help the interpreting process.
- *If there are any difficulties, address these immediately* and be prepared to change interpreter if needed.
- *Talk to your interpreter after each session to seek and give feedback*. Interpreting traumatic material can be distressing, and your interpreter may have experienced negative life events too, so check how they are coping.
- *Remember every interpreted encounter is also culturally laden*, and your interpreter is not just a translator, but a professional 'cultural broker' who can help you and your client bridge gaps.

For people from minority groups who experience systematic discrimination and/or ongoing harassment, some threat-related appraisals and behaviours may be adaptive from their perspective, while perhaps not from ours where we are a member of the contrasting majority. Sometimes, threat-related beliefs have been accurate and adaptive in the past, but the threat has passed or lessened, and they are maintained by trauma memories. Similarly, coping strategies such as avoidance, vigilance, rumination, confrontation, and defensive pessimism may have been, or continue to be, adaptive. Rather than assume that all such coping is unhelpful, or that all threat-focused appraisals are inaccurate, we need to work together to fully understand the threats our clients face, and how best to deal with them.

As a transgender woman, Michelle had faced bullying, harassment, and abuse throughout her life, in addition to a serious assault. She was understandably wary when out of her house, and avoided eye contact and interactions with strangers as much as possible. Her therapist validated her experiences, and they discussed how Michelle could cope with the discrimination she faced, without needing to hide away. To build her resources, Michelle decided to engage more with the transgender community online, sharing her experiences, and received an outpouring of support and encouragement. Michelle also learnt that experiences of serious assault, while not unheard of, were rare and that people who made comments on the street would not in all likelihood attack her.

Some of our clients find it helpful to discuss and explore discrimination to better understand its lingering impact. For example, we may discuss concepts from social psychology such as 'in-group/out-group' prejudice, not to justify the behaviour of others who have mistreated our clients but to help understand and therefore depersonalise it.

Another focus of diversity-responsive interventions is to draw on the strengths and skills which arise from certain cultural norms or membership of particular groups. For example, social support may be more readily available in close-knit communities, whether in physical or virtual domains. Spirituality and religion can offer numerous resources, including community (e.g. church groups), coping strategies (such as meditation or prayer), access to advice from faith leaders, metaphors and stories from religious texts, and other sources of positive beliefs (e.g. 'the person who died is now peaceful/reunited with loved ones in the afterlife', 'things happen for a reason; even if I don't understand yet why I survived, it must be part of a greater plan for me').

Hot cognitions

- My therapist can't relate to what I have been through
- People in my community think I am mad/to blame/will reject me because of my experiences
- I will be discriminated against so I need to keep my guard up and expect the worst
- It's not safe to talk about these things with someone inside/outside my community

OBSTACLES IN THE THERAPEUTIC RELATIONSHIP

One common obstacle is where differences in characteristics of the therapist and client lead to gaps in understanding or create threats for the client. A client may not feel fully understood by a therapist that does not have shared lived experience and all therapists will have 'blind spots' relating to their own diversity characteristics. For example, we may make assumptions based on our personal norms (such as what would be distressing about a particular trauma), without fully exploring it with our client. Alternatively, the therapist may inadvertently be a trigger for a client because of characteristics that match a trauma perpetrator or past aggressor (e.g. their appearance, gender, or accent). Lastly, therapists and clients can fall into familiar roles linked to their characteristics. For example, a younger therapist working with an older person may assume a more deferential stance in the therapeutic relationship and hold back from challenging them.

We discuss issues in the therapeutic relationship in Chapter 24. When they arise from issues of difference, it can help to map our diversity characteristics and those of our clients, looking for crossovers that can lead to over-identification, and differences which can lead to gaps in our understanding (El-Leithy, 2014). We need to be curious and open with our clients and ask about their identity and values, as well as actively educate ourselves about their cultural backgrounds.

FAQ: How can I best work with women affected by gender-based violence as a man?

An example of a matching feature between the therapist and trauma perpetrator is when male therapists treat female clients who have been affected by gender-based violence. We usually give our clients a choice about the gender of their therapist, making clear that it is understandable if they prefer not to work with a man, and that they can opt to change at any point in treatment. However, having a male therapist can be therapeutically beneficial for women in this situation, by offering an alternative experience of a man who is not abusive.

There are additional steps that can help in forming the therapeutic relationship. As with other areas of difference between us and the client, we make it clear from the start that the male therapist will not fully understand aspects of a woman's experience, and ask to be corrected and informed if we get something wrong. We are honest and open about the fact that most perpetrators of violence are men. We also name and discuss societal biases linked to violence against women, including victim-blaming and 'slut-shaming'.

It can be helpful to learn and practise stimulus discrimination and acknowledge possible triggers to trauma memories that may occur during sessions. We discuss and agree the language we will use to talk about the trauma, such as preferred terms for body parts if we are talking about a physical or sexual assault. As much as possible, we want our clients to feel in control and safe in our sessions; this in itself can be an important part of therapy.

Another obstacle can occur when cultural beliefs conflict with treatment engagement, for example, due to mistrust of the therapist, difficulties with the structure of CBT, or certain techniques. We have already discussed how to flex and adapt our intervention in response to an individual's needs but, when this is insufficient, we need to directly tackle any impasse to avoid the client dropping out.

Chrissie struggled to engage in treatment for PTSD following a car accident. Some of Chrissie's family had been involved in crime and Chrissie felt that she was 'tarred with the same brush' as them. She also felt that she was 'looked down on' because she had grown up on a council estate, and was a single mother who claimed benefits. Chrissie often became angry in therapy if she perceived her therapist as patronising or demeaning her. Chrissie's therapist was concerned she would drop out, so asked Chrissie if they could spend a session talking about their differences. Chrissie talked at length about the discrimination she and her family had faced, including from the NHS, police, and social services. Her therapist validated that, given her experiences, it would be understandable for Chrissie to expect further mistreatment and have learnt ways of dealing with this. Chrissie called this her 'guard dog' and agreed she could turn this on very quickly if she needed to defend herself or her family. Chrissie's therapist asked how therapy could be helpful, what might trigger her 'guard dog', and what they should do if it arose. They also added Chrissie's experiences of discrimination to her formulation and discussed how they had affected her appraisals about the trauma.

Notes from the therapy room: Col

Col grew up in Grenada in the Caribbean and joined the British Army following an overseas recruitment drive. Col experienced racist bullying from his first days as a cadet, which continued when he joined his regiment. Two fellow soldiers were particularly instrumental in this, bullying Col in various subtle and more obvious ways, including spreading rumours about him, alienating him socially, trolling him on social media, hiding or breaking his possessions, using racist language, and making racist jokes. This culminated in them attacking Col after a night out, leaving him with a severe shoulder injury and ending his career in the army. The military police were involved and the men were convicted of common assault. Col believed the charge would have been more serious if the same assault had been carried out by a Black soldier on a white one. His senior officers refused to acknowledge that the attack was racially motivated, or that there was a problem with racism in the regiment. Col was understandably bitter about the response to the assault, about the way that his career had ended, and spent a lot of time brooding on the injustice.

As well as re-experiencing symptoms of PTSD relating to the assault, Col was hypervigilant for danger, and also for discriminatory or racist behaviour. For example, he had been pulled over by the police on several occasions for no good reason, adding to his belief that 'all white people are racist' and 'people want to bring me down'. He also reported negative experiences with mental health services, including being sectioned when he reported suicidal ideation. He said that doctors saw him as a 'mad, bad Black man'.

In therapy, Col explained these experiences, and his therapist validated how difficult they must have been, and that Col's treatment had been unacceptable and indefensible. Col's therapist was white and asked if they could discuss this, given Col's experiences and his belief that white people were racist and untrustworthy. Col was given the option of seeing a non-white therapist at the service but decided to continue with his existing one as he had already explained his situation. They discussed how to build trust between them, and how Col could tell her if he was unhappy about anything she said or did. She acknowledged that there would be 'blind spots' due to their different backgrounds, and asked Col to let her know when she showed gaps in her understanding. She also disclosed that she had heard numerous accounts from other clients of experiences of racism in many contexts, including the army and health service. Together, they worked on a formulation (Figure 25.1).

Col's treatment included reliving, updating, and rescripting his memories of the assault, which related to his primary goal of improving his nightmares. As these improved, they moved on to a

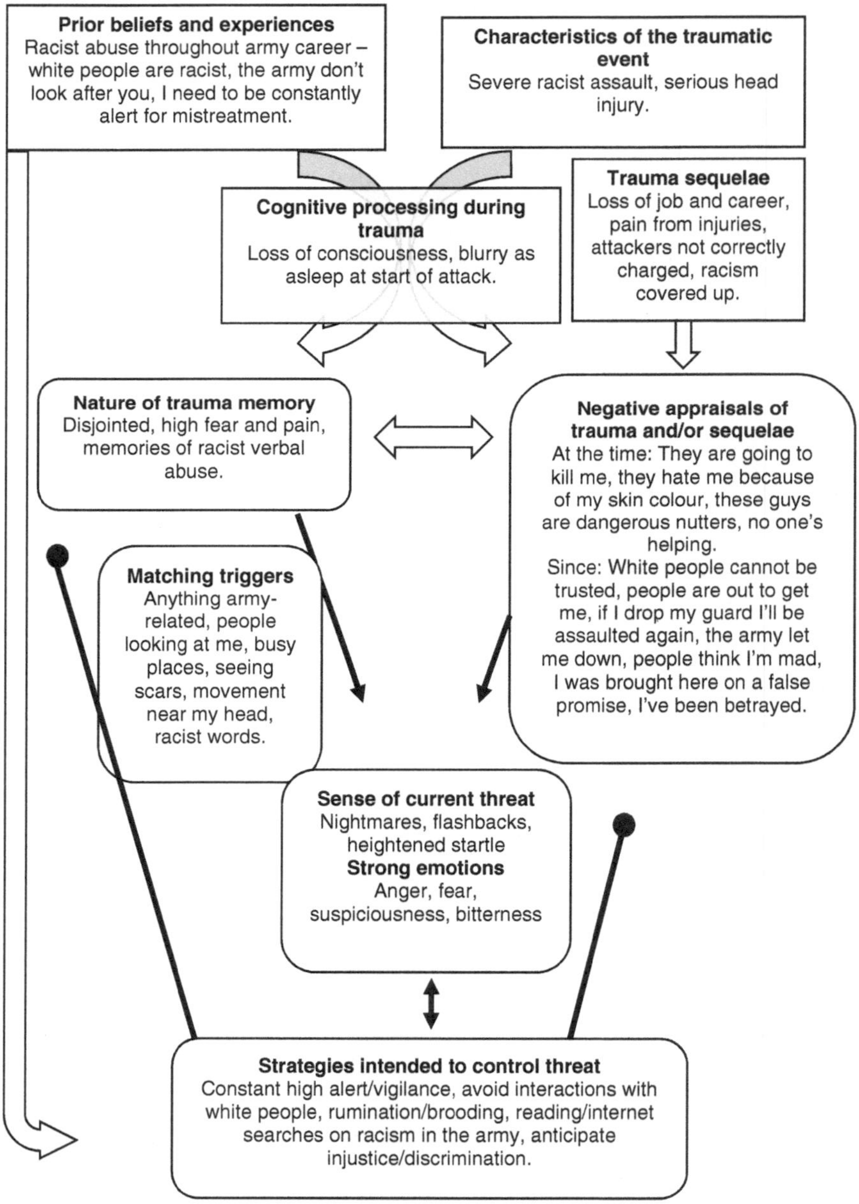

Figure 25.1 Col's formulation

secondary goal of 'getting past' his bitterness at how he had been mistreated. Col felt betrayed by the army, who had promised him a good career and had let him down personally, as well as other recruits from ethnic minorities, by allowing racism to flourish. Col and his therapist used techniques for addressing betrayal-based moral injury, such as having a conversation in imagery with a senior figure who Col respected, to explain the situation and ask how he could move forward. In imagery, he also confronted the senior officer who had denied racism in the regiment and imagined him being court-martialled and dishonourably discharged. After these conversations, Col decided he wanted to stop brooding about the past and prioritise his well-being until he had recovered from PTSD and could challenge the army again about his treatment.

This in turn motivated Col to engage in more 'reclaiming your life' activities including exercise, spending time with family, and looking for a new job. As Col increased his range of activities, he began to spend more time with white people, and therapy turned to addressing his beliefs about discrimination. Col had some positive experiences of these interactions, although he remained aware of, and distressed by, experiences of discrimination as well. They discussed how Col could live with the reality of racism, without assuming that he would be discriminated against by all white people he met. He planned to speak to Black friends to seek their views on this issue, and to check out ambiguous situations where Col was unsure if he was being discriminated against or not. By the end of therapy, Col reported that his belief 'all white people are racist' had shifted to 'some white people are racist', and this was easier to live with. He also fed back that he was glad he had received treatment from a white therapist because the experience of opening up about his experiences, being taken seriously, and respected had helped him feel more trusting of white people.

Recommended reading

Beck, A., Naz, S., Brooks, M., & Jankowska, M. (2019). *Improving access to psychological therapies (IAPT): Black, Asian and minority ethnic service user positive practice guide*. Available at: https://babcp.com/Therapists/BAME-Positive-Practice-Guide-PDF

d'Ardenne, P., Farmer, E., Ruaro, L., & Priebe, S. (2007). Not lost in translation: Protocols for interpreting trauma-focused CBT. *Behavioural and Cognitive Psychotherapy*, *35*, 303–316.

El-Leithy, S. (2014). Working with diversity in CBT. In A. Whittington & N. Grey (Eds.). *How to become a more effective CBT therapist: Mastering metacompetence in clinical practice* (pp. 44–62). John Wiley & Sons.

Livingston, N. A., Berke, D., Scholl, J., Ruben, M., & Shipherd, J. C. (2020). Addressing diversity in PTSD treatment: Clinical considerations and guidance for the treatment of PTSD in LGBTQ populations. *Current Treatment Options in Psychiatry*, *7*, 53–69.

CHAPTER TWENTY SIX
Looking after yourself

Jamie realised he was showing signs of compassion fatigue when he noticed he was dreading going to work and couldn't stop worrying about one of his clients. With the support of his manager, Jamie made changes to his caseload and supervision arrangements. He also reflected on his own thoughts, feelings, and behaviours about working with trauma and applied some CBT strategies to himself.

Treating PTSD can be an immensely rewarding experience. It is also challenging. We hear details of intensely traumatic events and, in doing so, imagine them ourselves. Empathy can be painful; we absorb some of the distress that our clients feel, and their stories may trigger our own painful memories. We may face ethical, moral, and legal dilemmas with our clients. Our work is only one part of our life; we may also be dealing with other stressors, traumas, mental and physical health issues. We may be battling with self-worth and imposter syndrome. Stress can also come from the systems we are working within, such as over-stretched services, tensions with co-workers or bosses, and unhealthy workplaces.

Considering all these pressures, it is understandable that psychological therapists working with trauma often experience burnout, compassion fatigue, and secondary traumatic stress symptoms. In this chapter, we will discuss these concepts, and the challenges we face with this work. There aren't easy solutions, but we will review the evidence on what helps and our top tips on taking care of yourself when you work with trauma.

The impact of working with trauma

Several different, overlapping terms are used to describe the psychological impact of working with trauma. 'Vicarious traumatisation' often refers to changes in beliefs and schemas, while 'secondary traumatic stress' (Figley, 1995) refers to the development of PTSD symptoms in those who work with traumatised clients. Indeed, the inclusion of indirect exposure to trauma as a criterion A event in DSM-5 means that psychological therapists are considered at risk of PTSD due to their repeated exposure to traumatic material. 'Compassion fatigue' (Figley, 2002) was initially described as a form of secondary traumatic stress reaction but the term is now used more broadly, to mean the emotional exhaustion and reduced capacity for empathy that can arise in professionals working with traumatised groups. 'Burnout' is another common term, describing the utter physical and mental exhaustion caused by chronic stress and frustration. Although theoretically different, these terms represent overlapping constructs that are used fairly interchangeably in the literature. As compassion fatigue represents the overarching concept, we will use this term.

The flipside of compassion fatigue is compassion satisfaction: the sense of fulfilment, pleasure, and accomplishment that therapists experience. Many trauma therapists report this experience in

DOI: 10.4324/9781003288329-32

their work (Sodeke-Gregson et al., 2013), highlighting the potential positives of working with PTSD. Akin to the concept of post-traumatic growth, compassion satisfaction can arise from many aspects of trauma work, not least witnessing the extraordinary courage and resilience our clients show to endure and recover from horrendous traumatic experiences. Compassion fatigue and compassion satisfaction can fluctuate for us all at different points in our working lives and it is possible, even likely, to experience both at the same time. Our goal is to minimise or mend the former and maximise the latter.

SELF-ASSESSMENT

Given the risk of compassion fatigue, therapists need to regularly 'check-in' with how we are feeling and actively monitor for any 'red flags'. Ideally, this should be a standing item in supervision. Over time, this can help us develop an understanding of our personal 'fatigue signatures' so that we can more readily identify in ourselves the onset of compassion fatigue. Several standardised measures are available as a starting point, including the Professional Quality of Life Scale (ProQol-III; Stamm, 2005).

Warning signs can fall in various domains, including:

- *Emotional*: Feeling detached or overly involved with clients, irritability, feeling guilty about clients or therapy outcomes, feeling sad or hopeless, feeling flat, drained, overwhelmed, feelings of dread about going to work, anxiety.
- *Physiological*: Feeling constantly tired, difficulty sleeping, poor concentration, headaches, nausea, digestive and bowel symptoms, increased startle response, muscle tension, heart palpitations.
- *Cognitive*: Self-doubt and self-criticism, pessimism and loss of hope, preoccupation with particular clients which persists outside work, safety fears.
- *Behavioural*: Working long hours, over-preparing for sessions, ruminating about work, avoiding working with certain clients or aspects of treatment (e.g. memory work with certain traumas), concealing during supervision, hypervigilance or other safety precautions, excessive use of alcohol or drugs.

As part of a check-in, therapists should regularly ask themselves reflective questions about their well-being, including the following (Meichenbaum, 2007):

- How am I doing?
- What would I like to change?
- What is hardest about this work? What worries me?
- Are there any aspects of my job that I dread? If so, why and what can I do about them?
- How have I changed since I began this work? (Both positively and negatively?)
- Am I showing any signs of compassion fatigue/burnout? If so, what am I doing to address these?
- What work barriers reduce my satisfaction or increase my stress and how can these be addressed?
- What do I find rewarding about my work?
- What helps me to do this work?
- What are my personal resources and strengths?

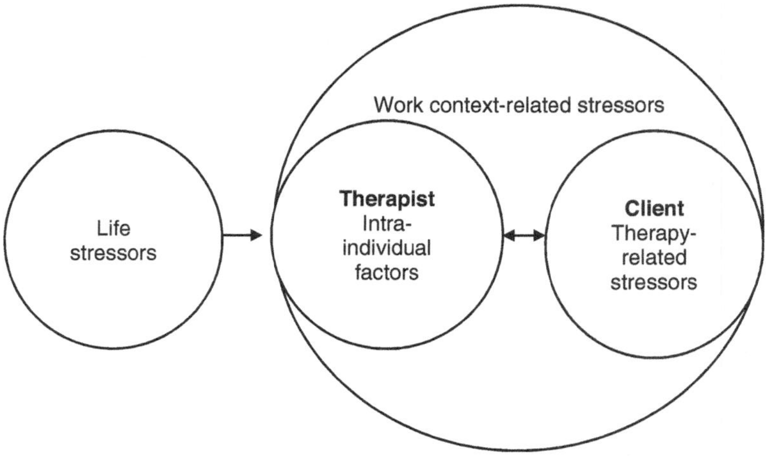

Figure 26.1 Sources of potential stress for therapists

- How can I use social supports more effectively?
- What resources in my workplace can I draw on to help me with this work?

These questions allow us to monitor our well-being, stimulate reflections about how to build our resilience, and tackle difficulties as early as possible.

THE PRESSURES WE FACE AND HOW TO COPE

The pressures on therapists come from a variety of sources, illustrated in Figure 26.1. These sources of stress interact with each other and the effects can multiply. For example, we may be coping well with stress in one domain, but when it also arises in another, our resources become overwhelmed.

INTRA-INDIVIDUAL STRESSORS

Each of us brings personal qualities and characteristics to our job. Some of these will improve our resilience to stress, but many qualities that make us good therapists also leave us vulnerable to compassion fatigue. For example, being an empathic therapist brings warmth, compassion, and commitment to a therapy relationship, but it can also make us more sensitive to taking on our clients' distress and more protective of our clients, perhaps meaning we avoid elements of therapy they will find upsetting. Many of us have our own experiences of mental health problems or trauma. This can confer strengths in trauma work and is often a strong motivator to work with traumatised clients, but can introduce challenges too.

FAQ: How can I work with PTSD if I have my own trauma history?

Many therapists have experienced trauma themselves, and some will have personal experience of PTSD or other mental health issues. Lived experience is a potential strength as a therapist, conferring empathy, authenticity, motivation, and compassion. However, several research studies have shown it is a risk factor for compassion fatigue (Turgoose, & Maddox,

2017); perhaps increased personal identification takes an emotional toll, or working with some clients or traumas can trigger our own trauma memories, making it harder to keep the boundaries between professional and personal life.

As therapists in this position, we need to be especially self-aware and prioritise our well-being in all the ways recommended in this chapter, avoiding what might be a strong drive to care for others to the detriment of ourselves. We need to be particularly mindful of our own 'emotional buttons' and signs they have been activated, as well as our underlying negative beliefs and unhelpful compensatory strategies. At times, we may need to put on the 'empathy brakes' if we find ourselves over-identifying with a client. It is preferable to make supervisors aware of lived experience, to allow open conversations about the impact of the work on us and elicit support. For example, there may be clients with similar traumas to ours that may be too difficult to work with; services should allow therapists the option of declining a case if so.

Personal therapy can be worthwhile to help us reflect on our work, the personal–professional interface, and any secondary traumatic stress symptoms which emerge. Where PTSD symptoms are ongoing, therapists should seek evidence-based treatment.

Working with PTSD can be anxiety-provoking for therapists, especially early in our careers. Clients are frequently very distressed in sessions and many therapists worry about 'retraumatising' them. This can sometimes lead therapists to hold back from the more challenging parts of treatment, such as reliving the trauma memories, out of office behavioural experiments, and visiting the trauma site, all of which are powerful interventions. Overcoming this anxiety is therefore important, for the benefit of both therapist and client. Luckily, as CBT therapists, we know about effective treatments for anxiety! Addressing our therapist cognitions and behaviours, ideally with the help of a supervisor or personal therapist, can be immensely helpful.

Many therapists are also prone to perfectionist standards and can be self-critical. Unfortunately, not all our clients will recover and this is true for every therapist. When we take this as an indicator of our personal effectiveness, it can knock our confidence. We may suffer from imposter syndrome, doubting our adequacy and worrying we will be 'found out'. In this book, we have mostly given examples where treatment has gone well, but we could easily fill another book with examples where it has not. We have often made mistakes, and we have also had disappointing experiences of trying very hard, with a committed client, who has still not recovered.

Awareness of our strengths and vulnerabilities is important, as is engaging in reflective practice. The following principles are important throughout our working life, whether or not we are suffering from compassion fatigue.

To look after others, we need to look after ourselves

Many therapists put others' needs before their own. But, to be effective, compassionate therapists, we also need to look after ourselves. Self-care is different for everybody. The key is to balance the emotional energy that we expend at work with activities that replenish us. For some, this is exercise, for others it is rest. Some therapists have personal therapy, others prefer to have a drink with a friend, keep a journal, or do something creative. One thing we all need is time off, so make sure to take your holiday time allocation, especially when you notice the signs of fatigue kicking in.

Maintaining boundaries and balance

Compassion fatigue can occur when we let work permeate all aspects of our life. If you find yourself thinking about your clients at the weekend, working late into the evening, or taking on your client's difficulties as if they are your own, then think carefully about re-setting your boundaries. It's a cliché, but getting a work–life balance is critical. Work smarter, not harder and don't work at your maximum capacity for long periods. Rather, aim to operate at about 80% of your full capacity, so you have room for unplanned workplace demands.

Remember to share the responsibility for recovery with your client by keeping treatment collaborative and doing things with your client, not for them. If we take on all the pressure of a successful outcome, it will feel like a personal failure if treatment does not go to plan.

FAQ: How do I maintain boundaries if I work from home?

With the rise of digital therapies, working from home may become increasingly commonplace. Treating PTSD from our homes can blur work–life boundaries, so we need to take practical steps to maintain them. For example, ideally, find a workspace that does not double as a living or sleeping space. If you don't have a spare room to use as an office, try to demarcate an area for your workspace. Ensure you have fixed breaks and mark a clear end to the working day by closing down your computer and closing the door to, or clearing away, your workspace at a set time, without letting the working day blur into your free time. It often helps to create a 'buffer' task, like taking a walk or run at the end of the working day, to replicate the effect of a commute and create some mental distance from work. During client session time, reduce the potential distractions in your workspace, by turning off phones and email and asking co-habitants not to disturb you (although child and pet-related interruptions are sometimes unavoidable!).

Working from home can also be more isolating, so we need to plan to keep connected with our team and maintain our morale. Arrange with colleagues to speak regularly, and have the option to arrange a call with a peer or supervisor if you need to talk through a difficult session. Consider setting up a text/email 'group chat' so you can replicate the casual 'check-ins' with each other throughout the day, and share 'distraction files' (e.g. pictures of cute animals or landscapes; Rees, 2017).

Holding onto the positives

Remaining optimistic and hopeful can be challenging when working with trauma, so find ways to regularly remind yourself of the positives. Think about what you are most proud of achieving in your work and keep a reminder of it nearby. Keep a folder of nice emails/cards/letters from grateful clients and re-read them when you are feeling discouraged. Where progress is slow, remind yourself of previous clients where treatment has had its ups and downs but ultimately been effective – stay relentlessly hopeful!

It can also help to remind yourself why you like working with trauma (if you are reading this book, we assume that you do!) and what gives you compassion satisfaction. Our clients frequently inspire us with their courage and strength. Our work allows us a unique insight into experiences we will never have. Being trusted with the personal and painful memories and inner worlds of our clients is a privilege that we don't take lightly.

Remembering our strengths is also important. We are all different and bring our own experiences and personal qualities to our work. You might be the one who cheers up a colleague at the end of a tough day, keeps everyone calm during a team discussion, bakes the best cakes for meetings, or makes clients feel truly heard for the first time. It's easy to notice our faults, but pay attention to your strengths too!

Using our therapy skills on ourselves

As therapists, we don't always practice what we preach. When we are struggling, we should ask ourselves the classic CBT question 'what would you say to someone else about this?'. It probably wouldn't be 'just get on with it' or 'work even harder'. Other therapy skills can be useful too. We can formulate our reactions (see the case at the end of the chapter), use thought records, activity diaries, 'worry time' or 'worry tree' interventions, update or rescript difficult memories or work-related nightmares, weigh up risk probabilities, and use behavioural experiments to address our problematic thoughts and behaviours. There is also preliminary evidence that dispositional mindfulness is negatively correlated with compassion fatigue; it may follow that mindfulness is a useful skill for therapists to use (Turgoose, & Maddox, 2017).

Asking for help

It won't be a surprise to learn that social support is negatively correlated with compassion fatigue (MacRitchie, & Leibowitz, 2010). Building up, and calling on, our support networks is important to protect our well-being and to turn to if we are struggling. Some therapists feel ashamed to admit they are experiencing compassion fatigue but, as Meichenbaum (2007) suggests, it is a sign of a committed and sensitive therapist. As we tell our clients, it is a strength to know when to ask for help. This may be from your supervisor, colleagues, personal therapist, or peer networks.

Isla had a history of depression. She was passionate about her work as a CBT therapist, but at times she struggled with her mental health. Isla had undergone treatment herself in the past and had developed a detailed coping plan, which enabled her to monitor the warning signs that her mood was deteriorating and to implement strategies that had worked for her in the past. Isla and a work colleague who also had lived experience of mental health problems met for coffee once a fortnight and checked in with each other about how they were coping. Isla's supervisor was also aware of her depression and was supportive when Isla needed time off or to make changes to her work patterns.

Hot cognitions

- I'm not good at my job/as good as my peers and others will find out
- It's down to me to rescue/save my clients – if I don't, I've failed
- The more hours I work/the more I prepare, the better a therapist I will be
- Working with trauma has made realise the world is full of pain and suffering
- Bad things can happen at any time – I need to protect my loved ones

LIFE STRESSORS

At different times in our professional lives, we face significant stressors in other areas of our life, such as health problems, family demands, relationship breakdowns, bereavements, or caring responsibilities. Working with trauma means there is little emotional respite at work from distress we are facing at home. Some therapists choose to take time out when competing demands become unmanageable, or to manage their time differently, such as shorter hours, reduced caseload, or avoiding certain clients or traumas. Such occupational changes rely on support from managers and sometimes discussions with occupational health.

If you continue working as usual during a period of life stress, be kind to yourself and reflective about what you need. Think through what does and doesn't help. You may not be able to control all aspects of your life, but your ways of coping are within your control. The previous section on self-care is particularly important.

Jenny's partner Susie became seriously unwell with cancer. Initially, Jenny found work a welcome distraction from the sadness and worry of supporting her but, as Susie became more ill, Jenny decided to request a period of compassionate leave to care for her. After Susie died, Jenny returned to work but agreed with her manager that she would initially carry a smaller caseload, and not work with any cases of traumatic bereavement or medically related traumas.

THERAPY-RELATED STRESSORS

Some of the stressors facing therapists arise from the work itself. We may find ourselves struggling to switch off at the end of the day; for example, after hearing particularly horrific stories, working with clients who are suicidal or present a risk to others, or those who have perpetrated violence. We may face challenging ethical, moral, or legal dilemmas in our work. For example, deciding whether to break confidentiality brings two ethical principles into conflict; our client's rights to privacy and control over their personal information, and the rights of others to be protected from harm. When clients make prejudiced or derogatory comments, this can introduce a conflict between our beliefs around fairness and respect, and our wish to maintain positive regard for our client. These conflicts can be stressful to resolve.

To cope with difficult therapy situations, good supervision is essential. If you are a supervisor, read our 'top tips' box. Having an 'open door' culture within a team is invaluable, where therapists can informally 'decompress' after a tough session, discuss a thorny issue, or seek support in managing risk when their supervisor is unavailable. For therapists working alone, remotely, or in private practice, finding a way to replicate these informal support networks (whilst maintaining client confidentiality) is advisable.

Training also helps. Specialist training in working with trauma is protective against compassion fatigue (Sprang et al., 2007) as is evidence-based practice (Craig, & Sprang, 2010). Feeling competent and confident in the therapy we are delivering increases our resilience when facing challenges.

Shireen was treating a client who had problems with anger and had previously been violent to others. In sessions, she occasionally became angry with Shireen. Shireen took the issue to supervision and found it helpful to list what she was finding challenging: maintaining empathy with a client who had perpetrated violence and was sometimes rude to Shireen, managing the risk the client posed to others, and evaluating the risk within therapy sessions. Formulating the client helped Shireen with the first issue, as she had a long and complex history of multiple abuses and had difficulty regulating her emotions, which Shireen could empathise with. Nevertheless, her supervisor reminded her that verbal abuse towards Shireen was unacceptable and they agreed how Shireen could discuss this with the client, setting clear boundaries around abusive behaviour. They also used a risk assessment tool to review the risk the client posed to others and Shireen decided to develop a violence safety plan with the client.

Top tips: How to be an effective and compassionate PTSD supervisor

Whole books have been written on good supervisory practice, which we won't repeat here. Instead, we want to highlight some principles which are especially pertinent when supervising PTSD therapists:

- *Provide a secure attachment*: Be warm, hopeful, cheerful, and even-tempered. Show gratitude, demonstrate you 'have their back', celebrate their success, and give positive feedback wherever you can.
- *Model 'calmness under fire'*: Encourage a 'we can get through this together' attitude when supervisees are anxious or things go wrong. Help them step back and formulate problems in therapy, then make action plans.
- *Review and normalise the impact of the work*: A standing item on a supervision agenda should be a well-being check. We normalise the likelihood of compassion fatigue and discuss it openly so there is no shame. Use the questions on page 301–2 for sporadic but regular reviews.
- *Make time to listen*: When you are under a lot of pressure, it is difficult to give time and space to supervision. Supervisees may not disclose that they are struggling if supervision time feels rushed.
- *Model self-care and help-seeking*: Supervisees will follow your example, so make sure you are prioritising self-care. Take a lunch break. Leave on time. Show vulnerability and ask for support when needed.
- *Balance supervisory elements*: Supervision has multiple functions. Generally, a mix of didactic, experiential, and reflective practice is optimal (Bennett-Levy, 2006). Supervision should not be therapy for the supervisee but, if they are struggling, allocate time to discuss their needs.
- *Formulate*: The supervisor has the potential to 'hover above' therapy and observe what the therapist may not. Figure 24.1 (page 285) can be useful in supervision to formulate the therapeutic relationship.
- *Promote safe feedback*: It is hard for supervisees to give honest feedback due to the power imbalance in the supervisory relationship. We need to create opportunities for receiving feedback and actively engage in our development as supervisors.

WORK CONTEXT PRESSURES

Stress can arise from pressures on services, both at team level and more broadly within organisations. Many services face high demands for psychological therapy in the context of limited resources. This often translates into hard-to-meet targets for waiting lists, caseloads, and recovery rates. Services offering treatment via the NHS and other public sector organisations can experience periodic 'restructures' which often include cuts to staffing capacity. One of the enemies of compassion is time pressure so, unsurprisingly, compassion fatigue can arise in such stressful circumstances. Stressors can also arise within teams. Bullying, harassment, and poor managerial behaviours have an enormous impact on the well-being of staff. Working in private practice is not immune from pressure either; many therapists work alone or have limited team support, and face the challenge of generating referrals and income.

For therapists working with trauma, we need the same conditions for delivering treatment as our clients who are receiving it: social support, control, predictability and safety. Unfortunately, our work context may not always support these needs, and we may have limited power to make changes. Here are some strategies that may help:

- *Control the controllable*: There will be some aspects of your work context that will be within your control. For example, you may be able to negotiate with managers about your supervision needs, caseloads, hours, and training. If you feel that you are developing compassion fatigue, this is an important step. You may need to re-think your working patterns, including taking a break from trauma work entirely if needed. Task-focused coping is inversely related to compassion fatigue (Zeidner et al., 2013).
- *Seek support*: Especially if you do not feel supported by your supervisor and/or manager, seek support from elsewhere. Build peer support networks within your organisation but also speak to others outside your system, who can often provide a valuable external perspective.
- *Know your red lines*: Some work circumstances are unacceptable. For example, bullying or harassment should never be tolerated. It is important to know your rights and who to speak to when a red line has been crossed; this may be a senior manager, your human resources department, union, or professional bodies. Document any treatment you are unhappy with and seek support.
- *Build your personal resources*: Building personal resilience can help you to cope with external stressors, but the concept of resilience can be a double-edged sword, as it can locate the blame for compassion fatigue in the affected party. Being affected by stress, and struggling at points in your life does not mean you are not resilient! We talk to our clients about self-compassion and ask them which teacher would get better results from their students: a critical one or a supportive, encouraging one. We should follow our own advice. Resilience is about self-care and compassion, utilising our strengths, and building the support that we need to face difficult situations.

Top tips: Creating a psychologically healthy work-place

There is an ethical imperative to create a psychologically healthy workplace, and a financial one too: stressed employees take more time off work, are less effective, and hand in their notice sooner. We all have the power to contribute to a psychologically healthy workplace and a supportive culture, although most responsibility lies with team leaders and the wider organisation.

- *Foster cohesion*: Promote a positive workplace culture where everyone shares a way of working, pulls together to get the job done, and has each other's back. Model an 'open door' policy, check in with each other, show appreciation, and be considerate of others' feelings.
- *Bolster team spirit*: Encourage positive relationships by making the workplace an enjoyable social environment, including through optional social activities. Make time to celebrate workplace successes and important personal days. Allow staff time to support each other through activities and discussions unrelated to work.
- *Equip and train adequately*: Make sure everyone has the resources to do their job safely and effectively, including a suitable physical working environment that reduces, rather than contributes to, stress. Provide the support, supervision, and training people need to master their skills.
- *Increase involvement*: Staff who are strongly engaged with their work, team, and organisation are more motivated, productive, and achieve better outcomes. Involve staff

in decision making. Create a dynamic where everyone is listened to, respected, and has their needs considered.
- *Focus on strengths*: Engagement also increases when we focus on strengths. Find out what your colleagues are interested in, value, and are good at. Tailor job plans to capitalise on strengths and encourage staff to develop specialisms.
- *Promote well-being*: Support colleagues to achieve work–life balance, particularly if they have personal stressors. Consider offering flexible working, tailoring caseloads, or rotating roles and functions. Promote self-care by making it part of the team culture to take breaks, leave on time, and rest when needed.
- *Support staff who are struggling*: Proactively identify colleagues who may be struggling, including reaching out to those who appear 'too busy'. If someone you manage reports difficulties, offer them time to reflect, recharge, and develop an action plan. Have a low threshold for referring to support services.
- *Read up*: There are plenty of resources on what makes a psychologically healthy workplace. Try the British Psychological Society (BPS, 2017) guidance for a start.

Notes from the therapy room: Jamie

Jamie is a CBT therapist working in a busy NHS psychology service. He had an interest in trauma and agreed with his manager to take on extra PTSD clients to learn more. However, Jamie noticed after a while that he was starting to dread his sessions with PTSD clients, especially one young woman who had been abducted and raped. She regularly experienced suicidal ideation and Jamie found himself worrying about her between sessions. Jamie realised that he wasn't sleeping well and had become anxious about his girlfriend El going out at night. If El went out without him, Jamie would wait up until she got home, and preferred to pick her up from the train station so that she didn't walk alone to their flat. Jamie also felt unsupported by his supervisor, who was very busy and regularly cancelled supervision.

One morning, Jamie felt overwhelmingly anxious about going to work. He called in sick and, after thinking for a few days, decided that he needed to tell his manager that he was struggling. His manager took Jamie's concerns seriously, and together they agreed that Jamie should reduce the number of PTSD clients on his caseload temporarily. He also planned his work schedule so that he would see his PTSD clients just before his lunch break, so that he had time to de-stress if needed. Jamie explained that he was not receiving regular supervision, so his manager allocated him to another supervisor, who had more time.

At the start of his new supervision arrangement, Jamie opened up about the difficulties he was having with trauma work and asked that each supervision session included a 'check-in' on how he was coping. Jamie also filled in a questionnaire on compassion fatigue and they discussed his answers together and created a 'hot cross bun' diagram to summarise the cognitive, behavioural, emotional, and physiological elements of how he was feeling (Figure 26.2).

This exercise made Jamie realise that his increased anxiety for his girlfriend was probably due to working with several trauma cases involving attacks on young women which had heightened his awareness of potential harm. Jamie had worked with his clients on calculating the probability of such an attack happening (which was very low) and he realised that, just like his clients, his experiences had skewed his perception of the likelihood of threat. Reminding himself that such attacks are extremely infrequent helped Jamie, and he decided to speak to his girlfriend about what was an appropriate level of caution.

Jamie's supervisor also helped him address his other anxious thoughts, including his fear that his client may attempt suicide. His supervisor normalised this as a concern that many clinicians have,

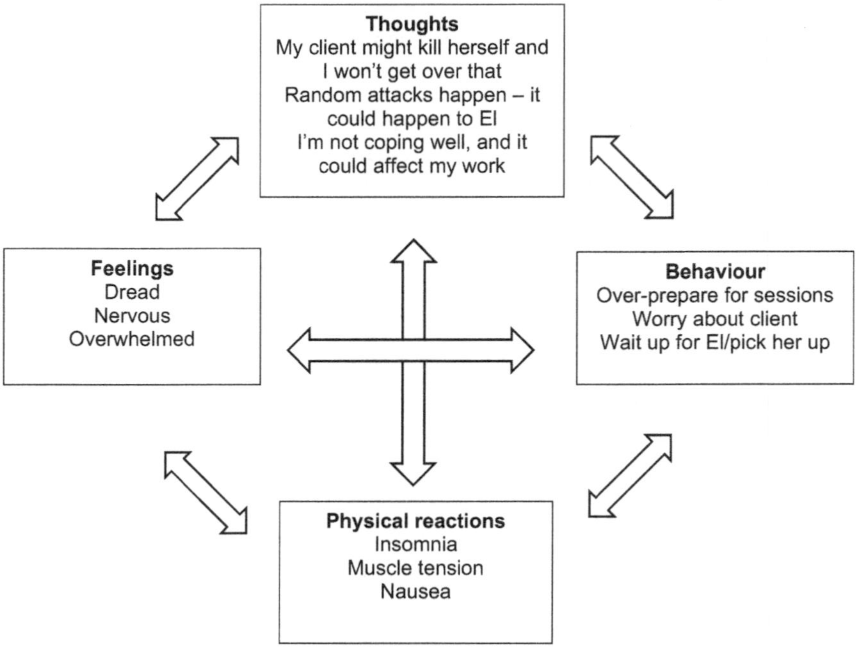

Figure 26.2 Jamie's hot cross bun

and together they reviewed the risk protocols for the service and the client's safety plans. This helped reassure Jamie that he was doing everything he could to keep his clients safe and that the responsibility was not his alone, but shared with the service, his supervisor, and the clients themselves.

Jamie also reviewed his self-care strategies and made some changes. He found running was an effective stress management strategy, so he planned to finish work on time every day and go for a run. He also reduced the amount of time he spent preparing for sessions and reviewing them afterwards, which gave him more time during the working day. He made sure he took a lunch break and between sessions he went outside for a short walk with a colleague. He also made efforts to improve his sleep hygiene including taking some time to read or listen to music before bed and cutting down on caffeine.

Over the next few months, Jamie felt less stressed. He continued to check in with his supervisor about how he was feeling. Jamie attended further training on working with PTSD, and gradually increased his caseload again, monitoring any signs of compassion fatigue, and maintaining his self-care.

Recommended reading

Billings, J., Kember, T., Greene, T., Grey, N., El-Leithy, S., Lee, D., & Bloomfield, M. (2020). Guidance for planners of the psychological response to stress experienced by hospital staff associated with COVID: Early interventions. *Occupational Medicine*, 70(5), 327–329.

Meichenbaum, D. (2007). Self-care for trauma psychotherapists and caregivers: Individual, social and organizational interventions. www.melissainstitute.org/documents/Meichenbaum_SelfCare_11th-conf. pdf

Turgoose, D., & Maddox, L. (2017). Predictors of compassion fatigue in mental health professionals: A narrative review. *Traumatology*, 23(2), 172–185.

References

Alpert, J. L., Brown, L. S., & Courtois, C. A. (1998). Symptomatic clients and memories of childhood abuse: What the trauma and child sexual abuse literature tells us. *Psychology, Public Policy, and Law*, 4(4), 941–995.

American Psychiatric Association. (2013). *Diagnostic and statistical manual of mental disorders* (5th ed.).

Arch, J. J., & Craske, M. G. (2009). First-line treatment: A critical appraisal of cognitive behavioral therapy developments and alternatives. *Psychiatric Clinics*, 32(3), 525–547.

Armour, C., Fried, E. I., Deserno, M. K., Tsai, J., & Pietrzak, R. H. (2017). A network analysis of DSM-5 posttraumatic stress disorder symptoms and correlates in US military veterans. *Journal of Anxiety Disorders*, 45, 49–59.

Armour, C., Greene, T., Contractor, A. A., Weiss, N., Dixon-Gordon, K., & Ross, J. (2020). Posttraumatic stress disorder symptoms and reckless behaviors: A network analysis approach. *Journal of Traumatic Stress*, 33(1), 29–40.

Arntz, A. (2012). Imagery rescripting as a therapeutic technique: Review of clinical trials, basic studies, and research agenda. *Journal of Experimental Psychopathology*, 3(2), 189–208.

Arntz, A., & Van Genderen, H. (2020). *Schema therapy for borderline personality disorder*. John Wiley & Sons.

Arntz, A., & Weertman, A. (1999). Treatment of childhood memories: Theory and practice. *Behaviour Research and Therapy*, 37(8), 715–740.

Australian Psychological Society. (1994). *Guidelines relating to the reporting of recovered memories*. Carlton, South Victoria.

Baas, M. A., van Pampus, M. G., Braam, L., Stramrood, C. A., & de Jongh, A. (2020). The effects of PTSD treatment during pregnancy: systematic review and case study. *European Journal of Psychotraumatology*, 11(1), 1762310.

Babor, T. F., Higgins-Biddle, J. C., Saunders, J. B., & Monteiro, M. G. (2001). *The alcohol use disorders identification test: Guidelines for use in Primary Care*. World Health Organization.

Back, S. E., Foa, E. B., & Killeen, T. K. (2014). *Concurrent treatment of PTSD and substance use disorders using prolonged exposure (COPE): Therapist guide*. Treatments That Work.

Barlow, D. H., Farchione, T. J., Bullis, J. R., Gallagher, M. W., Murray-Latin, H., Sauer-Zavala, S., Bentley, K. H., Thompson-Hollands, J., Conklin, L. R., Boswell, J. F., Ametaj, A., Carl, J. R., Boettcher, H., & Cassiello-Robbins, C. (2017). The unified protocol for transdiagnostic treatment of emotional disorders compared with diagnosis-specific protocols for anxiety disorders: A randomized clinical trial. *JAMA Psychiatry*, 74(9), 875–884.

Barton, S., Armstrong, P., Wicks, L., Freeman, E., & Meyer, T. D. (2017). Treating complex depression with cognitive behavioural therapy. *The Cognitive Behaviour Therapist*, 10, E17.

Bass, E., & Davis, L. (2002). *The courage to heal: A guide for women survivors of child sexual abuse*. Random House.

Beck, A. (2019). Understanding Black and Minority Ethnic service user's experience of racism as part of the assessment, formulation and treatment of mental health problems in cognitive behaviour therapy. *The Cognitive Behaviour Therapist*, 12, E8.

Beck, A., & Naz, S. (2019). The need for service change and community outreach work to support trans-cultural cognitive behaviour therapy with Black and Minority Ethnic communities. *The Cognitive Behaviour Therapist*, 12, E1.

Beck, A., Naz, S., Brooks, M., & Jankowska, M. (2019). Improving Access to Psychological Therapies (IAPT): Black, Asian and Minority Ethnic service user positive practice guide. Available at: https://babcp.com/Therapists/BAME-Positive-Practice-Guide-PDF

Beck, A. T. (Ed.). (1979). *Cognitive therapy of depression*. Guilford Press.

Beck, A. T. (1987). Cognitive models of depression. *Journal of Cognitive Psychotherapy*, 1(1), 5–37.

Beck, J. G., & Clapp, J. D. (2011). A different kind of comorbidity: Understanding posttraumatic stress disorder and chronic pain. *Psychological Trauma: Theory, Research, Practice, and Policy*, 3(2), 101–108.

Beck, J. G., Coffey, S. F., Foy, D. W., Keane, T. M., & Blanchard, E. B. (2009). Group cognitive behavior therapy for chronic posttraumatic stress disorder: An initial randomized pilot study. *Behavior Therapy*, 40(1), 82–2.

Bedard-Gilligan, M., Garcia, N., Zoellner, L. A., & Feeny, N. C. (2018). Alcohol, cannabis, and other drug use: Engagement and outcome in PTSD treatment. *Psychology of Addictive Behaviors*, 32(3), 277–288.

Beierl, E. T., Böllinghaus, I., Clark, D. M., Glucksman, E., & Ehlers, A. (2020). Cognitive paths from trauma to posttraumatic stress disorder: A prospective study of Ehlers and Clark's model in survivors of assaults or road traffic collisions. *Psychological Medicine*, 1–10.

Bellet, B. W., Jones, P. J., & McNally, R. J. (2020). Self-triggering? An exploration of individuals who seek reminders of trauma. *Clinical Psychological Science*, 8(4), 739–755.

Bendall, S., Jackson, H. J., Hulbert, C. A., & McGorry, P. D. (2008). Childhood trauma and psychotic disorders: A systematic, critical review of the evidence. *Schizophrenia Bulletin*, 34(3), 568–579.

Bennett, H., & Wells, A. (2010). Metacognition, memory disorganization and rumination in posttraumatic stress symptoms. *Journal of Anxiety Disorders*, 24(3), 318–325.

Bennett-Levy, J. (2006). Therapist skills: A cognitive model of their acquisition and refinement. *Behavioural and Cognitive Psychotherapy*, 34(1), 57–78.

Bennett-Levy, J. E., Butler, G. E., Fennell, M. E., Hackman, A. E., Mueller, M. E., & Westbrook, D. E. (2004). *Oxford guide to behavioural experiments in cognitive therapy*. Oxford University Press.

Ben-Zur, H., & Zeidner, M. (2009). Threat to life and risk-taking behaviors: A review of empirical findings and explanatory models. *Personality and Social Psychology Review*, 13(2), 109–128.

Berntsen, D., & Rubin, D. C. (2006). The centrality of event scale: A measure of integrating a trauma into one's identity and its relation to post-traumatic stress disorder symptoms. *Behaviour Research and Therapy*, 44(2), 219–231.

Birchwood, M., Michail, M., Meaden, A., Tarrier, N., Lewis, S., Wykes, T., Davies, L., Dunn, G., & Peters, E. (2014). Cognitive behaviour therapy to prevent harmful compliance with command hallucinations (COMMAND): A randomised controlled trial. *The Lancet Psychiatry*, 1(1), 23–33.

Black, M., Hitchcock, C., Bevan, A., Leary, C. O., Clarke, J., Elliott, R., Watson, P., LaFortune, L., Rae, S., Gilbody, S., & Kuyken, W. (2018). The HARMONIC trial: Study protocol for a randomised controlled feasibility trial of Shaping Healthy Minds – a modular transdiagnostic intervention for mood, stressor-related and anxiety disorders in adults. *BMJ Open*, 8(8), e024546.

Blakey, S. M., Love, H., Lindquist, L., Beckham, J. C., & Elbogen, E. B. (2018). Disentangling the link between posttraumatic stress disorder and violent behavior: Findings from a nationally representative sample. *Journal of Consulting and Clinical Psychology*, 86(2), 169–178.

Blanchard, E. B., Hickling, E. J., Mitnick, N., Taylor, A. E., Loos, W. R., & Buckley, T. C. (1995). The impact of severity of physical injury and perception of life threat in the development of post-traumatic stress disorder in motor vehicle accident victims. *Behaviour Research and Therapy*, 33(5), 529–534.

Blasco-Fontecilla, H., Fernández-Fernández, R., Colino, L., Fajardo, L., Perteguer-Barrio, R., & De Leon, J. (2016). The addictive model of self-harming (non-suicidal and suicidal) behavior. *Frontiers in Psychiatry*, 7, 8.

Boals, A., & Ruggero, C. (2016). Event centrality prospectively predicts PTSD symptoms. *Anxiety, Stress, & Coping*, 29(5), 533–541.

Boelen, P. A., de Keijser, J., van den Hout, M. A., & van den Bout, J. (2007). Treatment of complicated grief: A comparison between cognitive-behavioral therapy and supportive counseling. *Journal of Consulting and Clinical Psychology*, 75(2), 277–284.

Boelen, P. A., Van Den Hout, M. A., & Van Den Bout, J. (2006). A cognitive-behavioral conceptualization of complicated grief. *Clinical Psychology: Science and Practice*, 13(2), 109–128.
Bordin, E. S. (1979). The generalizability of the psychoanalytic concept of the working alliance. *Psychotherapy: Theory, Research and Practice*, 16, 252–260.
Brady, F., Warnock-Parkes, E., Barker, C., & Ehlers, A. (2015). Early in-session predictors of response to trauma-focused cognitive therapy for posttraumatic stress disorder. *Behaviour Research and Therapy*, 75, 40–47.
Brake, C., Adams, T., Hood, C., & Badour, C. (2019). Posttraumatic mental contamination and the interpersonal psychological theory of suicide: Effects via DSM-5 PTSD symptom clusters. *Cognitive Therapy and Research*, 43, 259–271.
Brand, R. M., Hardy, A., Bendall, S., & Thomas, N. (2020). A tale of two outcomes: Remission and exacerbation in the use of trauma-focused imaginal exposure for trauma-related voice-hearing. Key learnings to guide future practice. *Clinical Psychologist*, 24(2), 195–205.
Brand, R. M., McEnery, C., Rossell, S., Bendall, S., & Thomas, N. (2018). Do trauma-focussed psychological interventions have an effect on psychotic symptoms? A systematic review and meta-analysis. *Schizophrenia Research*, 195, 13–22.
Brandon, S., Boakes, J., Glaser, D., & Green, R. (1998). Recovered memories of childhood sexual abuse: Implications for clinical practice. *The British Journal of Psychiatry*, 172(4), 296–307.
Breslau, N., Davis, G. C., Peterson, E. L., & Schultz, L. (1997). Psychiatric sequelae of posttraumatic stress disorder in women. *Archives of General Psychiatry*, 54(1), 81–87.
Brewin, C. R. (2006). Understanding cognitive behaviour therapy: A retrieval competition account. *Behaviour Research and Therapy*, 44(6), 765–784.
Brewin, C. R., & Andrews, B. (2014). Why it is scientifically respectable to believe in repression: A response to Patihis, Ho, Tingen, Lilienfeld, and Loftus (2014). *Psychological Science*, 25(10), 1964–1966.
Brewin, C. R., Dalgleish, T., & Joseph, S. (1996). A dual representation theory of posttraumatic stress disorder. *Psychological Review*, 103(4), 670–686.
Brewin, C. R., Gregory, J. D., Lipton, M., & Burgess, N. (2010). Intrusive images in psychological disorders: Characteristics, neural mechanisms, and treatment implications. *Psychological Review*, 117(1), 210–232.
Brewin, C. R., & Patel, T. (2010). Auditory pseudohallucinations in United Kingdom war veterans and civilians with posttraumatic stress disorder. *The Journal of Clinical Psychiatry*, 71(4), 419–425.
Briere, J. (2019). *Treating risky and compulsive behavior in trauma survivors*. Guilford Press.
British Psychological Society. (2016). *Guidance on the Management of Disclosures of Non-Recent (Historic) Child Sexual Abuse*. www.bps.org.uk/news-and-policy/guidance-management-disclosures-non-recent-historic-child-sexual-abuse-2016
British Psychological Society. (2017). *Psychology at work: Improving wellbeing and productivity in the workplace*. www.bps.org.uk/news-and-policy/sychology-work-improving-wellbeing-and-productivity-workplace
Brown, R. J., & Reuber, M. (2016a). Towards an integrative theory of psychogenic non-epileptic seizures (PNES). *Clinical Psychology Review*, 47, 55–70.
Brown, R. J., & Reuber, M. (2016b). Psychological and psychiatric aspects of psychogenic non-epileptic seizures (PNES): A systematic review. *Clinical Psychology Review*, 45, 157–182.
Brown, T. A., Campbell, L. A., Lehman, C. L., Grisham, J. R., & Mancill, R. B. (2001). Current and lifetime comorbidity of the DSM-IV anxiety and mood disorders in a large clinical sample. *Journal of Abnormal Psychology*, 110(4), 585.
Bryan, A. O., Bryan, C. J., Morrow, C. E., Etienne, N., & Ray-Sannerud, B. (2014). Moral injury, suicidal ideation, and suicide attempts in a military sample. *Traumatology*, 20(3), 154–160.
Bryan, C. J. (2016). Treating PTSD within the context of heightened suicide risk. *Current Psychiatry Reports*, 18(8), 73.
Bryan, C. J., & Rudd, M. D. (2018). *Brief cognitive-behavioral therapy for suicide prevention*. Guilford Press.
Bryant, R. A. (2019). Post-traumatic stress disorder: A state-of-the-art review of evidence and challenges. *World Psychiatry*, 18(3), 259–269.

Burnham, J. (2012). Developments in Social GGRRAAACCEEESSS: Visible–invisible, voiced–unvoiced. In I. Krause (Ed.), *Culture and reflexivity in systemic psychotherapy* (pp. 139–160). Karnac.

Burns, D. (2008). *Feeling good:The new mood therapy*. Harper.

Buswell, G., Haime, Z., Lloyd-Evans, B., & Billings, J. (2021). A systematic review of PTSD to the experience of psychosis: prevalence and associated factors. *BMC psychiatry*, *21*(1), 1–13.

Cadman, L., Waller, J., Ashdown-Barr, L., & Szarewski, A. (2012). Barriers to cervical screening in women who have experienced sexual abuse: An exploratory study. *Journal of Family Planning and Reproductive Health Care*, *38*(4), 214–220.

Carey, M., & Wells, C. (2019). Cognitive Behavioural Therapy Suicide Prevention (CBT-SP) imagery intervention: A case report. *Cognitive Behaviour Therapist*, *12*. Cambridge University Press.

Carlson, E. B., Dalenberg, C., & McDade-Montez, E. (2012). Dissociation in posttraumatic stress disorder part I: Definitions and review of research. *Psychological Trauma:Theory, Research, Practice, and Policy*, *4*(5), 479–489.

Carmassi, C., Akiskal, H. S., Yong, S. S., Stratta, P., Calderani, E., Massimetti, E., Akiskal, K. K., Rossi, A., & Dell'Osso, L. (2013). Post-traumatic stress disorder in DSM-5: Estimates of prevalence and criteria comparison versus DSM-IV-TR in a non-clinical sample of earthquake survivors. *Journal of Affective Disorders*, *151*(3), 843–848.

Carragher, N., Sunderland, M., Batterham, P. J., Calear, A. L., Elhai, J. D., Chapman, C., & Mills, K. (2016). Discriminant validity and gender differences in DSM-5 posttraumatic stress disorder symptoms. *Journal of Affective Disorders*, *190*, 56–67.

Carrigan, N., & Allez, K. (2017). Cognitive behaviour therapy for post-traumatic stress disorder in a person with an autism spectrum condition and intellectual disability: A case study. *Journal of Applied Research in Intellectual Disabilities*, *30*(2), 326–335.

Casey, B. J., Craddock, N., Cuthbert, B. N., Hyman, S. E., Lee, F. S., & Ressler, K. J. (2013). DSM-5 and RDoC: progress in psychiatry research?. *Nature Reviews Neuroscience*, *14*(11), 810–814.

Černis, E., Cooper, M., & Chan, C. (2018). Developing a new measure of dissociation: The Dissociative Experiences Measure, Oxford. *Psychiatry Research*, *269*, 229–236.

Chard, K. M., Ricksecker, E. G., Healy, E. T., Karlin, B. E., & Resick, P. A. (2012). Dissemination and experience with cognitive processing therapy. *Journal of Rehabilitation Research & Development*, *49*(5), 667–678.

Chemtob, C. M., Novaco, R. W., Hamada, R. S., & Gross, D. M. (1997). Cognitive-behavioral treatment for severe anger in posttraumatic stress disorder. *Journal of Consulting and Clinical Psychology*, *65*(1), 184–189.

Chilcoat, H. D., & Breslau, N. (1998). Posttraumatic stress disorder and drug disorders: Testing causal pathways. *Archives of General Psychiatry*, *55*(10), 913–917.

Christianson, S. Å., & Safer, M. A. (1996). Emotional events and emotions in autobiographical memories. In D. C. Rubin (Ed.), *Remembering our past: Studies in autobiographical memory* (pp. 218–243). Cambridge University Press.

Chu, J., & Leino, A. (2017). Advancement in the maturing science of cultural adaptations of evidence-based interventions. *Journal of Consulting and Clinical Psychology*, *85*(1), 45–57.

Clapp, J. D., & Beck, J. G. (2012). Treatment of PTSD in older adults: Do cognitive-behavioral interventions remain viable?. *Cognitive and Behavioral Practice*, *19*(1), 126–135.

Clark, D. M. (1986). A cognitive approach to panic. *Behaviour Research and Therapy*, *24*(4), 461–470.

Clark, D. M. (1999). Anxiety disorders: Why they persist and how to treat them. *Behaviour Research and Therapy*, *37*(1), 5–27.

Clohessy, S., & Ehlers, A. (1999). PTSD symptoms, response to intrusive memories and coping in ambulance service workers. *British Journal of Clinical Psychology*, *38*(3), 251–265.

Cloitre, M. (2020). ICD-11 complex post-traumatic stress disorder: Simplifying diagnosis in trauma populations. *The British Journal of Psychiatry*, *216*(3), 129–131.

Cloitre, M. (2021). Complex PTSD: assessment and treatment. *European Journal of Psychotraumatology*, *12*(sup1), 1866423.

Cloitre, M., Garvert, D. W., Weiss, B., Carlson, E. B., & Bryant, R. A. (2014). Distinguishing PTSD, complex PTSD, and borderline personality disorder: A latent class analysis. *European Journal of Psychotraumatology*, *5*(1), 25097.

Cloitre, M., Koenen, K. C., Cohen, L. R., & Han, H. (2002). Skills training in affective and interpersonal regulation followed by exposure: A phase-based treatment for PTSD related to childhood abuse. *Journal of Consulting and Clinical Psychology*, 70(5), 1067–1074.

Cloitre, M., Shevlin, M., Brewin, C. R., Bisson, J. I., Roberts, N. P., Maercker, A., Karatzias, T., & Hyland, P. (2018). The International Trauma Questionnaire: Development of a self-report measure of ICD-11 PTSD and complex PTSD. *Acta Psychiatrica Scandinavica*, 138(6), 536–546.

Coffey, S. F., Schumacher, J. A., Nosen, E., Littlefield, A. K., Henslee, A. M., Lappen, A., & Stasiewicz, P. R. (2016). Trauma-focused exposure therapy for chronic posttraumatic stress disorder in alcohol and drug dependent patients: A randomized controlled trial. *Psychology of Addictive Behaviors*, 30(7), 778–790.

Compean, E., & Hamner, M. (2019). Posttraumatic stress disorder with secondary psychotic features (PTSD-SP): Diagnostic and treatment challenges. *Progress in Neuro-Psychopharmacology and Biological Psychiatry*, 88, 265–275.

Conner, K. R., Lathrop, S., Caetano, R., Wiegand, T., Kaukeinen, K., & Nolte, K. B. (2017). Presence of alcohol, cocaine, and other drugs in suicide and motor vehicle crash decedents ages 18 to 54. *Alcoholism: clinical and experimental research*, 41(3), 571–575.

Contractor, A. A., & Weiss, N. H. (2019). Typologies of PTSD clusters and reckless/self-destructive behaviors: A latent profile analysis. *Psychiatry Research*, 272, 682–691.

Contractor, A. A., Weiss, N. H., Dranger, P., Ruggero, C., & Armour, C. (2017). PTSD's risky behavior criterion: Relation with DSM-5 PTSD symptom clusters and psychopathology. *Psychiatry Research*, 252, 215–222.

Contractor, A. A., Weiss, N. H., Kearns, N. T., Caldas, S. V., & Dixon-Gordon, K. L. (2020). Assessment of posttraumatic stress disorder's E2 criterion: Development, pilot testing, and validation of the Posttrauma Risky Behaviors Questionnaire. *International Journal of Stress Management*, 27(3), 292–303.

Conway, M. A., & Loveday, C. (2015). Remembering, imagining, false memories & personal meanings. *Consciousness and cognition*, 33, 574–581.

Coons, P. M. (1994). Confirmation of childhood abuse in child and adolescent cases of multiple personality disorder and dissociative disorder not otherwise specified. *Journal of Nervous and Mental Disease*, 182, 461–464.

Cordon, I. M., Pipe, M. E., Sayfan, L., Melinder, A., & Goodman, G. S. (2004). Memory for traumatic experiences in early childhood. *Developmental Review*, 24(1), 101–132.

Coughtrey, A. E., Shafran, R., Knibbs, D., & Rachman, S. J. (2012). Mental contamination in obsessive–compulsive disorder. *Journal of Obsessive-Compulsive and Related Disorders*, 1(4), 244–250.

Coventry, P. A., Meader, N., Melton, H., Temple, M., Dale, H., Wright, K., Cloitre, M., Karatzias, T., Bisson, J., Roberts, N. P., Brown, J. V. E., Barbui, C., Churchill, R., Lovell, K., McMillan, D., & Gilbody, S. (2020). Psychological and pharmacological interventions for posttraumatic stress disorder and comorbid mental health problems following complex traumatic events: Systematic review and component network meta-analysis. *PLoS medicine*, 17(8), e1003262.

Craig, C. D., & Sprang, G. (2010). Compassion satisfaction, compassion fatigue, and burnout in a national sample of trauma treatment therapists. *Anxiety, Stress, & Coping*, 23(3), 319–339.

Craske, M. G. (2012). Transdiagnostic treatment for anxiety and depression. *Depression and Anxiety*, 29(9), 749–753.

Craske, M. G., & Mystkowski, J. L. (2006). Exposure therapy and extinction: Clinical studies. In M. G. Craske, D. Hermans, & D. Vansteenwegen (Eds.). *Fear and learning: From basic processes to clinical implications* (pp. 217–233). American Psychological Association.

Craske, M. G., Treanor, M., Conway, C. C., Zbozinek, T., & Vervliet, B. (2014). Maximizing exposure therapy: An inhibitory learning approach. *Behaviour Research and Therapy*, 58, 10–23.

Crime Prosecution Service. (2020). *Guidance on Pre-Trial Therapy*. www.cps.gov.uk/publication/guidance-pre-trial-therapy

Crombag, H. F., Wagenaar, W. A., & Van Koppen, P. J. (1996). Crashing memories and the problem of 'source monitoring'. *Applied Cognitive Psychology*, 10(2), 95–104.

Cunningham, K. C. (2020). Shame and guilt in PTSD. In M. Tull & N. Kimbrel (Eds.) *Emotion in posttraumatic stress disorder* (pp. 145–171). Academic Press.

Dalenberg, C. J. (2004). Maintaining the safe and effective therapeutic relationship in the context of distrust and anger: Countertransference and complex trauma. *Psychotherapy: Theory, Research, Practice, Training*, 41(4), 438–447.

Davidson, K. M. (2014). CBT for people with personality disorders. In A. Whittington, & N. Grey. (Eds.). *How to become a more effective CBT therapist: Mastering metacompetence in clinical practice*. John Wiley & Sons.

Deary, V., Chalder, T., & Sharpe, M. (2007). The cognitive behavioural model of medically unexplained symptoms: a theoretical and empirical review. *Clinical Psychology Review*, 27(7), 781–797.

de Bont, P. A. J. M., van den Berg, D. P. G., van der Vleugel, B. M., de Roos, C. J. A. M., de Jongh, A., van der Gaag, M., & van Minnen, A. M. (2016). Prolonged exposure and EMDR for PTSD v. a PTSD waiting-list condition: Effects on symptoms of psychosis, depression and social functioning in patients with chronic psychotic disorders. *Psychological Medicine*, 46(11), 2411–2421.

de Jongh, A., Groenland, G. N., Sanches, S., Bongaerts, H., Voorendonk, E. M., & Van Minnen, A. (2020). The impact of brief intensive trauma-focused treatment for PTSD on symptoms of borderline personality disorder. *European Journal of Psychotraumatology*, 11(1), 1721142.

de Jongh, A., Resick, P. A., Zoellner, L. A., van Minnen, A., Lee, C. W., Monson, C. M., Foa, E. B., Wheeler, K., Broeke, E. T., Feeny, N., Rauch, S. A., Chard, K. M., Mueser, K. T., Sloan, D. M., van der Gaag, M., Rothbaum, B. O., Neuner, F., de Roos, C., Hehenkamp, L. M. J., … Bicanic, I. A. E. (2016). Critical analysis of the current treatment guidelines for complex PTSD in adults. *Depression and Anxiety*, 33(5), 359–369.

Deliramich, A. N., & Gray, M. J. (2008). Changes in women's sexual behavior following sexual assault. *Behavior Modification*, 32(5), 611–621.

Department of Health. (2003). *Confidentiality: NHS code of practice*. www.gov.uk/government/publications/confidentiality-nhs-code-of-practice

Derogatis, L. R. (1993). *Brief Symptom Inventory. Administration, scoring, and procedures manual* (4th ed.). National Computer Systems.

Dixon, L. E., Ahles, E., & Marques, L. (2016). Treating posttraumatic stress disorder in diverse settings: recent advances and challenges for the future. *Current Psychiatry Reports*, 18(12), 107–117.

Dougall, A. L., & Baum, A. (2004). Psychoneuroimmunology and trauma. In P. P. Schnurr & B. L. Green (Eds.), *Trauma and health: Physical health consequences of exposure to extreme stress* (pp. 129–155). American Psychological Association.

Drescher, K. D., Rosen, C. S., Burling, T. A., & Foy, D. W. (2003). Causes of death among male veterans who received residential treatment for PTSD. *Journal of Traumatic Stress*, 16(6), 535–543.

Duffy, M., & Wild, J. (2017). A cognitive approach to persistent complex bereavement disorder (PCBD). *The Cognitive Behaviour Therapist*, 10, 1–19.

Dunmore, E., Clark, D. M., & Ehlers, A. (2001). A prospective investigation of the role of cognitive factors in persistent posttraumatic stress disorder (PTSD) after physical or sexual assault. *Behaviour Research and Therapy*, 39(9), 1063–1084.

Eccles, J. A., Owens, A. P., Mathias, C. J., Umeda, S., & Critchley, H. D. (2015). Neurovisceral phenotypes in the expression of psychiatric symptoms. *Frontiers in Neuroscience*, 9, 4.

Egede, L. E., & Osborn, C. Y. (2010). Role of motivation in the relationship between depression, self-care, and glycemic control in adults with type 2 diabetes. *The Diabetes Educator*, 36(2), 276–283.

Ehlers, A., & Clark, D. M. (2000). A cognitive model of posttraumatic stress disorder. *Behaviour Research and Therapy*, 38(4), 319–345.

Ehlers, A., Clark, D. M., Hackmann, A., McManus, F., & Fennell, M. (2005). Cognitive therapy for post-traumatic stress disorder: development and evaluation. *Behaviour Research and Therapy*, 43(4), 413–431.

Ehlers, A., Clark, D. M., Hackmann, A., McManus, F., Fennell, M., Herbert, C., & Mayou, R. (2003). A Randomized controlled trial of cognitive therapy, a self-help booklet, and repeated assessments as early interventions for posttraumatic stress disorder. *Archives of General Psychiatry*, 60(10), 1024–1032.

Ehlers, A., Grey, N., Wild, J., Stott, R., Liness, S., Deale, A., Handley, R., Albert, I., Cullen, D., Hackman, A., Manley, J., McManus, F., Brady, F., Salkovskis, P., & Clark, D. M. (2013). Implementation of cognitive therapy for PTSD in routine clinical care: Effectiveness and moderators of outcome in a consecutive sample. *Behaviour Research and Therapy*, 51(11), 742–752.

Ehlers, A., Hackmann, A., Grey, N., Wild, J., Liness, S., Albert, I., Deale, A., Stott, R., & Clark, D. M. (2014). A randomized controlled trial of 7-day intensive and standard weekly cognitive therapy for PTSD and emotion-focused supportive therapy. *American Journal of Psychiatry*, 171(3), 294–304.

Ehlers, A., Maercker, A., & Boos, A. (2000). Posttraumatic stress disorder following political imprisonment: The role of mental defeat, alienation, and perceived permanent change. *Journal of Abnormal Psychology*, 109(1), 45–55.

Ehring, T., Kleim, B., & Ehlers, A. (2012). Cognition and emotion in posttraumatic stress disorder. In M. D. Robinson, E. Watkins, & E. Harmon-Jones (Eds.), *Handbook of cognition and emotion* (pp. 401–420). Guilford Press.

Elbogen, E. B., Fuller, S., Johnson, S. C., Brooks, S., Kinneer, P., Calhoun, P. S., & Beckham, J. C. (2010). Improving risk assessment of violence among military veterans: An evidence-based approach for clinical decision-making. *Clinical psychology review*, 30(6), 595–607.

Elbogen, E. B., Johnson, S. C., Wagner, H. R., Sullivan, C., Taft, C. T., & Beckham, J. C. (2014). Violent behaviour and post-traumatic stress disorder in US Iraq and Afghanistan veterans. *The British Journal of Psychiatry*, 204(5), 368–375.

Ellard, K. K., Fairholme, C. P., Boisseau, C. L., Farchione, T. J., & Barlow, D. H. (2010). Unified protocol for the transdiagnostic treatment of emotional disorders: Protocol development and initial outcome data. *Cognitive and Behavioral Practice*, 17(1), 88–101.

El-Leithy, S. (2014). Working with diversity in CBT. In A. Whittington, & N. Grey. (Eds.). *How to become a more effective CBT therapist: Mastering metacompetence in clinical practice* (pp. 44–62). Routledge.

Ellis, A. E., Simiola, V., Brown, L., Courtois, C., & Cook, J. M. (2018). The role of evidence-based therapy relationships on treatment outcome for adults with trauma: A systematic review. *Journal of Trauma & Dissociation*, 19(2), 185–213.

Elrassas, H. H., Elsayed, Y. A., El Nagar, Z. M., Abdeen, M. S., & Mohamed, A. T. (2020). Cognitive impairment in patients diagnosed with tramadol dependence compared to healthy controls. *International Clinical Psychopharmacology*, 36(1), 38–44.

Elwood, L. S., Hahn, K. S., Olatunji, B. O., & Williams, N. L. (2009). Cognitive vulnerabilities to the development of PTSD: A review of four vulnerabilities and the proposal of an integrative vulnerability model. *Clinical Psychology Review*, 29(1), 87–100.

Engelbrecht, A., & Jobson, L. (2016). Exploring trauma associated appraisals in trauma survivors from collectivistic cultures. *Springerplus*, 5(1), 1–11.

Espay, A. J., Aybek, S., Carson, A., Edwards, M. J., Goldstein, L. H., Hallett, M., LaFaver, K., LaFrance, W. C., Lang, A. E., Nicholson, T., Nielsen, G., Reuber, M., Voon, V., Stone, J., & Morgante, F. (2018). Current concepts in diagnosis and treatment of functional neurological disorders. *JAMA Neurology*, 75(9), 1132–1141.

Fairbrother, N., & Rachman, S. (2004). Feelings of mental pollution subsequent to sexual assault. *Behaviour Research and Therapy*, 42(2), 173–189.

Faw, B. (2009). Conflicting intuitions may be based on differing abilities: Evidence from mental imaging research. *Journal of Consciousness Studies*, 16(4), 45–68.

Feinstein, A., & Phil, M. (2006). *Journalists under fire: The psychological hazards of covering war*. JHU Press.

Figley, C. R. (1995). Compassion fatigue: Toward a new understanding of the costs of caring. In B. H. Stamm (Ed.), *Secondary traumatic stress: Self-care issues for clinicians, researchers, and educators* (pp. 3–28). The Sidran Press.

Figley, C. R. (Ed.). (2002). *Treating compassion fatigue*. Routledge.

First, M. B., & Williams, J. B. W. (2021). *Quick Structured Clinical Interview for DSM-5 Disorders (QuickSCID-5)*. American Psychiatric Association.

First, M. B., Williams, J. B. W., Karg, R. S., & Spitzer, R. L. (2016). *Structured Clinical Interview for DSM-5 Disorders, Clinician Version (SCID-5-CV)*. American Psychiatric Association.

Fisher, J. (1999). The work of stabilization in trauma treatment. *Trauma Center Lecture Series, Boston, Massachusetts*. https://janinafisher.com/pdfs/stabilize.pdf

Flood, A. M., Boyle, S. H., Calhoun, P. S., Dennis, M. F., Barefoot, J. C., Moore, S. D., & Beckham, J. C. (2010). Prospective study of externalizing and internalizing subtypes of posttraumatic stress disorder and their relationship to mortality among Vietnam veterans. *Comprehensive Psychiatry, 51*(3), 236–242.

Foa, E. B., Ehlers, A., Clark, D. M., Tolin, D. F., & Orsillo, S. M. (1999). The posttraumatic cognitions inventory (PTCI): Development and validation. *Psychological Assessment, 11*(3), 303–314.

Foa, E. B., Gillihan, S. J., & Bryant, R. A. (2013). Challenges and successes in dissemination of evidence-based treatments for posttraumatic stress: Lessons learned from prolonged exposure therapy for PTSD. *Psychological Science in the Public Interest, 14*(2), 65–111.

Foa, E. B., Hembree, E. A., & Rothbaum, B. O. (2007). *Prolonged exposure therapy for PTSD: Emotional processing of traumatic experiences: Therapist guide*. Oxford University Press.

Foa, E. B., & Rothbaum, B. O. (1998). *Treating the trauma of rape*. Guilford Press.

Foa, E. B., Steketee, G., & Rothbaum, B. O. (1989). Behavioral/cognitive conceptualizations of post-traumatic stress disorder. *Behavior Therapy, 20*(2), 155–176.

Focht-New, G., Clements, P. T., Barol, B., Faulkner, M. J., & Service, K. P. (2008). Persons with developmental disabilities exposed to interpersonal violence and crime: Strategies and guidance for assessment. *Perspectives in Psychiatric Care, 44*(1), 3–13.

Forbes, D., Creamer, M., Bisson, J. I., Cohen, J. A., Crow, B. E., Foa, E. B., Friedman, M. J., Keane, T. M., Kudler, H. S., & Ursano, R. J. (2010). A guide to guidelines for the treatment of PTSD and related conditions. *Journal of Traumatic Stress, 23*(5), 537–552.

Forbes, D., Parslow, R., Creamer, M., Allen, N., McHugh, T., & Hopwood, M. (2008). Mechanisms of anger and treatment outcome in combat veterans with posttraumatic stress disorder. *Journal of Traumatic Stress, 21*(2), 142–149.

Frankland, A., & Cohen, L. (1999). Working with recovered memories. *Psychologist, 12*(2), 82–83.

French, C. (2006). Recovered and false memories. *Psychologist, 19*(6), 352–355.

Frewen, P. A., Dozois, D. J., Neufeld, R. W., & Lanius, R. A. (2008). Meta-analysis of alexithymia in posttraumatic stress disorder. *Journal of Traumatic Stress, 21*(2), 243–246.

Friedman, M. J., Schnurr, P., & Keane, T. M. (Eds.). (2021). *Handbook of PTSD: Science and practice* (3rd ed.). Guilford Press.

Galovski, T. E., Monson, C., Bruce, S. E., & Resick, P. A. (2009). Does cognitive-behavioral therapy for PTSD improve perceived health and sleep impairment?. *Journal of Traumatic Stress, 22*(3), 197–204.

Gauntlett-Gilbert, J., Keegan, A., & Petrak, J. (2004). Drug-facilitated sexual assault: Cognitive approaches to treating the trauma. *Behavioural and Cognitive Psychotherapy, 32*(2), 215–223.

Gawande, A. (2010). *Complications: A surgeon's notes on an imperfect science*. Profile Books.

Ghomi, M., Wrightman, M., Ghaemian, A., Grey, N., Pickup, T., & Richardson, T. (2020). Development and validation of the Readiness for Therapy Questionnaire (RTQ). *Behavioural and Cognitive Psychotherapy*, 1–13.

Gillespie, K., Duffy, M., Hackmann, A., & Clark, D. M. (2002). Community based cognitive therapy in the treatment of post-traumatic stress disorder following the Omagh bomb. *Behaviour Research and Therapy, 40*(4), 345–357.

Giourou, E., Skokou, M., Andrew, S. P., Alexopoulou, K., Gourzis, P., & Jelastopulu, E. (2018). Complex posttraumatic stress disorder: The need to consolidate a distinct clinical syndrome or to reevaluate features of psychiatric disorders following interpersonal trauma?. *World Journal of Psychiatry, 8*(1), 12–19.

Glass, K., Flory, K., Hankin, B. L., Kloos, B., & Turecki, G. (2009). Are coping strategies, social support, and hope associated with psychological distress among Hurricane Katrina survivors?. *Journal of Social and Clinical Psychology, 28*(6), 779–795.

Gradus, J. L., Qin, P., Lincoln, A. K., Miller, M., Lawler, E., Sørensen, H. T., & Lash, T. L. (2010). Post-traumatic stress disorder and completed suicide. *American Journal of Epidemiology, 171*(6), 721–727.

Granello, D. H. (2010). The process of suicide risk assessment: Twelve core principles. *Journal of Counseling & Development, 88*(3), 363–370.

Gray, M. J., Nash, W. P., & Litz, B. T. (2017). When self-blame is rational and appropriate: The limited utility of Socratic questioning in the context of moral injury: Commentary on Wachen et al. (2016). *Cognitive and Behavioral Practice, 24*(4), 383–387.

Greenberger, D., & Padesky, C. A. (1995). *Mind over mood: A cognitive therapy treatment manual for clients*. Guilford Press.

Grey, N. (2007). Post-traumatic stress disorder: Investigation. *The Handbook of Clinical Adult Psychology* (pp. 82–102). Routledge.

Grey, N. (2009). Imagery and psychological threat in PTSD. In Stopa, L. (Ed.). *Imagery and the threatened self: Perspectives on mental imagery and the self in cognitive therapy*. Routledge.

Groschwitz, R. C., & Plener, P. L. (2012). The neurobiology of non-suicidal self-injury (NSSI): A review. *Suicidology Online*, 3(1), 24–32.

Grossman, D. (1996). *On killing: The psychological cost of learning to kill in war and society*. Black Boy Books.

Guarnaccia, P. J., Lewis-Fernández, R., & Marano, M. R. (2003). Toward a Puerto Rican popular nosology: Nervios and ataque de nervios. *Culture, Medicine and Psychiatry*, 27(3), 339–366.

Gwozdziewycz, N., & Mehl-Madrona, L. (2013). Meta-analysis of the use of narrative exposure therapy for the effects of trauma among refugee populations. *The Permanente Journal*, 17(1), 70–76.

Hagengimana, A., & Hinton, D. E. (2009). 'Ihahamuka', a Rwandan syndrome of response to the genocide. In D. E. Hinton, & B. J. (Eds.), *Culture and panic disorder* (pp. 204–229). Stanford University Press.

Haney, C., Banks, C., & Zimbardo, P. (1973). Study of prisoners and guards in a simulated prison. *Naval Research Reviews*, 26(9), 1–17.

Hardy, A. (2017). Pathways from trauma to psychotic experiences: A theoretically informed model of posttraumatic stress in psychosis. *Frontiers in Psychology*, 8, 697.

Hardy, A., Emsley, R., Freeman, D., Bebbington, P., Garety, P. A., Kuipers, E. E., Dunn, G., & Fowler, D. (2016). Psychological mechanisms mediating effects between trauma and psychotic symptoms: the role of affect regulation, intrusive trauma memory, beliefs, and depression. *Schizophrenia Bulletin*, 42, S34–S43.

Hardy, A., Fowler, D., Freeman, D., Smith, B., Steel, C., Evans, J., Garety, P., Kuipers, E., Bebbington, P., & Dunn, G. (2005). Trauma and hallucinatory experience in psychosis. *The Journal of Nervous and Mental Disease*, 193(8), 501–507.

Harned, M. S. (2014). The combined treatment of PTSD with borderline personality disorder. *Current Treatment Options in Psychiatry*, 1(4), 335–344.

Harned, M. S., Korslund, K. E., Foa, E. B., & Linehan, M. M. (2012). Treating PTSD in suicidal and self-injuring women with borderline personality disorder: Development and preliminary evaluation of a dialectical behavior therapy prolonged exposure protocol. *Behaviour Research and Therapy*, 50(6), 381–386.

Harvey, M. R. (1999). Memory research and clinical practice: A critique of three paradigms and a framework for psychotherapy with trauma survivors. In L. Williams, & V.L. Banyard. (Eds.), *Trauma and memory*. Sage.

Herman, J. L. (1992). Complex PTSD: A syndrome in survivors of prolonged and repeated trauma. *Journal of Traumatic Stress*, 5(3), 377–391.

Hinton, D., Hinton, S., Um, K., Chea, A., & Sak, S. (2002). The Khmer 'weak heart' syndrome: Fear of death from palpitations. *Transcultural Psychiatry*, 39(3), 323–344.

Hinton, D. E., & Lewis-Fernández, R. (2011). The cross-cultural validity of posttraumatic stress disorder: Implications for DSM-5. *Depression and Anxiety*, 28(9), 783–801.

Hinton, D. E., Rivera, E. I., Hofmann, S. G., Barlow, D. H., & Otto, M. W. (2012). Adapting CBT for traumatized refugees and ethnic minority patients: Examples from culturally adapted CBT (CA-CBT). *Transcultural Psychiatry*, 49(2), 340–365.

Hoeboer, C. M., de Kleine, R. A., Oprel, D. A., Schoorl, M., van der Does, W., & van Minnen, A. (2021). Does complex PTSD predict or moderate treatment outcomes of three variants of exposure therapy?. *Journal of Anxiety Disorders*, 102388.

Hoeboer, C. M., De Kleine, R. A., Molendijk, M. L., Schoorl, M., Oprel, D. A. C., Mouthaan, J., Van der Does, W., & Van Minnen, A. (2020). Impact of dissociation on the effectiveness of psychotherapy for post-traumatic stress disorder: Meta-analysis. *BJPsych Open*, 6(3), e53.

Holmes, E. A., Brown, R. J., Mansell, W., Fearon, R. P., Hunter, E. C. M., Frasquilho, F., & Oakley, D. A. (2005). Are there two qualitatively distinct forms of dissociation? A review and some clinical implications. *Clinical Psychology Review*, 25(1), 1–23.

Horowitz, M. J. (1975). Intrusive and repetitive thoughts after experimental stress: A summary. *Archives of General Psychiatry*, 32(11), 1457–1463.

Hyland, P., Shevlin, M., Karatzias, T., & Cloitre, M. (2020). *The International Trauma Exposure Measure (ITEM)*. Unpublished measure. www.traumameasuresglobal.com/item.

Imel, Z. E., Laska, K., Jakupcak, M., & Simpson, T. L. (2013). Meta-analysis of dropout in treatments for posttraumatic stress disorder. *Journal of Consulting and Clinical Psychology*, 81(3), 394–404.

International Society for Traumatic Stress Studies Guidelines Committee. (2019). ISTSS guidelines position paper on complex PTSD in adults. *International Society for Traumatic Stress Studies*.

Jacobsen, L. K., Southwick, S. M., & Kosten, T. R. (2001). Substance use disorders in patients with posttraumatic stress disorder: A review of the literature. *American Journal of Psychiatry*, 158(8), 1184–1190.

Jaffe, A. E., DiLillo, D., Gratz, K. L., & Messman-Moore, T. L. (2019). Risk for revictimization following interpersonal and noninterpersonal trauma: Clarifying the role of posttraumatic stress symptoms and trauma-related cognitions. *Journal of Traumatic Stress*, 32(1), 42–55.

James, E. L., Lau-Zhu, A., Clark, I. A., Visser, R. M., Hagenaars, M. A., & Holmes, E. A. (2016). The trauma film paradigm as an experimental psychopathology model of psychological trauma: Intrusive memories and beyond. *Clinical Psychology Review*, 47, 106–142.

James, L. M., Strom, T. Q., & Leskela, J. (2014). Risk-taking behaviors and impulsivity among veterans with and without PTSD and mild TBI. *Military Medicine*, 179(4), 357–363.

Janoff-Bulman, R. (1989). Assumptive worlds and the stress of traumatic events: Applications of the schema construct. *Social Cognition*, 7(2), 113–136.

Janoff-Bulman, R. (1992). *Shattered assumptions: Towards a new psychology of trauma*. Free Press.

Janoff-Bulman, R. (2010). *Shattered assumptions*. Simon & Schuster.

Jones, R. S., & Banks, R. (2007). Behavioural treatment of PTSD in a person with Intellectual Disability. *European Journal of Behavior Analysis*, 8(2), 251–256.

Jung, K., & Steil, R. (2012). The feeling of being contaminated in adult survivors of childhood sexual abuse and its treatment via a two-session program of cognitive restructuring and imagery modification: A case study. *Behavior Modification*, 36(1), 67–86.

Jung, K., & Steil, R. (2013). A randomized controlled trial on cognitive restructuring and imagery modification to reduce the feeling of being contaminated in adult survivors of childhood sexual abuse suffering from posttraumatic stress disorder. *Psychotherapy and Psychosomatics*, 82(4), 213–220.

Karatzias, T., Howard, R., Power, K., Socherel, F., Heath, C., & Livingstone, A. (2017). Organic vs. functional neurological disorders: The role of childhood psychological trauma. *Child Abuse and Neglect*, 63, 1–6.

Kaysen, D., Atkins, D. C., Moore, S. A., Lindgren, K. P., Dillworth, T., & Simpson, T. (2011). Alcohol use, problems, and the course of posttraumatic stress disorder: A prospective study of female crime victims. *Journal of Dual Diagnosis*, 7(4), 262–279.

Keane, T. M., Zimering, R. T., & Caddell, J. M. (1985). A behavioral formulation of posttraumatic stress disorder in Vietnam veterans. *Behavior Therapist*, 8(1), 9–12.

Keen, N., Hunter, E., & Peters, E. (2017). Integrated trauma-focused cognitive-behavioural therapy for post-traumatic stress and psychotic symptoms: A case-series study using imaginal reprocessing strategies. *Frontiers in Psychiatry*, 8, 92.

Keller, S. M., Zoellner, L. A., & Feeny, N. C. (2010). Understanding factors associated with early therapeutic alliance in PTSD treatment: Adherence, childhood sexual abuse history, and social support. *Journal of Consulting and Clinical Psychology*, 78(6), 974–979.

Kessler, R. C., Chiu, W. T., Demler, O., & Walters, E. E. (2005). Prevalence, Severity, and Comorbidity of 12-Month DSM-IV Disorders in the National Comorbidity Survey Replication. *Archives of General Psychiatry*, 62(6), 617–627.

Killgore, W. D., Cotting, D. I., Thomas, J. L., Cox, A. L., McGurk, D., Vo, A. H., Castro, C. A., & Hoge, C. W. (2008). Post-combat invincibility: Violent combat experiences are associated with increased risk-taking propensity following deployment. *Journal of Psychiatric Research*, 42(13), 1112–1121.

Killikelly, C., Zhou, N., Merzhvynska, M., Stelzer, E. M., Dotschung, T., Rohner, S., Han Sun, L., & Maercker, A. (2020). Development of the International Prolonged Grief Disorder Scale for the

ICD-11: Measurement of core symptoms and culture items adapted for Chinese and German-speaking samples. *Journal of Affective Disorders*, 277, 568–576.
Kircanski, K., Lieberman, M. D., & Craske, M. G. (2012). Feelings into words: Contributions of language to exposure therapy. *Psychological Science*, 23(10), 1086–1091.
Kleim, B., Ehlers, A., & Glucksman, E. (2007). Early predictors of chronic post-traumatic stress disorder in assault survivors. *Psychological Medicine*, 37(10), 1457–1467.
Kleim, B., Grey, N., Wild, J., Nussbeck, F. W., Stott, R., Hackmann, A., Clark, D. M., & Ehlers, A. (2013). Cognitive change predicts symptom reduction with cognitive therapy for posttraumatic stress disorder. *Journal of Consulting and Clinical Psychology*, 81(3), 383–393.
Klonsky, E. D., Saffer, B. Y., & Bryan, C. J. (2018). Ideation-to-action theories of suicide: A conceptual and empirical update. *Current Opinion in Psychology*, 22, 38–43.
Kopelman, M. D. (2002). Disorders of memory. *Brain*, 125(10), 2152–2190.
Kozlowska, K., Walker, P., McLean, L., & Carrive, P. (2015). Fear and the defense cascade: Clinical implications and management. *Harvard Review of Psychiatry*, 23(4), 263–287.
Krakow, B., & Zadra, A. (2010). Imagery rehearsal therapy: Principles and practice. *Sleep Medicine Clinics*, 5(2), 289–298.
Kubany, E. S., & Manke, F. P. (1995). Cognitive therapy for trauma-related guilt: Conceptual bases and treatment outlines. *Cognitive and Behavioral Practice*, 2(1), 27–61.
Kubany, E. S., & Ralston, T. (2008). *Treating PTSD in battered women: A step-by-step manual for therapists and counselors*. New Harbinger Publications.
Kulkarni, J. (2017). Complex PTSD: A better description for borderline personality disorder?. *Australasian Psychiatry*, 25(4), 333–335.
Lang, P. J. (1977). Imagery in therapy: An information processing analysis of fear. *Behavior Therapy*, 8(5), 862–886.
Leahy, R. L. (2002). A model of emotional schemas. *Cognitive and Behavioral Practice*, 9(3), 177–190.
Leahy, R. L. (2003). Emotional Schemas and Resistance. In R. L. Leahy (Ed.), *Roadblocks in cognitive-behavioral therapy: Transforming challenges into opportunities for change* (pp. 91–115). Guilford Press.
Leahy, R. L. (2007). Emotional Schemas and Resistance to Change in Anxiety Disorders. *Cognitive and Behavioral Practice*, 14(1), 36–45.
Lechner-Meichsner, F., & Steil, R. (2021). A clinician rating to diagnose CPTSD according to ICD-11 and to evaluate CPTSD symptom severity: Complex PTSD Item Set additional to the CAPS (COPISAC). *European Journal of Psychotraumatology*, 12(1), 1891726.
Lee, D. A. (2005). The perfect nurturer: A model to develop a compassionate mind within the context of cognitive therapy. In P. Gilbert (Ed.), *Compassion: Conceptualisations, research and use in psychotherapy* (pp. 338–363). Routledge.
Lee, D. A., Scragg, P., & Turner, S. (2001). The role of shame and guilt in traumatic events: A clinical model of shame-based and guilt-based PTSD. *British Journal of Medical Psychology*, 74(4), 451–466.
Lillie, M., & Strelan, P. (2016). Careful what you wish for: Fantasizing about revenge increases justice dissatisfaction in the chronically powerless. *Personality and Individual Differences*, 94, 290–294.
Linehan, M. M. (1987). Dialectical behavior therapy for borderline personality disorder: Theory and method. *Bulletin of the Menninger Clinic*, 51(3), 261–276.
Linehan, M. M. (2014). *DBT? Skills Training Handouts and Worksheets*. Guilford Press.
Linehan, M. M., Bohus, M., & Lynch, T. R. (2007). Dialectical behavior therapy for pervasive emotion dysregulation. *Handbook of Emotion Regulation*, 1, 581–605.
Litz, B. T., Lebowitz, L., Gray, M. J., & Nash, W. P. (2017). *Adaptive disclosure: A new treatment for military trauma, loss, and moral injury*. Guilford Press.
Litz, B. T., Stein, N., Delaney, E., Lebowitz, L., Nash, W. P., Silva, C., & Maguen, S. (2009). Moral injury and moral repair in war veterans: A preliminary model and intervention strategy. *Clinical Psychology Review*, 29(8), 695–706.
Livingston, N. A., Berke, D., Scholl, J., Ruben, M., & Shipherd, J. C. (2020). Addressing diversity in PTSD treatment: Clinical considerations and guidance for the treatment of PTSD in LGBTQ populations. *Current Treatment Options in Psychiatry*, 7, 53–69.

Loewenstein, R. J. (2018). Dissociation debates: Everything you know is wrong. *Dialogues in Clinical Neuroscience*, 20(3), 229–242.

Loftus, E. F. (1993). The reality of repressed memories. *American Psychologist*, 48(5), 518–537.

Loftus, E. F., & Pickrell, J. E. (1995). The formation of false memories. *Psychiatric Annals*, 25(12), 720–725.

Lombardo, M. (2012). EMDR target time line. *Journal of EMDR Practice and Research*, 6(1), 37–46.

Looney, K., El-Leithy, S., & Brown, G. (2021). The role of simulation in imagery rescripting for post-traumatic stress disorder: a single case series. *Behavioural and Cognitive Psychotherapy*, 49(3), 257–271.

Lukowiak, K. (1993). *A Soldier's Song*. Harvill Secker.

Lundorff, M., Holmgren, H., Zachariae, R., Farver-Vestergaard, I., & O'Connor, M. (2017). Prevalence of prolonged grief disorder in adult bereavement: A systematic review and meta-analysis. *Journal of Affective Disorders*, 212, 138–149.

Lusk, J. D., Sadeh, N., Wolf, E. J., & Miller, M. W. (2017). Reckless self-destructive behavior and PTSD in veterans: The mediating role of new adverse events. *Journal of Traumatic Stress*, 30(3), 270–278.

Maccallum, F., & Bryant, R. A. (2013). A cognitive attachment model of prolonged grief: Integrating attachments, memory, and identity. *Clinical Psychology Review*, 33(6), 713–727.

MacRitchie, V., & Leibowitz, S. (2010). Secondary traumatic stress, level of exposure, empathy and social support in trauma workers. *South African Journal of Psychology*, 40, 149–158.

Maguen, S., Lucenko, B. A., Reger, M. A., Gahm, G. A., Litz, B. T., Seal, K. H., Knight, S. J., & Marmar, C. R. (2010). The impact of reported direct and indirect killing on mental health symptoms in Iraq war veterans. *Journal of Traumatic Stress*, 23(1), 86–90.

Marks, E. M., & Hunter, M. S. (2015). Medically unexplained symptoms: An acceptable term?. *British Journal of Pain*, 9(2), 109–114.

Maslow, A. H. (1943). A theory of human motivation. *Psychological Review*, 50(4), 370–396.

McCann, I. L., & Pearlman, L. A. (1990). Vicarious traumatization: A framework for understanding the psychological effects of working with victims. *Journal of Traumatic Stress*, 3(1), 131–149.

McDonald, S. (2000). *Five steps to tyranny*. Available for free viewing at www.youtube.com/watch?v=PeBisBQblFM (January 2022)

McFarlane, A. C. (2017). Post-traumatic stress disorder is a systemic illness, not a mental disorder: Is Cartesian dualism dead. *Medical Journal of Australia*, 206(6), 248–249.

McFetridge, M., Hauenstein Swan, A., Heke, S., & Karatzias, T. (2017). *UK Psychological Trauma Society (UKPTS) guideline for the treatment and planning of services for complex Post-Traumatic Stress Disorder in adults*. UKPTS (United Kingdom Post Traumatic Stress Society).

McLaughlin, A. A., Keller, S. M., Feeny, N. C., Youngstrom, E. A., & Zoellner, L. A. (2014). Patterns of therapeutic alliance: Rupture–repair episodes in prolonged exposure for posttraumatic stress disorder. *Journal of Consulting and Clinical Psychology*, 82(1), 112–121.

McNally, R. J. (2018). Recovered memories of childhood sexual abuse. In R. Rogers, & S. D. Bender. (Eds.), *Clinical assessment of deception and malingering* (pp. 387–400). Guildford Press.

McNally, R. J., Lasko, N. B., Clancy, S. A., Macklin, M. L., Pitman, R. K., & Orr, S. P. (2004). Psychophysiological responding during script-driven imagery in people reporting abduction by space aliens. *Psychological Science*, 15(7), 493–497.

McNally, R. J., Litz, B. T., Prassas, A., Shin, L. M., & Weathers, F. W. (1994). Emotional priming of autobiographical memory in post-traumatic stress disorder. *Cognition and Emotion*, 8(4), 351–367.

McNeil, J. E. (1996). Can PTSD occur with amnesia for the precipitating event?. *Cognitive Neuropsychiatry*, 1(3), 239–246.

Meichenbaum, D. (2007, May). Self-care for trauma psychotherapists and caregivers: Individual, social and organizational interventions. In *11th Annual Conference of the Melissa Institute for Violence Prevention and Treatment of Victims of Violence, Miami, FL*. www. Melissainstitute. org/documents/Meichenbaum_SelfCare_11thconf. pdf

Merckelbach, H., Muris, P., Horselenberg, R., & Rassin, E. (1998). Traumatic intrusions as worse case scenarios. *Behaviour Research and Therapy*, 36(11), 1075–1079.

Messman-Moore, T. L., & Long, P. J. (2003). The role of childhood sexual abuse sequelae in the sexual revictimization of women: An empirical review and theoretical reformulation. *Clinical Psychology Review*, 23(4), 537–571.

Milgram, S. (1963). Behavioral study of obedience. *The Journal of Abnormal and Social Psychology, 67*(4), 371–378.
Miller, M. W., & Resick, P. A. (2007). Internalizing and externalizing subtypes in female sexual assault survivors: Implications for the understanding of complex PTSD. *Behavior Therapy, 38*(1), 58–71.
Miller, W. R., & Rollnick, S. (2012). *Motivational interviewing: Helping people change*. Guilford Press.
Millgram, Y., Joormann, J., Huppert, J. D., & Tamir, M. (2015). Sad as a matter of choice? Emotion-regulation goals in depression. *Psychological Science, 26*(8), 1216–1228.
Monson, C. M., & Fredman, S. J. (2012). *Cognitive-behavioral conjoint therapy for PTSD: Harnessing the healing power of relationships*. Guilford Press.
Moorey, S. (2013). Cognitive Interpersonal Worksheet. Downloaded from: www.cognitiveconnections.co.uk/
Moorey, S. (2014). Transference and counter-transference. In A. Whittington, & N. Grey (Eds.), *How to become a more effective CBT therapist: Mastering metacompetence in clinical practice* (pp. 132–145). John Wiley & Sons.
Moorey, S., & Lavender, A. (2018). The therapeutic alliance: Building a collaborative relationship and managing challenges. In S. Moorey, & A. Lavender (Eds.), *The therapeutic relationship in cognitive behavioural therapy* (pp. 16–31). Sage.
Morey, L. C. (2003). *Essentials of PAI assessment*. John Wiley & Sons.
Morrison, A. P. (2017). A manualised treatment protocol to guide delivery of evidence-based cognitive therapy for people with distressing psychosis: Learning from clinical trials. *Psychosis, 9*(3), 271–281.
Morrison, A. P., Frame, L., & Larkin, W. (2003). Relationships between trauma and psychosis: A review and integration. *British Journal of Clinical Psychology, 42*(4), 331–353.
Moulds, M. L., Bisby, M. A., Wild, J., & Bryant, R. A. (2020). Rumination in posttraumatic stress disorder: A systematic review. *Clinical Psychology Review*, 101910.
Mowrer, O. (1947). On the dual nature of learning—a re-interpretation of 'conditioning' and 'problem-solving.' *Harvard Educational Review, 17*, 102–148.
Mowrer, O. (1960). *Learning theory and behavior*. John Wiley & Sons.
Mullins, J. A. (1996). Has time rewritten every line?: Recovered-memory therapy and the potential expansion of psychotherapist liability. *Washington and Lee Law Review, 53*(2), 763–802.
Murray, H., & El-Leithy, S. (2021). Behavioural experiments in cognitive therapy for posttraumatic stress disorder: Why, when, and how?. *Verhaltenstherapie*, 1–11.
Murray, H., Merritt, C., & Grey, N. (2015). Returning to the scene of the trauma in PTSD treatment: Why, how and when? *The Cognitive Behaviour Therapist, 8*, e28.
Murray, H., Merritt, C., & Grey, N. (2016). Clients' experiences of returning to the trauma site during PTSD treatment: An exploratory study. *Behavioural and Cognitive Psychotherapy, 44*(4), 420–430.
Murray, H., Pethania, Y., & Medin, E. (2021). Survivor guilt: A cognitive approach. *The Cognitive Behaviour Therapist, 14*.
Murray, J., Ehlers, A., & Mayou, R. A. (2002). Dissociation and post-traumatic stress disorder: Two prospective studies of road traffic accident survivors. *The British Journal of Psychiatry, 180*(4), 363–368.
Najavits, L. (2002). *Seeking safety: A treatment manual for PTSD and substance abuse*. Guilford Press.
Najavits, L. M., Schmitz, M., Gotthardt, S., & Weiss, R. D. (2005). Seeking safety plus exposure therapy: An outcome study on dual diagnosis men. *Journal of Psychoactive Drugs, 37*(4), 425–435.
Nandi, C., Crombach, A., Bambonye, M., Elbert, T., & Weierstall, R. (2015). Predictors of posttraumatic stress and appetitive aggression in active soldiers and former combatants. *European Journal of Psychotraumatology, 6*(1), 26553.
National Institute for Health and Care Excellence. (2009). Borderline personality disorder: recognition and management. Clinical guideline [CG78].
National Institute for Health and Care Excellence. (2014). Psychosis and schizophrenia in adults: Prevention and management. Clinical guideline [CG178].
National Institute for Health and Care Excellence. (2018). Posttraumatic stress disorder. NICE guideline [NG116].

Neimeyer, R. A. (2001). The language of loss: Grief therapy as a process of meaning reconstruction. In R. A. Neimeyer (Ed.), *Meaning reconstruction and the experience of loss* (pp. 261–292). American Psychological Association.

Neimeyer, R. A. (2017). Complicated grief: Assessment and intervention. In S. N. Gold (Ed.), *APA handbook of trauma psychology: Trauma practice* (pp. 343–362). American Psychological Association.

Nijs, J., Roussel, N., Van Oosterwijck, J., De Kooning, M., Ickmans, K., Struyf, F., Meeus, M., & Lundberg, M. (2013). Fear of movement and avoidance behaviour toward physical activity in chronic-fatigue syndrome and fibromyalgia: State of the art and implications for clinical practice. *Clinical Rheumatology*, *32*(8), 1121–1129.

Norman, S., Allard, C., Browne, K., Capone, C., Davis, B., & Kubany, E. (2019). *Trauma informed guilt reduction therapy: Treating guilt and shame resulting from trauma and moral injury*. Academic Press.

Novakova, B. (2019). *The mechanisms of imagery rescripting for post-traumatic stress disorder in asylum seekers and refugees* [Unpublished doctoral thesis]. Royal Holloway, University of London.

O'Cleirigh, C., Safren, S. A., Taylor, S. W., Goshe, B. M., Bedoya, C. A., Marquez, S. M., Boroughs, M. S., & Shipherd, J. C. (2019). Cognitive behavioral therapy for trauma and self-care (CBT-TSC) in men who have sex with men with a history of childhood sexual abuse: A randomized controlled trial. *AIDS and Behavior*, *23*(9), 2421–2431.

Olff, M., Amstadter, A., Armour, C., Birkeland, M. S., Bui, E., Cloitre, M., Ehlers, A., Ford, J. D., Greene, T., Hansen, M., Lanius, R., Roberts, N., Rosner, R., & Thoresen, S. (2019). A decennial review of psychotraumatology: What did we learn and where are we going?. *European Journal of Psychotraumatology*, *10*(1), 1672948.

Orcutt, H. K., Erickson, D. J., & Wolfe, J. (2002). A prospective analysis of trauma exposure: The mediating role of PTSD symptomatology. *Journal of Traumatic Stress*, *15*(3), 259–266.

Otto, M. W., & Hinton, D. E. (2006). Modifying exposure-based CBT for Cambodian refugees with posttraumatic stress disorder. *Cognitive and Behavioral Practice*, *13*(4), 261–270.

Oulton, J. M., Strange, D., Nixon, R. D., & Takarangi, M. K. (2018). PTSD and the role of spontaneous elaborative "nonmemories". *Psychology of Consciousness: Theory, Research, and Practice*, *5*(4), 398–413.

Pacella, M. L., Hruska, B., & Delahanty, D. L. (2013). The physical health consequences of PTSD and PTSD symptoms: A meta-analytic review. *Journal of Anxiety Disorders*, *27*(1), 33–46.

Padesky, C. A. (1993). Socratic questioning: Changing minds or guiding discovery. In *A keynote address delivered at the European Congress of Behavioural and Cognitive Therapies, London* (Vol. 24).

Padesky, C. A. (1994). Schema change processes in cognitive therapy. *Clinical Psychology & Psychotherapy*, *1*(5), 267–278.

Panagioti, M., Gooding, P., & Tarrier, N. (2009). Post-traumatic stress disorder and suicidal behavior: A narrative review. *Clinical Psychology Review*, *29*(6), 471–482.

Patihis, L., Lilienfeld, S. O., Ho, L., & Loftus, E. F. (2014). Unconscious repressed memory is scientifically questionable. *Psychological Science*, *25*(10), 1968–1969.

Paulik, G., Newman-Taylor, K., Steel, C., & Arntz, A. (2020). Managing dissociation in imagery rescripting for voice hearers with trauma: Lessons from a case series. *Cognitive and Behavioral Practice*. https://doi.org/10.1016/j.cbpra.2020.06.009.

Paulik, G., Steel, C., & Arntz, A. (2019). Imagery rescripting for the treatment of trauma in voice hearers: A case series. *Behavioural and Cognitive Psychotherapy*, *47*(6), 709–725.

Pearson, D. G., Deeprose, C., Wallace-Hadrill, S. M., Heyes, S. B., & Holmes, E. A. (2013). Assessing mental imagery in clinical psychology: A review of imagery measures and a guiding framework. *Clinical Psychology Review*, *33*(1), 1–23.

Perkonigg, A., Kessler, R. C., Storz, S., & Wittchen, H. U. (2000). Traumatic events and post-traumatic stress disorder in the community: Prevalence, risk factors and comorbidity. *Acta Psychiatrica Scandinavica*, *101*(1), 46–59.

Piaget, J. (1970). Piaget's theory. In P. H. Mussen (Ed.), *Carmichael's manual of child psychology, third edition, Vol. 1*. John Wiley & Co.

Possis, E., Bui, T., Gavian, M., Leskela, J., Linardatos, E., Loughlin, J., & Strom, T. (2014). Driving difficulties among military veterans: clinical needs and current intervention status. *Military Medicine*, *179*(6), 633–639.

Prigerson, H. G., Kakarala, S., Gang, J., & Maciejewski, P. K. (2021). History and status of prolonged grief disorder as a psychiatric diagnosis. *Annual Review of Clinical Psychology*, *17*, 109–126.

Psychotherapy and Counselling Federation of Australia. (2017). *Consensus guidelines for working with recovered memory*. www.pacfa.org.au/consensus-guidelines-for-working-with-recovered-memory/

Pugh, M. (2018). Cognitive behavioural chairwork. *International Journal of Cognitive Therapy*, *11*(1), 100–116.

Rees, G. (2017). *Handling traumatic imagery: Developing a standard operating procedure*. Dart Centre for Trauma and Journalism. https://dartcenter.org/resources/handling-traumatic-imagery-developing-standard-operating-procedure

Resick, P. A., Monson, C. M., & Chard, K. M. (2016). *Cognitive processing therapy for PTSD: A comprehensive manual*. Guilford Press.

Resick, P. A., & Schnicke, M. K. (1992). Cognitive processing therapy for sexual assault victims. *Journal of Consulting and Clinical Psychology*, *60*(5), 748–756.

Resick, P. A., & Schnicke, M. K. (1993). *Cognitive processing therapy for rape victims: A treatment manual* (Vol. 4). Sage.

Reynolds, M., & Brewin, C. R. (1998). Intrusive cognitions, coping strategies and emotional responses in depression, post-traumatic stress disorder and a non-clinical population. *Behaviour Research and Therapy*, *36*(2), 135–147.

Richards, L. (2009). Domestic abuse, stalking and harassment and honour based violence (DASH, 2009) risk identification and assessment and management model. *Association of Police Officers (ACPO)*.

Rizvi, S. L., & Ritschel, L. A. (2014). Mastering the art of chain analysis in dialectical behavior therapy. *Cognitive and Behavioral Practice*, *21*(3), 335–349.

Robichaud, M., Koerner, N., & Dugas, M. J. (2019). *Cognitive behavioral treatment for generalized anxiety disorder: From science to practice*. Routledge.

Rubin, D. C., & Umanath, S. (2015). Event memory: A theory of memory for laboratory, autobiographical, and fictional events. *Psychological Review*, *122*(1), 1–23.

Runeson, B., Odeberg, J., Pettersson, A., Edbom, T., Adamsson, I. J., & Waern, M. (2017). Instruments for the assessment of suicide risk: A systematic review evaluating the certainty of the evidence. *PLoS one*, *12*(7), e0180292.

Salkovskis, P. M., Warwick, H. M., & Deale, A. C. (2003). Cognitive-behavioral treatment for severe and persistent health anxiety (hypochondriasis). *Brief Treatment & Crisis Intervention*, *3*(3), 353–367.

Salmon, K., & Bryant, R. A. (2002). Posttraumatic stress disorder in children: The influence of developmental factors. *Clinical Psychology Review*, *22*(2), 163–188.

Salomons, T. V., Osterman, J. E., Gagliese, L., & Katz, J. (2004). Pain flashbacks in posttraumatic stress disorder. *The Clinical Journal of Pain*, *20*(2), 83–87.

Schauer, M., & Elbert, T. (2010). Dissociation following traumatic stress. *Zeitschrift Für Psychologie*, *218*(2), 109–127.

Schauer, M., Neuner, F., & Elbert, T. (2011). *Narrative exposure therapy: A short-term treatment for traumatic stress disorders*. Hogrefe.

Schnyder, U., & Cloitre, M. (Eds.). (2015). *Evidence based treatments for trauma-related psychological disorders: A practical guide for clinicians*. Springer.

Schnyder, U., Ehlers, A., Elbert, T., Foa, E. B., Gersons, B. P. R., Resick, P. A., Shapiro, F., & Cloitre, M. (2015). Psychotherapies for PTSD: What do they have in common? *European Journal of Psychotraumatology*, *6*(1), 28186.

Schottenbauer, M. A., Glass, C. R., Arnkoff, D. B., Tendick, V., & Gray, S. H. (2008). Nonresponse and dropout rates in outcome studies on PTSD: Review and methodological considerations. *Psychiatry: Interpersonal and Biological Processes*, *71*(2), 134–168.

Schry, A. R., Rissling, M. B., Gentes, E. L., Beckham, J. C., Kudler, H. S., Straits-Tröster, K., & Calhoun, P. S. (2015). The relationship between posttraumatic stress symptoms and physical health in a survey of US veterans of the Iraq and Afghanistan era. *Psychosomatics*, *56*(6), 674–684.

Seebauer, L., Froß, S., Dubaschny, L., Schönberger, M., & Jacob, G. A. (2014). Is it dangerous to fantasize revenge in imagery exercises? An experimental study. *Journal of Behavior Therapy and Experimental Psychiatry*, *45*(1), 20–25.

Sharp, T. J., & Harvey, A. G. (2001). Chronic pain and posttraumatic stress disorder: Mutual maintenance?. *Clinical Psychology Review*, 21(6), 857–877.

Shay, J. (1994). *Achilles in Vietnam: Combat trauma and the undoing of character*. Simon & Schuster.

Shear, K., Frank, E., Houck, P. R., & Reynolds, C. F. (2005). Treatment of complicated grief: A randomized controlled trial. *Jama*, 293(21), 2601–2608.

Shear, K., & Shair, H. (2005). Attachment, loss, and complicated grief. *Developmental Psychobiology*, 47(3), 253–267.

Sheehy, K., Noureen, A., Khaliq, A., Dhingra, K., Husain, N., Pontin, E. E., Cawley, R., & Taylor, P. J. (2019). An examination of the relationship between shame, guilt and self-harm: A systematic review and meta-analysis. *Clinical Psychology Review*, 73, 101779.

Sippel, L. M., & Marshall, A. D. (2011). Posttraumatic stress disorder symptoms, intimate partner violence perpetration, and the mediating role of shame processing bias. *Journal of Anxiety Disorders*, 25(7), 903–910.

Smith, D. W., Davis, J. L., & Fricker-Elhai, A. E. (2004). How does trauma beget trauma? Cognitions about risk in women with abuse histories. *Child Maltreatment*, 9(3), 292–303.

Smith, K. V., & Ehlers, A. (2021). Prolonged grief and posttraumatic stress disorder following the loss of a significant other: An investigation of cognitive and behavioural differences. *PLos One*, 16(4), e0248852.

Smith, K. V., Wild, J., & Ehlers, A. (2020). The masking of mourning: Social disconnection after bereavement and its role in psychological distress. *Clinical Psychological Science*, 8(3), 464–476.

Smith, S. M., & Greaves, D. H. (2017). Recovered memories. In M. P. Toglia, J. D. Read, D. F. Ross, & R. C. L. Lindsay (Eds.), *The handbook of eyewitness psychology: Volume I: Memory for events* (pp. 299–320). Psychology Press.

Sodeke-Gregson, E. A., Holttum, S., & Billings, J. (2013). Compassion satisfaction, burnout, and secondary traumatic stress in UK therapists who work with adult trauma clients. *European Journal of Psychotraumatology*, 4(1), 21869.

Southwick, S. M., Morgan, C. A., Nicolaou, A. L., & Charney, D. S. (1997). Consistency of memory for combat-related traumatic events in veterans of Operation Desert Storm. *American Journal of Psychiatry*, 154(2), 173–177.

Spiller, T. R., Schick, M., Schnyder, U., Bryant, R. A., Nickerson, A., & Morina, N. (2017). Symptoms of posttraumatic stress disorder in a clinical sample of refugees: a network analysis. *European Journal of Psychotraumatology*, 8(sup3), 1318032.

Sprang, G., Clark, J. J., & Whitt-Woosley, A. (2007). Compassion fatigue, compassion satisfaction, and burnout: Factors impacting a professional's quality of life. *Journal of Loss and Trauma*, 12(3), 259–280.

Stamm, B. H. (2005). *The ProQOL manual: The professional quality of life scale: Compassion satisfaction, burnout & compassion fatigue/secondary trauma scales*. Sidran.

Steel, C., Fowler, D., & Holmes, E. A. (2005). Trauma-related intrusions and psychosis: An information processing account. *Behavioural and Cognitive Psychotherapy*, 33(2), 139–152.

Stott, R. (2007). When head and heart do not agree: a theoretical and clinical analysis of rational-emotional dissociation (RED) in cognitive therapy. *Journal of Cognitive Psychotherapy*, 21(1), 37.

Stott, R. (2009). Tripping into trauma: Cognitive-behavioural treatment for a traumatic stress reaction following recreational drug use. In N. Grey (Ed.), *A casebook of cognitive therapy for traumatic stress reactions* (pp. 65–76). Routledge.

Stott, R., Mansell, W., Salkovskis, P., Lavender, A., & Cartwright-Hatton, S. (2010). *Oxford guide to metaphors in CBT: Building cognitive bridges*. Oxford University Press.

Strange, D., & Takarangi, M. K. (2012). False memories for missing aspects of traumatic events. *Acta Psychologica*, 141(3), 322–326.

Strange, D., & Takarangi, M. K. T. (2015). Investigating the variability of memory distortion for an analogue trauma. *Memory*, 23(7), 991–1000.

Tarrier, N., Harwood, S., Yusopoff, L., Beckett, R., & Baker, A. (1990). Coping strategy enhancement (CSE): A method of treating residual schizophrenic symptoms. *Behavioural and Cognitive Psychotherapy*, 18(4), 283–293.

Taylor, S., Fedoroff, I. C., Koch, W. J., Thordarson, D. S., Fecteau, G., & Nicki, R. M. (2001). Posttraumatic stress disorder arising after road traffic collisions: Patterns of response to cognitive-behavior therapy. *Journal of Consulting and Clinical Psychology*, 69(3), 541–551.

Taylor, S., Frueh, B. C., & Asmundson, G. J. (2007). Detection and management of malingering in people presenting for treatment of posttraumatic stress disorder: Methods, obstacles, and recommendations. *Journal of Anxiety Disorders*, 21(1), 22–41.

Terheggen, M. A., Stroebe, M. S., & Kleber, R. J. (2001). Western conceptualizations and Eastern experience: A cross-cultural study of traumatic stress reactions among Tibetan refugees in India. *Journal of Traumatic Stress*, 14(2), 391–403.

Terr, L. (1988). What happens to early memories of trauma? A study of twenty children under age five at the time of documented traumatic events. *Journal of the American Academy of Child & Adolescent Psychiatry*, 27(1), 96–104.

Testa, M., Hoffman, J. H., & Livingston, J. A. (2010). Alcohol and sexual risk behaviors as mediators of the sexual victimization-revictimization relationship. *Journal of Consulting and Clinical Psychology*, 78(2), 249–259.

Testa, R. J., Habarth, J., Peta, J., Balsam, K., & Bockting, W. (2015). Development of the gender minority stress and resilience measure. *Psychology of Sexual Orientation and Gender Diversity*, 2(1), 65–77.

Thompson, C. T., Vidgen, A., & Roberts, N. P. (2018). Psychological interventions for post-traumatic stress disorder in refugees and asylum seekers: A systematic review and meta-analysis. *Clinical Psychology Review*, 63, 66–79.

Thompson-Hollands, J., Jun, J. J., & Sloan, D. M. (2017). The association between peritraumatic dissociation and PTSD symptoms: The mediating role of negative beliefs about the self. *Journal of Traumatic Stress*, 30(2), 190–194.

Tomasulo, D. J., & Razza, N. J. (2007). Posttraumatic stress disorders. In R. Fletcher, E. Loschen, C. Stavrakaki, & M. First (Eds.), *Diagnostic manual–intellectual disability: A textbook of diagnosis of mental disorders in persons with intellectual disability* (pp. 365–378). National Association for the Dually Diagnosed.

Turgoose, D., & Maddox, L. (2017). Predictors of compassion fatigue in mental health professionals: A narrative review. *Traumatology*, 23(2), 172–185.

van den Berg, D. P., de Bont, P. A., van der Vleugel, B. M., De Roos, C., de Jongh, A., van Minnen, A., & van der Gaag, M. (2015). Trauma-focused treatment in PTSD patients with psychosis: Symptom exacerbation, adverse events, and revictimization. *Schizophrenia Bulletin*, 42(3), 693–702.

van den Berg, D. P., van de Giessen, I., & Hardy, A. (2020). Trauma therapies in psychosis. In J. Badcock, & G. Paulik (Eds.), *A clinical introduction to psychosis* (pp. 447–463). Academic Press.

van den Berk-Clark, C., Secrest, S., Walls, J., Hallberg, E., Lustman, P. J., Schneider, F. D., & Scherrer, J. F. (2018). Association between posttraumatic stress disorder and lack of exercise, poor diet, obesity, and co-occurring smoking: A systematic review and meta-analysis. *Health Psychology*, 37(5), 407–416.

van der Kolk, B. A. (2003). The neurobiology of childhood trauma and abuse. *Child and Adolescent Psychiatric Clinics of North America*, 12(2) 292–317.

van der Kolk, B. A., & Fisler, R. (1995). Dissociation and the fragmentary nature of traumatic memories: Overview and exploratory study. *Journal of Traumatic Stress*, 8(4), 505–525.

van Voorhees, E. E., Dennis, P. A., Neal, L. C., Hicks, T. A., Calhoun, P. S., Beckham, J. C., & Elbogen, E. B. (2016). Posttraumatic stress disorder, hostile cognitions, and aggression in Iraq/Afghanistan era veterans. *Psychiatry*, 79(1), 70–84.

Varese, F., Smeets, F., Drukker, M., Lieverse, R., Lataster, T., Viechtbauer, W., Read, J., van Os, J., & Bentall, R. P. (2012). Childhood adversities increase the risk of psychosis: A meta-analysis of patient-control, prospective-and cross-sectional cohort studies. *Schizophrenia Bulletin*, 38(4), 661–671.

Vlaeyen, J. W., & Linton, S. J. (2000). Fear-avoidance and its consequences in chronic musculoskeletal pain: a state of the art. *Pain*, 85(3), 317–332.

Vogt, D. S., Shipherd, J. C., & Resick, P. A. (2012). Posttraumatic maladaptive beliefs scale: evolution of the personal beliefs and reactions scale. *Assessment*, 19(3), 308–317.

Ward-Brown, J., Keane, D., Bhutani, G., Malkin, D., Sellwood, B., & Varese, F. (2018). TF-CBT and EMDR for young people with trauma and first episode psychosis (using a phasic treatment approach): Two early intervention service case studies. *The Cognitive Behaviour Therapist*, 11.

Waszczuk, M. A., Ruggero, C., Li, K., Luft, B. J., & Kotov, R. (2019). The role of modifiable health-related behaviors in the association between PTSD and respiratory illness. *Behaviour Research and Therapy, 115*, 64–72.

Watkins, J. G. (1971). The affect bridge: A hypnoanalytic technique. *The International Journal of Clinical and Experimental Hypnosis, 19*(1), 21–27.

Watson, H., Rapee, R., & Todorov, N. (2016). Imagery rescripting of revenge, avoidance, and forgiveness for past bullying experiences in young adults. *Cognitive Behaviour Therapy, 45*(1), 73–89.

Weathers, F. W., Blake, D. D., Schnurr, P. P., Kaloupek, D. G., Marx, B. P., & Keane, T. M. (2013a). *The Life Events Checklist for DSM-5 (LEC-5)*. Instrument available from the National Center for PTSD at www.ptsd.va.gov

Weathers, F. W., Blake, D. D., Schnurr, P. P., Kaloupek, D. G., Marx, B. P., & Keane, T. M. (2013c). *The Clinician-Administered PTSD Scale for DSM-5 (CAPS-5)*. American Psychological Association.

Weathers, F. W., Litz, B. T., Keane, T. M., Palmieri, P. A., Marx, B. P., & Schnurr, P. P. (2013b). *The PTSD Checklist for DSM-5 (PCL-5)*. National Center for PTSD.

Webster, C., & Kingston, S. (2014). *Poverty and crime*. Joseph Rowntree Foundation.

Weingardt, K. R., Loftus, E. F., & Lindsay, D. S. (1995). Misinformation revisited: New evidence on the suggestibility of memory. *Memory & Cognition, 23*(1), 72–82.

Weiss, N. H., Sullivan, T. P., & Tull, M. T. (2015). Explicating the role of emotion dysregulation in risky behaviors: A review and synthesis of the literature with directions for future research and clinical practice. *Current Opinion in Psychology, 3*, 22–29.

Westbrook, D. (2014). The central pillars of CBT. In A. Whittington, & N. Grey (Eds), *How to become a more effective CBT therapist: Mastering metacompetence in clinical practice* (pp. 17–30). Routledge.

Westbrook, D., Kennerley, H., & Kirk, J. (2011). *An introduction to cognitive behaviour therapy: Skills and applications*. Sage.

Westra, H. A., Dozois, D. J., & Marcus, M. (2007). Expectancy, homework compliance, and initial change in cognitive-behavioral therapy for anxiety. *Journal of Consulting and Clinical Psychology, 75*(3), 363–373.

Wheatley, J., Brewin, C. R., Patel, T., Hackmann, A., Wells, A., Fisher, P., & Myers, S. (2007). 'I'll believe it when I can see it': Imagery rescripting of intrusive sensory memories in depression. *Journal of Behavior Therapy and Experimental Psychiatry, 38*(4), 371–385.

Whisman, M. A. (1999). Marital dissatisfaction and psychiatric disorders: Results from the national comorbidity survey. *Journal of Abnormal Psychology, 108*(4), 701–706.

White, M. (1998). Notes on externalizing problems. In C. White & D. Denborough (Eds.), *Introducing narrative therapy: A collection of practice-based writings* (pp. 219–224). Dulwich Centre Publications.

Whittington, A. (2014). Working with co-morbid depression and anxiety disorders. In A. Whittington, & N. Grey. (Eds.). *How to become a more effective CBT therapist: Mastering metacompetence in clinical practice* (pp. 65–82). John Wiley & Sons.

Whittington, A., & Grey, N. (2014). Mastering metacompetnece: The science and art of CBT. In A. Whittington, & N. Grey (Eds.), *How to become a more effective CBT therapist: Mastering metacompetence in clinical practice* (pp. 3v16). John Wiley & Sons.

Wild, J. (2009). Cognitive therapy for post-traumatic stress disorder and permanent physical injury. In N. Grey (Ed.), *A casebook of cognitive therapy for traumatic stress reactions* (pp. 147–162). Routledge.

Wild, J., & Clark, D. M. (2011). Imagery rescripting of early traumatic memories in social phobia. *Cognitive and Behavioral Practice, 18*(4), 433–443.

Wilker, S., Kleim, B., Geiling, A., Pfeiffer, A., Elbert, T., & Kolassa, I. T. (2017). Mental defeat and cumulative trauma experiences predict trauma-related psychopathology: Evidence from a postconflict population in northern Uganda. *Clinical Psychological Science, 5*(6), 974–984.

Williams, D. R., Yu, Y., Jackson, J. S., & Anderson, N. B. (1997). Racial differences in physical and mental health: Socio-economic status, stress and discrimination. *Journal of Health Psychology, 2*(3), 335–351.

Williams, L. M. (1995). Recovered memories of abuse in women with documented child sexual victimization histories. *Journal of Traumatic Stress, 8*(4), 649–673.

Williamson, V., Murphy, D., Phelps, A., Forbes, D., & Greenberg, N. (2021). Moral injury: the effect on mental health and implications for treatment. *The Lancet Psychiatry*, 8(6), 453–455.

Williamson, V., Murphy, D., Stevelink, S. A. M., Jones, E., Wessely, S., & Greenberg, N. (2020). Confidentiality and psychological treatment of moral injury: The elephant in the room. *BMJ Military Health*, 167(6), 451–453.

World Health Organisation. (2018). *International Classifications of Diseases: 11th Revision*.

Yeterian, J. D., Berke, D. S., Carney, J. R., McIntyre-Smith, A., St. Cyr, K., King, L., Kline, K., Phelps, A., Litz, B. T., & Moral Injury Outcomes Project Consortium. (2019). Defining and measuring moral injury: Rationale, design, and preliminary findings from the moral injury outcome scale consortium. *Journal of Traumatic Stress*, 32(3), 363–372.

Young, J. E., Klosko, J. S., & Weishaar, M. E. (2006). *Schema therapy: A practitioner's guide*. Guilford Press.

Young, K., Chessell, Z., Chisholm, A., Brady, F., Akbar, S., Vann, M., Rouf, K., & Dixon, L. (2021). A cognitive behavioural therapy (CBT) approach for working with strong feelings of guilt after traumatic events. *The Cognitive Behaviour Therapist*, 14, E26.

Zayfert, C., & Becker, C. B. (2019). *Cognitive-behavioral therapy for PTSD: A case formulation approach*. Guilford Press.

Zayfert, C., & DeViva, J. C. (2004). Residual insomnia following cognitive behavioral therapy for PTSD. *Journal of Traumatic Stress*, 17(1), 69–73.

Zeidner, M., Hadar, D., Matthews, G., & Roberts, R. D. (2013). Personal factors related to compassion fatigue in health professionals. *Anxiety, Stress & Coping*, 26(6), 595–609.

Zimmerman, M., Rothschild, L., & Chelminski, I. (2005). The prevalence of DSM-IV personality disorders in psychiatric outpatients. *American Journal of Psychiatry*, 162(10), 1911–1918.

Zlotnick, C., Mattia, J. I., & Zimmerman, M. (1999). Clinical correlates of self-mutilation in a sample of general psychiatric patients. *The Journal of Nervous and Mental Disease*, 187(5), 296–301.

Zoellner, L., Graham, B., Marks, E., Feeny, N., Bentley, J., Franklin, A., & Lang, D. (2018). Islamic trauma healing: Initial feasibility and pilot data. *Societies*, 8, 47.

Zortea, T. C., Cleare, S., Melson, A. J., Wetherall, K., & O'Connor, R. C. (2020). Understanding and managing suicide risk. *British Medical Bulletin*, 134(1), 73–84.

Index

Note: Bold page numbers refer to tables; *italic* page numbers refer to figures.